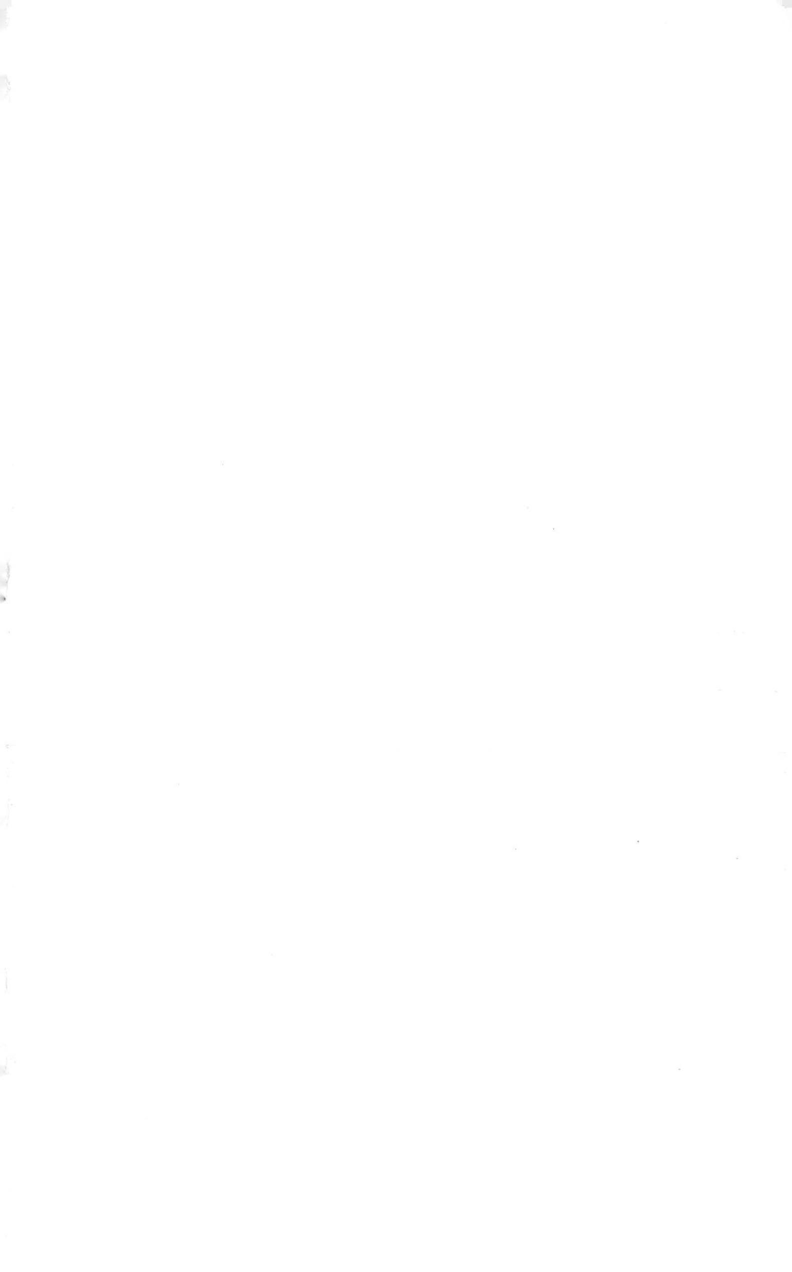

Compendium of Animal Reproduction

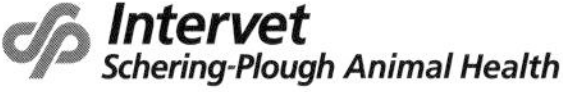

Preface

It is with great pleasure that I would like to present to you the new edition of the Compendium of Animal Reproduction. It is already the 10th edition of this book that has found its place on shelves and in the hearts of our colleagues, veterinary practitioners, academic teachers and students of veterinary medicine. They made the management of reproduction in domestic animals a part of their daily practice and share my never failing passion for reproduction science.

The mission of this book is not only to bring the latest scientific discoveries but also to help translating them into solutions applicable to the everyday work of a vet for the benefit of the veterinary profession and its clients, the animal owners.

It was a great experience to work on the Compendium again, however it would not be possible to accomplish it without help of my colleagues who devoted their time and enthusiasm to this project. I would like to express my gratitude and appreciation to Dr. Linda Horspool who reviewed and up-dated chapters 7, 8 and 11 and to Dr. Marc Martens for his revision of chapter 4.
I am also indebted to Dr. David Pepper for his help in correcting and editing the English text.
I hope that you will find the Compendium to be a useful source of information on this fascinating subject both from the scientific and practical point of view.

Monika Ptaszynska, editor 10th edition

ISBN 90-801886-6-2
Publisher Intervet International bv

060200.12.09
10th revised edition, 2009

Table of Contents

1. Physiology of Reproduction in Mammals

1.1 Introduction

Two regulatory systems govern the reproductive process in mammals. The endocrine system and the nervous system each has a specific role, and a subtle interplay between the two is essential for the cascade of events that results in the birth and successful rearing of healthy offspring. This first chapter will provide some basic theory about the way in which the reproductive processes function, using a brief glimpse of what happens in the cow to illustrate the relationships between the different parts of the process. More detailed information about the reproductive cycle in cattle and other animals can be found in the chapters on the various species. Short sections at the end of this chapter discuss the endocrine process in the male, and some aspects of seasonality.

1.2 Nervous system, hormone system and cell messengers

Nervous system: Stimuli from the environment are received by the senses and transmitted to the brain. With respect to reproduction, examples of sensory input from the environment include information received via the eyes (light, other animals of the same species), the nose (sexually significant odours), and touch (proximity of other animals), and the optic, olfactory and sensory nerves transmit the messages to the brain. The brain translates the information and, as necessary, reacts by sending impulses along nerve fibres to a target organ. Hormone system: A hormone can be defined as a chemical substance, produced in a gland or tissue in the body, which evokes a specific reaction in hormone-sensitive tissue. The hormone system exerts its influence by means of these chemical messengers. It is regulated by a complex of feedback loops, and impulses from the nervous system and various organs. Its activity can be subdivided according to the way the hormones reach the target cells (Norman and Litwack 1997).

Systemic hormones-endocrine hormones
In the endocrine system, the hormone is synthesized and stored in specialized cells of an anatomically defined endocrine gland. These hormones are released into the blood stream and carried (frequently by specific transport proteins) to a target organ, often distant from the source.
The endocrine system includes secretory glands that release their hormones into the general circulation (e.g. insulin), as well as into closed circulatory systems (e.g. GnRH).

Paracrine hormones
So-called paracrine hormones influence cells or organs in their immediate neighbourhood. For example, the production of testosterone by the interstitial Leydig cells of the testes, acting on the adjacent seminiferous tubules.

Autocrine hormones
Autocrine describes the process in which the producing cell is also the target cell. The prostaglandins are good examples.

Neurotransmitters
Nowadays, neurotransmitters are increasingly commonly considered to be hormones, i.e. they are hormone messengers. Neurotransmitters such as acetylocholine may be thought of as paracrine hormones.
To date, more is known about endocrine functions than about the rest of the hormone system. In the last decade, research workers have paid more attention to the paracrine and autocrine functions, but many details of these actions are still poorly understood.

Having reached a target cell the hormone needs to provoke a reaction, which is activated by the target cell's hormone-specific receptors - unique molecular structures, in or on the cell, with a highly specific affinity for a particular hormonal configuration.
The receptors therefore perform two important functions:
- Recognition of the specific hormone by the target cell.
- Translation of the signal into a cell-specific response.

The biochemical structure of hormone receptors can vary but, in general, each can recognise and interact with, a very specific hormone entity (by contrast with the lock-and-key model of the substrate-enzyme interaction).

Nonetheless all receptors have two key components:

a) a ligand binding domain that binds the matching hormone stereo-specifically
b) an effector domain that recognises the presence of the ligand domain-hormone complex and activates the cell-specific biological response, which usually involves activation or de-activation of enzymes in the target cells.

The receptors for steroid hormones are usually to be found in the cytosolic and nuclear compartments of the target cells where they interact directly with DNA. Receptors for peptide and protein hormones are usually located in the outer membrane of the cell. Most receptors, especially those in the cell membrane, require a second messenger to transmit the message. One of the best known second messengers is cyclic–AMP, as shown in Figure 1. After binding to the receptor, the hormone activates the adenylate-cyclase-system in the cell membrane. ATP is then converted into cyclic AMP. cAMP, the second messenger, in its turn, activates an inactive cAMP-protein-kinase-A that splits up into an active catalytic unit and a regulatory unit. The active catalytic unit of the protein-kinase stimulates the phosphorylation of a protein or enzyme, which then brings about the cellular effects, such as protein synthesis, growth or hormone secretion. Because of the generally low circulating concentrations of hormones, the receptor needs a very efficient capture mechanism for its matching hormone.

Figure 1 Cyclic AMP as second messenger

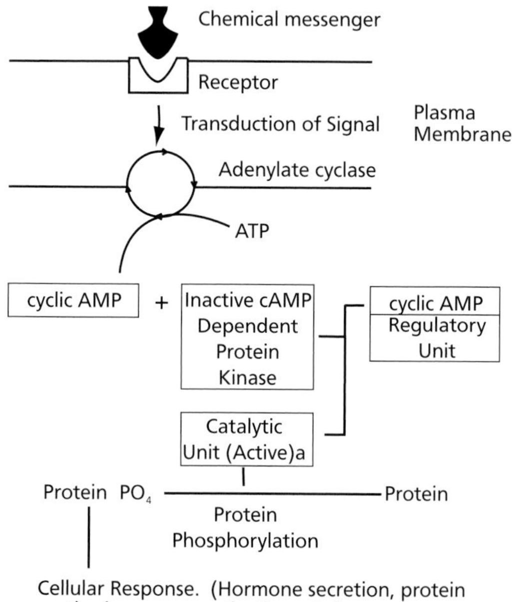

The effect of an endocrine hormone release can vary with particular circumstances. The number and type of receptors of a target cell are not fixed, and their formation and degradation is a dynamic process. The function of one hormone in a cell can be the induction or degradation of receptors for another messenger. Furthermore, receptors can be blocked by an excess of hormones. In this case, over-stimulation by a normally highly effective dose of hormones will cause no further effect. Many pathological conditions in the reproductive process are caused by disorders at the receptor level.

1.3 Regulation of reproduction in the female

For most of a normally fertile female's life, she experiences no regular cyclic activity (anoestrus). Taken together, the periods of inactivity in pre-puberty, pregnancy and lactation are much longer than the relatively short periods of cyclic activity. Nevertheless, most attention is focused on the latter, the periods when man most frequently interferes with the reproduction process (breeding/not breeding; choice of male/AI; control of oestrus; induction of ovulation etc.) and it is during these periods that most problems associated with breeding occur.

The principles of the hormonal control of reproduction are basically the same for all the domesticated animal species, though there are some differences between them. Some animals are poly-oestrus (cattle, swine) cycling throughout the year, others are only seasonally poly-oestrus (horse, sheep, cat). The dog is mono-oestrus.

There are also differences in the mechanism of ovulation. Most animals are spontaneous ovulators, but in the cat, rabbit and camel, ovulation is induced by the stimulation of sensory receptors in the vagina and cervix at coitus. The species-specific aspects of reproduction are covered in the chapters on the physiology of the different species. This section will only review the function and interaction of the most important hormones involved in reproduction (and their secretory and target tissues), using the sexual cycle of the cow as an example.

Figure 2 Inter-relationships in the control of female reproductive function

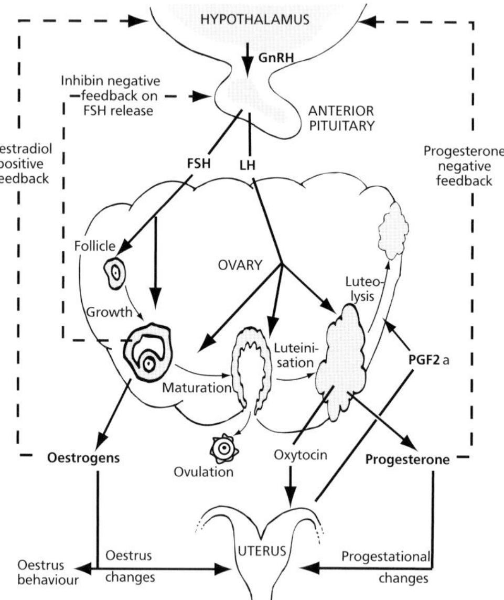

The reproductive process in mammals is regulated by a complex, and only partially understood, cascade of the combined activities of the central nervous system, a number of secretory tissues, target tissues and several hormones. Figure 2 is a schematic representation of the most important organs and hormones involved in reproduction in the female, with some of their functions and interactions.

The central nervous system (CNS) receives information from the animal's environment (visual, olfactory, auditory, and tactile stimuli) and conveys the information relevant for reproduction to the gonads via the Hypothalamo-Pituitary-Gonadal axis. The hypothalamus and the pituitary gland are closely attached to the ventral part of the brain. Both are not only hormone producers, but also target organs, constituting a sophisticated homeostatic feedback system by which they regulate their own rate of secretion.

Following a stimulus from the CNS, endocrine neurons in the hypothalamus produce one of its releasing hormones, Gonadotrophin Releasing Hormone (GnRH), a relatively simple 10-amino acid peptide (decapeptide). Since GnRH is highly conserved in mammals, technology for the control of fertility based on this hormone has a wide range of applications in different species.
GnRH is transported via the hypothalamo-hypophyseal portal system to the anterior lobe of the pituitary gland, its target organ. Here it stimulates specific cells of the pituitary gland to secrete Follicle Stimulating Hormone (FSH) and Luteinizing Hormone (LH). GnRH, FSH and LH are not released at a constant level, but in a series of pulses. In modulating the secretory activity of the pituitary gland, it is the amplitude and frequency of GnRH pulses that play a decisive role rather than a constant concentration of the hormone. Both internal factors (gonadal feedback mechanism) and external factors (photoperiod, pheromones, nutrition and metabolic status) exert their primary effect on the reproductive pattern through the modulation of GnRH secretion by the hypothalamus.

As already mentioned, GnRH stimulates the release of FSH and LH by pituitary cells. The gonadotrophins FSH and LH belong to the superfamily of glycoprotein hormones. They are composed of two different subunits, alpha and beta, which are non-covalently associated. These two hormones are not secreted synchronously *in vivo* since they are regulated independently. GnRH is of acute importance in controlling the secretion of LH. Hence, the pulsatile secretion of LH by the pituitary closely follows the pulsatile release of GnRH from the hypothalamus. GnRH stimulation rapidly triggers both the release and the biosynthesis of LH in order to replenish its resources. The LH content of the pituitary of most mammalian species is up to 10 times higher than that of FSH.
By contrast, FSH synthesis is modulated by various gonadal factors, though GnRH appears to be indispensable to its

maintenance. The pituitary stores of FSH are low and its secretion mirrors the rate and extent of its biosynthesis.
GnRH is released from the hypothalamus in a series of rapid bursts separated by a quiescent period. The pulsatile nature of GnRH secretion ensures that the target organ is always exposed to hormonal stimuli: constant stimulation by high concentrations would result in desensitisation of the target cells. It has been shown experimentally that continuous administration of high levels of GnRH leads to a progressive decrease in the pituitary's responsiveness to GnRH. This desensitisation is most probably caused by a decrease in the number of GnRH receptors on the cell membrane of pituitary cells.

One level down the Hypothalamo-pituitary-gonadal axis, FSH stimulates the development of ovarian follicles. In the theca interna of the follicle, LH stimulates the synthesis of androstenedione from cholesterol. Androstenedione is converted into testosterone which is aromatized into oestradiol-17β under the influence of FSH, in the granulosa cells of the follicle. Oestradiol exerts a positive feedback on the hypothalamus and pituitary gland, increasing the frequency of the GnRH pulses. Above a certain threshold level of oestradiol, the hypothalamus responds with a surge of GnRH which, in turn, induces an LH surge that initiates ovulation. Thus, with respect to ovarian function, FSH stimulates the growth of follicles, while LH stimulates their maturation, oestradiol production and ovulation. LH also supports the formation and the early function of the corpus luteum.

One of the principal effects of oestradiol is the induction of the signs of oestrus. Oestrus can be described as the behavioural and physical signs that signal to other animals that the female is in the fertile phase of her cycle, and will allow herself to be mated.

The granulosa cells also produce inhibin. Not all the effects of this hormone are understood, but its name is derived from its negative feedback on FSH release from the pituitary gland, thus controlling follicle development. After ovulation, the remnants of the follicle are remodelled into the corpus luteum, under the influence of LH. The cavity of the follicle is filled with blood vessels, and the granulosa cells increase in size. The corpus luteum is mainly a secretory organ producing progesterone and oxytocin.

Progesterone is essential for the normal cycle in the cow and, after conception, it is the hormone principally responsible for the maintenance of pregnancy. It reduces the GnRH pulse release, and therefore inhibits new ovulations. Furthermore, it prepares the endometrium for the nidation (in effect, the implantation) of the developing embryo, and inhibits uncontrolled contractions of the uterine wall which would be harmful to pregnancy. If the ovum released from the follicle during ovulation is not fertilized, no signal of pregnancy will be received from the embryo. At around day 16 after ovulation, the endometrium of the nonpregnant uterus will release prostaglandin $F_{2\alpha}$.

$PGF_{2\alpha}$ initiates the regression of the corpus luteum which is called luteolysis. The luteolytic mechanism of prostaglandins has not been completely elucidated, but it involves a reduction of the blood supply to the corpus luteum by vasoconstriction, as well as a direct effect on the luteal cells themselves. The primary site for the initiation of luteolysis is the large luteal cell of the ageing corpus luteum (Weem et al., 2006). Oxytocin produced in the corpus luteum is also thought to play a part in luteolysis. Binding of oxytocin to its receptor in the uterine endometrium of the non-pregnant ruminant stimulates the pulsatile secretion of $PGF_{2\alpha}$. Experimental evidence generated over the last 10 years indicates that oestrogens adjust the expression of uterine oxytocin receptors upwards, and progesterone, downwards. However, the way in which the intracellular dynamics in uterine target cells is affected by the changing exposure to oestrogens and progesterone during the oestrous cycle may be more complex than presently suspected. Endometrial $PGF_{2\alpha}$ secretion initiates luteolysis. Uterine venous $PGF_{2\alpha}$ begins to increase on days 11–13 in ewes, days 13–14 in sows, and days 16–17 post-oestrus in cows (reviewed in Weem et al., 2006).

Figure 3 Hormone levels during the oestrous cycle of a cow

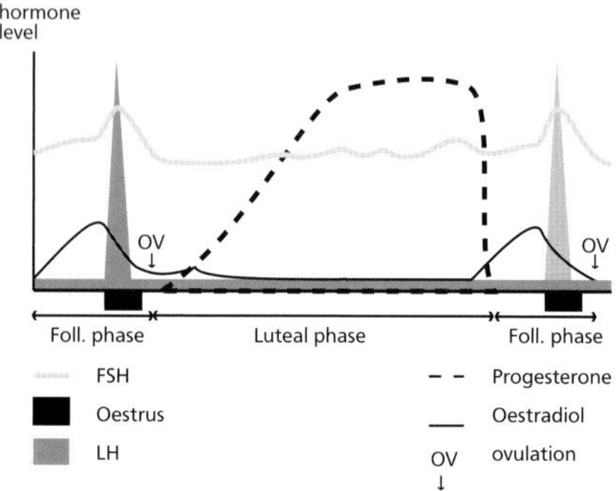

As a result of the regression of the corpus luteum, blood progesterone concentrations decline, removing the blocking effect on GnRH release from the hypothalamus. This initiates a new follicular phase and the final development of a pre-ovulatory follicle. The period of follicle ripening, oestrus and ovulation, characterized by the production of oestradiol, is called the follicular phase of the cycle. The progesterone-dominated phase, from ovulation to luteolysis, is called the luteal phase. See Figure 3.

The hormones involved in reproduction are listed in Table 1, along with the main function, origin and chemical structure of each. It is important to note that only some of the known actions of the individual hormones are included, and also that not all the functions of these hormones are understood. The table merely includes the known endocrine actions, but most also have various paracrine functions, which have not yet been sufficiently explored. Reproduction in the female and the male is regulated by the finely tuned interplay of actions and reactions of many of these hormones. Although much progress has been made in recent decades, a total understanding of these immensely complex processes is still to be attained.

Table 1 Biological activity of Follicle Stimulating Hormone (FSH) in the male *(Adapted from Norman& Litwak 1997)*

Name	**Origin**	**Main function**	**Chemical structure**
Melatonin	Pineal gland	Indicator day/night length	Indoleamin
GnRH	Hypothalamus	Stimulates FSH and LH release by the pituitary	Peptide (10 amino acids)
FSH	Anterior pituitary gland	Female: Stimulates ovarian follicle development and maturation Male: Stimulates spermatogenesis	Glycoprotein (> 200 amino acids)
LH	Anterior pituitary gland	Female: Stimulates maturation of ovarian follicles, induces ovulation, formation and maintenance of corpus luteum Male: Stimulates testosterone production	Glycoprotein (> 200 amino acids)
Oestrogens (oestradiol-17β)	Ovary (granulosa cells of the follicle)	Induces oestrus behaviour. Stimulates pre-ovulatory GnRH release	Steroid
Inhibin	Ovary (granulosa cells of the follicle) Male: Testis (Sertoli cells)	Female: Inhibitis FSH release by the pituitary gland (feedback mechanism)	Peptide
Progesterone	Ovary (corpus luteum)	Prepares the endometrium for nidation of an embryo Maintains pregnancy Decreases GnRH release, thus inhibits new ovulations	Steroid
Prostaglandin $F_{2\alpha}$	Uterus	Regression of the corpus luteum	Lipid-soluble acid

1.4 Regulation of reproduction in the male

The principles of reproduction in the male show a pattern similar to those of the female. The hormones responsible for the development and maintenance of the male phenotype are also the gonadotrophins: luteinizing hormone (LH, which in the male used to be called interstitial cell stimulating hormone ICSH) and follicle stimulating hormone (FSH) produced by pituitary gland; the androgenic steroid hormones, including testosterone, produced by the testes, and inhibin. The female steroid hormones, oestradiol and oestrone, also play an important part in the male in certain circumstances. Figure 4 represents the control of reproductive function in the male.

GnRH from the hypothalamus stimulates the release of FSH and LH. In the male, FSH in conjunction with testosterone, acts on the Sertoli cells of the seminiferous tubules of the testis at the time of puberty to initiate sperm production. Thereafter, throughout adult life, FSH acts directly on the seminiferous tubules (germ cells and Sertoli cells), stimulating spermatogenesis. The Sertoli cells produce inhibin, which has a negative feedback effect on FSH secretion by the pituitary gland. The biological activity of FSH in the male is summarised in Table 2.

Table 2 Biological activity of Follicle Stimulating Hormone (FSH) in the male

(Adapted from Norman& Litwak 1997)

Target cell	**Action**
Immature Sertoli cell	Stimulation of mitotic division
Mature Sertoli cell	Initiation of spermatogenesis Initiation of inhibin synthesis Stimulation of new protein production, including androgen-binding protein (ABP), GnRH-like peptide, Muellerian inhibiting factor (MIF)*, plasminogen activator and transferrin

** Muellerian inhibitory factor (MIF) is a gonadal peptide hormone that causes regression of the Muellerian ducts during male embryogenesis.*

LH stimulates the production of testosterone by the Leydig cells. The secretion of LH is inversely related to the blood levels of testosterone and oestradiol, as testosterone exerts a negative feedback effect on LH secretion by suppressing the pulsatile GnRH release from the hypothalamus.
Although LH is known to induce biological responses in both Leydig and Sertoli cells, LH-specific receptors have only been found on the Leydig cells. This would suggest that the action of LH on Sertoli cells is mediated through a paracrine mechanism. Receptors specific for FSH are present principally on Sertoli cells and to some extent on spermatogonia.

Testosterone (acting on the Sertoli cells) is also necessary for spermatogenesis. The presence of functional androgen nuclear receptors have been demonstrated in Leydig, Sertoli and peri-tubular cells in testicular tissue. Testosterone and other androgens are responsible for the differentiation and maturation of the male reproductive organs, the development of the male secondary characteristics, and the behaviour consistent with the male's role in reproduction.

Leydig cells therefore have the following main functions: production of testosterone and the initiation of complex paracrine interactions with the seminiferous tubules and Sertoli cells to influence the process of spermatogenesis. During sexual maturation, the Sertoli cells mature in terms of both their biochemical capability and their morphology. Thus the so-called blood-testis barrier is formed. The Sertoli cells are involved in five important functions: production of unique regulatory proteins such as the androgen-binding protein (ABP), nourishment of developing spermatozoa, phagocytosis of damaged spermatozoa, production of bicarbonate- and potassium-rich fluid used for the transport of mature sperm cells, and production of oestradiol from testosterone.

Figure 4 Inter-relationships in the control of male reproductive function

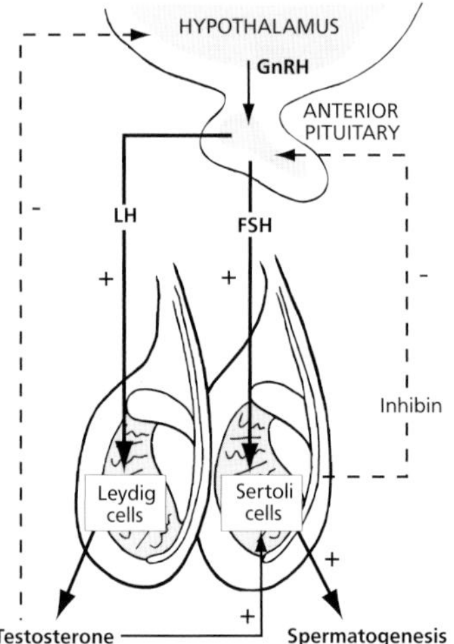

1.5 Seasonality

In temperate latitudes, animals are faced with recurrent, seasonal changes in temperature, climate and food availability, which can influence their reproductive activity. One of the common features of most wild, and some domesticated, species is the development of seasonal reproduction favouring birth at an optimal time of year, usually spring, which allows the new-born to grow under optimal conditions of climate and food availability before the following winter (Figure 5).

Figure 5 Timing of the seasons for breeding and birth in some mammalian species (adapted from Chemineau et al., 2008)

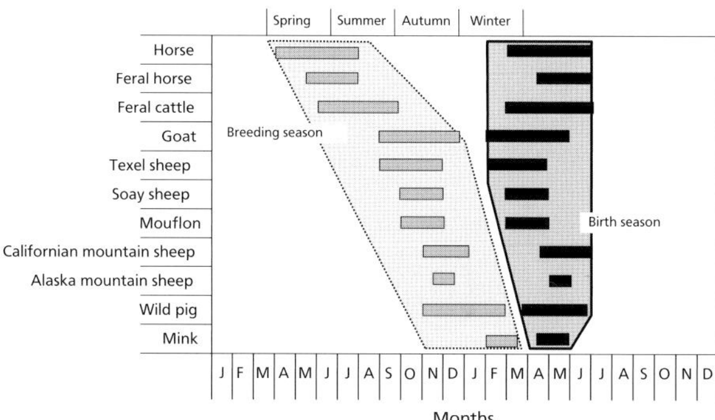

This means that periods of sexual activity (the oestrus season) alternate with periods of sexual inactivity (the anoestrus season). Among the domesticated species, sheep, goats and horses have retained the strongest seasonality in their reproductive processes. In sheep, for instance, sexual activity begins as the day length becomes shorter (short-day breeders), and in horses, sexual activity starts when day length increases (long-day breeders). In temperate and cold climates, this results in horses and sheep giving birth to their young in spring, when sufficient food is likely to give them the best chance of survival.

For any given species or breed, the breeding season is usually very stable throughout life, with relatively constant timing for the start and end of female ovulatory activity and a similarly consistent period of maximum sperm production in males. This precise and sustained timing is due to a complex mechanism which allows both sexes to synchronize the expression of their sexual activity and their breeding season, in alignment with external environmental factors.

The pineal gland is the main regulatory organ in the seasonality of breeding; it registers day length via the eyes and a complex of neural connections, see Figure 6. The pineal gland produces indoleamins, of which melatonin is the most important. Melatonin is produced and secreted during the night (dark).

As days become shorter, the animal's exposure to melatonin increases. By some means not yet fully elucidated, this exerts a stimulating effect on GnRH secretion by the hypothalamus in short-day breeders such as sheep. In long-day breeders, such as the horse, increased melatonin exposure has the opposite effect, inhibiting GnRH release by the hypothalamus. Thus differences in day length are recognised and translated into signals able to turn sexual activity on or off.

Generally speaking, photoperiod, which determines the endogenous circannual rhythm of reproductive activity, exerts its action through two different but complementary pathways, by adjusting the phases of gonadal development to external environmental changes, and by synchronizing the reproductive period between individuals of the same species (Chemineau et al., 2008).

Figure 6 Role of the pineal gland and melatonin in reproduction

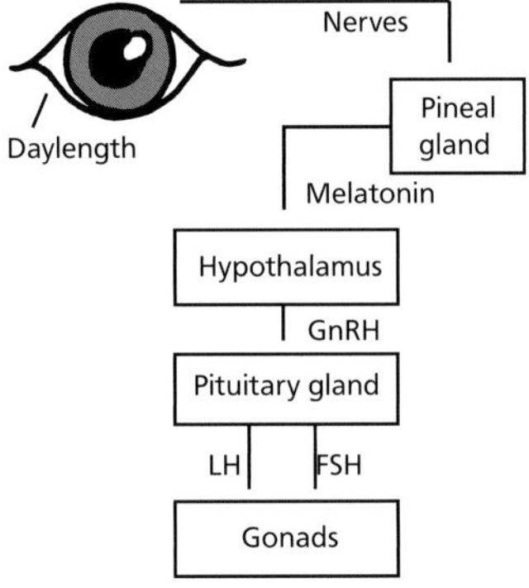

1.6 Further reading

Chemineau P., Guillaume D., Migaud M., Thiéry JC., Pellicer-Rubio MT., Malpaux B. Seasonality of Reproduction in Mammals: Intimate Regulatory Mechanisms and Practical Implications. Rerod Domest Anim 2008;43 (Suppl. 2): 40-47

Clarke IJ., Pompolo S. Synthesis and secretion of GnRH. Anim Reprod Sci 2005; 88: 29–55

Ginther OJ., Beg MA., Donadeu FX., Bergfelt DR. Mechanism of follicle deviation in monovular farm species. Anim Reprod Sci 2003;78:23 9–25 7

Herbert CA., Trigg TE. Applications of GnRH in the control and management of fertility in female animals. Animal Reproduction Science 2005; 88: 141-153

Mihm M., Bleach ECL. Endocrine regulation of ovarian antral follicle development in cattle. Anim Reprod Sci 2003;78:21 7–237

Norman AW and Litwack G. Hormones. 2nd Edn. Academic Press, 1997.

Thiéry JC., Chemineau P., Hernandez X., Migaud M., Malpaux B. Neuroendocrine interactions and seasonality. Dom Anim End 2002;23 :87–100

Weems CW., Weems YS., Randel RD. Prostaglandins and reproduction in female farm animals. Vet J 2006; 171: 206–228

2 Bovine Reproduction

2.1 Physiology

Nutritional influence

Numerous studies in dairy herds have clearly shown that a marked increase in milk production during early lactation increases the incidence of various reproductive problems (Grohn et al, 1994; Macmillan et al., 1996; Poso et al., 1996). Furthermore, the genetic capacity for extremely high levels of milk production in dairy cattle, together with changes in their nutritional management and larger herd sizes, have been associated with a gradual decline in fertility.

In late gestation, the nutritional requirements of the dairy cow inevitably place her in a catabolic state. Following parturition, milk production imposes additional high demands for glucose, fatty acids and proteins.

The inability to meet the high energy requirements for both maintenance and production in high yielding cows leads to a negative energy balance, particularly during the first few weeks after calving.

Decreased levels of glucose in the general circulation promote gluconeogenesis in the liver, and act as a potent trigger for lypolysis. The mobilised non-esterified fatty acids (NEFAs) serve as an alternative energy source in dairy cows to preserve the level of glucose which is utilized, preferentially, by the mammary gland, in the production of lactose.

It has been well documented that cows in too fat a condition at calving often have a reduced appetite and eventually develop a greater negative energy balance than that of their normal herd mates. These cows exhibit a more extensive mobilisation of body fat and a greater accumulation of triacylglycerols in the liver (Rukkwamsuk et al., 1998) leading to hepatic lipidosis which is associated, by many authors, with impaired fertility in the post partum period.

Energy balance during the first three weeks of lactation is highly correlated with the interval between calving and first ovulation (Butler et al., 2000). Moreover, it has been reported that severe negative energy balance may prolong the interval between calving and first ovulation. Low energy availability during the first few weeks of lactation impairs LH secretion, but it also reduces the responsiveness of the ovary to LH stimulation (Jolly et al., 1995; Butler 2000).

Endocrine environment in high-yielding dairy cows

Most available large data sets demonstrate an antagonistic relationship between milk production and fertility. Nonetheless the extent of this effect has been questioned, especially, as with many of the reproductive indices, no clear relationship with milk production has been established so far. However, observations in the field clearly indicate that high yielding dairy cows have much lower conception rates than heifers. The possible negative effect of high levels of milk production on the reproductive performance of high-yielders can be modulated through various aspects of reproductive function.

There is no uniform confirmation, in the literature, of a negative effect of high milk production levels on the intensity and duration of heat. However, both veterinary practitioners and farmers alike report that high-yielding dairy cows pose a problem with respect to oestrus detection. In a trial reported by Lopez et al. (2004) the duration of oestrus was correlated positively with peak oestradiol concentrations, and correlated negatively with milk production. Wiltbank et al. (2006) suggested that high levels of milk production lead to reduced circulating oestradiol concentrations, resulting in the decreased duration and intensity of oestrus. Decreased oestradiol concentrations could also cause increased follicular size because of the extended interval before the oestradiol-induced oestrus, GnRH-LH surge and ovulation of high yielding cows.

It now seems clear that very high-yielding cows may exhibit a different endocrine status to non-lactating cows, due to their high metabolic rate. Cows producing more milk develop larger follicles, but with lower circulating oestradiol concentrations (Lopes et al., 2004). Moreover, these high level producers have a greater volume of luteal tissue, but reduced circulating progesterone concentrations. The most likely explanation is

that the metabolism of steroid hormones increases as milk production increases in lactating dairy cows.
Wiltbank et al. (2006) proposed that some of the reproductive changes in lactating dairy cows are caused by a dramatic increase in steroid metabolism due to the enhanced feed intake and blood flow through the liver. In lactating dairy cows, a continuously high plane of nutrition leads to chronically elevated hepatic blood flow, and approximately double the rate of metabolism of steroid hormones observed in their non-lactating peers of similar size and age. Results of recent trials indicate that, even with a similar level of hormone production, the level of circulating concentrations of steroid hormones is lower during lactation (Sangsritavong et al., 2002; Wiltbank et al., 2006).
In addition to lower oestradiol concentrations at the start of oestrus, there is also likely to be a more rapid reduction in circulating oestradiol after LH surge due to the increased metabolism of this steroid. This would result in a shorter duration of oestrus in high-yielding cows. Elevated steroid metabolism due to high milk production levels can also have a more profound detrimental effect on fertility. The pre-ovulatory follicle and oocyte may be exposed to an extended period of elevated LH pulses, which in turn may lead to ovulation of an over-stimulated or prematurely-activated oocyte and thus to reduced fertility. Also the reduced rate of rise of progesterone following ovulation can reduce fertility because of the poorer survival of embryos.

Moreover, in high yielding dairy cows, at the ovarian level, follicular growth and development are most probably directly influenced by altered insulin, insulin-like growth factor I (IGF-I), leptin and levels of NEFAs. Since insulin stimulates follicular growth, maturation and steroidogenesis locally, its reduced concentrations post partum are linked with impaired follicular development.

It is important to recognise that the effects of the negative energy balance can still be observed even after cows begin to recover their body condition. Research workers have postulated the existence of a carry-over effect of the adverse metabolic conditions on the health of the pre-ovulatory follicle, during the early post partum period 2-3 months later. Such follicles may be less capable of producing adequate amounts of oestradiol, contain an oocyte of lower quality and, following ovulation, form a corpus luteum of reduced steroidogenic capacity.

Physiology of the oestrous cycle in cattle

The sexual cycle of the cow is generally independent of the season of the year. Oestrus or 'heat' is observed every 21 days on average, with a range of 18-24 days. Oestrus is taken as day zero of the cycle. It is of relatively short duration, lasting on average 18 hours, with a range of 4-24 hours. Ovulation takes place about 30 hours after the onset of oestrus, that is, after the end of behavioural oestrus. Fertilization of the ovum takes place in the oviduct. The blastocyst arrives in the uterus at around day 5. Pregnancy lasts for 279-290 days. The interval from calving to first ovulation varies greatly depending on the breed of cow, nutrition, milk yield, season and the presence of a sucking calf. The first ovulation after calving is frequently not accompanied by oestrus behaviour, and is known as a 'silent heat'. See also 2.4.1.

Follicular growth in cattle

Follicular growth and development in ruminants is characterized by two or three consecutive follicular waves per oestrous cycle. The coming of ultrasonography has allowed much information to be gathered about the stages of follicular growth and selection. Each wave involves the recruitment of a cohort of follicles from the total ovarian follicular stock, and the selection of a dominant follicle which continues to grow and mature to the pre-ovulatory stage while the others undergo atresia. Three distinct stages can be distinguished in follicular development: growth, selection and deviation phases.

Each wave consists of the simultaneous recruitment of three to six follicles to grow larger than 4–5 mm in diameter. Within a few days of the start of a wave, one follicle emerges as dominant. The dominant follicle continues to grow and differentiate, whereas its sister follicles stop growing, and regress. The dominant follicle of the first wave in two-wave cycles, and of the first and second waves in three-wave cycles, regresses. However, the dominant follicle of any follicular wave, including the first, can ovulate if the appropriate endocrine conditions are provided by the induction of luteolysis (by the injection of prostaglandin $F_{2\alpha}$) during its tenure of dominance.

The recruitment of waves of follicles

In cattle and other species, follicular waves are preceded or accompanied by a small rise in FSH.

All follicles growing as a cohort contain specific receptors for FSH and depend on this gonadotrophin for their growth. At this stage the growing follicles do not have a sufficient population of LH receptors to respond to an LH-like stimulation, which is why this stage of growth is sometimes called FSH-dependent. In cattle, sequential FSH rises of similar magnitude to the GnRH surge, associated with new waves of follicles, take place during the oestrous cycle, in the post partum period, during pregnancy and before puberty.

Selection of the dominant follicle

For reasons not yet properly understood, only one dominant follicle is selected from the cohort recruited by the small rise in FSH. A defining characteristic of the dominant follicle appears to be its greater capacity for oestradiol production. Secretion of oestradiol, and perhaps androgen, by the dominant follicle is associated with the cessation of the rise in FSH, and then its maintenance at basal levels (Ginther et al., 2000 a,b). The future dominant follicle acquires LH receptors which allow it to continue to grow in the environment of low FSH and increasing LH levels. This is confirmed by the enhanced binding ability of the granulosa cells of the newly selected dominant follicle.

By indirectly lowering the FSH level, the dominant follicle decreases the support crucial for the subordinate follicles by reducing the component vital for their growth, while at the same time benefiting from both the low FSH and increasing LH levels. At the time of deviation this dominant follicle can maintain follicular cell proliferation and enhance oestradiol production in spite of the declining FSH stimulation. It is possible that the dominant follicle has increased, or maintained, high FSH-receptor mRNA expression and FSH-binding, which allows it to pass the 8.5mm diameter threshold (Mihm and Evans 2008).

Recently, important information has emerged about the role of other modulators such as growth factors, inhibin and insulin in the differentiation and selection of the dominant follicle (Fortune et al., 2001; Mihm et al., 2003). The growth hormone causes an increase in the synthesis of insulin-like growth factor I (IGF-I) and its principal carrier protein and its binding protein.

It is now well accepted that the ovary is an important site of both IGF-I gene expression and reception. Most of the compounds of the IGF system are expressed in bovine follicles. Moreover, a recent review published by Silva et al. (2009) listed the following processes in which IGF-I is involved in cattle: stimulation of growth in primary and secondary follicles; oestradiol production by secondary and antral follicles; proliferation of granulosa cells in antral follicles; oocyte viability and maturation; increase in the sensitivity of follicles to gonadotrophins; follicle dominance; and multiple ovulation.
Since IGF-I has been demonstrated to enhance the FSH-induced granulosa cell differentiation, and especially LH receptor acquisition, the increased free IGF-I concentrations in the selected future dominant follicle may be responsible for its developmental advantage.

Selected dominant follicle
Following its selection, the growth, oestrogen activity and lifespan of the dominant follicle are controlled by the LH pulse pattern. Therefore any changes in the GnRH, and thus the LH, release pattern will have a profound effect on the continued growth of the dominant follicle and its ovulation. It is now well known that the increased frequency of LH pulses seen following progestagen treatments, for example, will prolong the period of dominance of this follicle from 2-7 days to more than 14 days, which affects the fertility of the oocyte (Diskin et al., 2002). Nutritional, environmental and even infectious factors, which directly and indirectly affect the GnRH/LH pattern in cattle, will have a considerable effect on the fate of the dominant follicle, and consequently on ovulation and fertility.

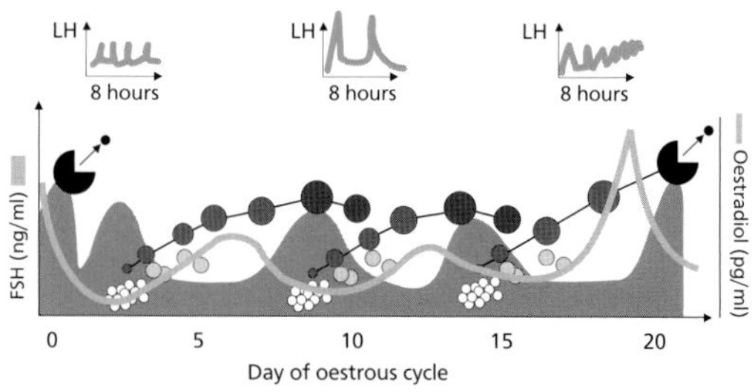

Formation and function of the corpus luteum

A very distinct structure is formed in place of an ovulated follicle called the corpus luteum. The corpus luteum is created by the process called luteinization involving both structural and functional changes in the granulosa and theca cells of the ovulated follicle which lead to the establishment of a transient secretory structure.

There are at least two types of cells with steroidogenic properties in the bovine corpus luteum: large and small luteal cells. The large luteal cells are formed from the granulosa cells, and the small ones from the thecal cells of the follicle, after ovulation has taken place. It is important to remember that the corpus luteum consists not only of steroidogenic luteal cells but also a multitude of other cells types, such as vascular endothelial cells, various immune cells and fibroblasts.

The formation of the corpus luteum is directly stimulated by the action of LH. However, there is clear evidence that steroidal and protein hormones, growth factors, eicosanoids and cytokines play important roles in the establishment of a functional corpus luteum (Berisha and Schams 2005).

In cattle and other domestic animals, it is the luteinizing hormone (LH) released from the pituitary gland that acts as the most potent regulator of the synthesis and secretion of progesterone by the corpus luteum (Skarzynski et al., 2008). LH stimulates the production of progesterone in small luteal cells via the specific LH receptor. Furthermore, intra-luteal progesterone concentrations have recently been demonstrated to be one of the most important factors supporting the maintenance of the function of the corpus luteum.

The newly formed corpus luteum is resistant to the action of exogenous $PGF_{2\alpha}$ until day 4-6 in cattle. It also seems that the sensitivity of the corpus luteum to extragonadal $PGF_{2\alpha}$ increases progressively towards the end of the luteal phase.

Luteolysis

In animals that have not become pregnant, regression of the corpus luteum, the process called luteolysis, is essential for sustained cyclicity and allows for the development of a new dominant follicle, giving the cow yet another chance to conceive. Luteolysis starts between days 16 and 17 post oestrus in the cow, initiated by prostaglandin $F_{2\alpha}$ ($PGF_{2\alpha}$) released from the uterus during the late luteal phase. Uterine venous $PGF_{2\alpha}$ increases initially on day 16-17 post oestrus in cows.

The luteolytic cascade can be summarised as follows: Oxytocin produced by the corpus luteum binds to specific oxytocin receptors in the endometrium (which have been induced by the limited amounts of oestradiol produced by the late luteal phase follicles), thus stimulating the release of $PGF_{2\alpha}$ from the endometrial cells. Prostaglandin is released into the uterine vein, reaches the ovary as previously described via the ovarian artery, and causes regression of the corpus luteum.
A rapid functional regression of the corpus luteum is characterised by a decrease in progesterone production, followed by a structural regression phase.
The mechanism of the luteolytic action of $PGF_{2\alpha}$ has not yet been completely elucidated, but two major mechanisms have been suggested:

1. Reduction of the blood flow in the corpus luteum
A rapid decrease in luteal blood flow has been proposed recently as one of the main luteolytic actions of $PGF_{2\alpha}$. The histological changes that take place during luteolysis include hypertrophy and hyperplasia of cells in the arteriolar wall, accumulation of elastic fibres in the media, mucoid degeneration of the intima, protrusion of some endothelial cells into the capillary lumen and the formation of adherent junctions across them, resulting in a decrease in the vascular diameter. Also, it has been recently demonstrated that an injection of a luteolytic dose of prostaglandin $F_{2\alpha}$ analogue in the mid-luteal phase increases the intraluteal production of vasoactive substances, which play an important part in the luteolytic cascade. It was shown that the reduction in luteal blood supply at 8 hours after prostaglandin injection was coincident with the onset of structural luteolysis, which was reflected in the initial significant decrease in CL volume.

2. Direct action on luteal cells
A direct action of prostaglandin on the luteal cells, resulting from both the decrease in cAMP synthesis, normally produced in response to LH, and the inhibition of the steroidogenic action of cAMP. These effects would be further amplified by a reduction in the number of LH receptors. During the structural phase of luteolysis, the luteal cells undergo a process of apoptosis (so-called 'programmed death').

This thesis is further supported by the results of a study that showed that a prostaglandin-induced reduction in plasma progesterone concentrations occurs before a detectable decrease in both the volume of the CL and the luteal blood flow.

2.2 Herd fertility management

For the optimal production of both milk and calves, the target is generally for every cow in the herd to produce a live healthy calf each year, i.e. to have a calving interval of 365 days. Numerous studies have documented that the period for which cows fail to become pregnant beyond the optimal interval post calving is expensive (Groenendaal et al., 2004; De Vries 2006). Many modern professional periodicals raise the question of whether a longer calving interval might benefit reproductive performance, especially in dairy cows, allowing longer for both energy resources and reproductive processes to be restored post partum. In spite of clear evidence that greater insemination efficiency is usually achieved around 70-90 days post calving than immediately following the voluntary waiting period, late breeding is generally not economically feasible in dairy and seasonal beef operations (Arbel et al., 2001).

The control of reproduction in the dairy herd is only one component of the whole farm management package, which should be the preserve of the veterinary practice. Reproductive performance on a dairy farm affects profitability directly through the milk production per cow per day, the number of replacements available, and voluntary and involuntary culling rates. It is important to recognise that reproductive management programs will differ because of varying on-farm costs, housing and handling facilities, farm targets and values, and management styles.

Communicating, to the farmer, the value of the cost-benefit of veterinary services is a key feature for the success of herd health programmes.

This chapter deals with the main aspects of herd fertility management.

2.2.1 Evaluation of fertility

Table 1 lists the parameters and targets commonly used to analyse and evaluate fertility in the dairy herd.

Table 1 Reproduction parameters and targets for diary herds

Parameter	Target
Calving-conception interval (av. number of days open)	< 90 days
Calving-1st insemination interval	< 70 days
Conception rate at 1st insemination	> 60%
Number of inseminations per conception	< 1.5
Abortions (between 45-265 days of pregnancy)	< 3%
Culling due to infertility	< 5%
Age at first calving	24 months

In the beef suckler herd, the weaned calf is the main source of income. The key figures for reproductive performance are shown in Table 2.

Table 2 Reproduction parameters and targets for beef herds

Parameter	Target
Length of the breeding period	< 63 days
Pregnancy rat (35 days after the end of the breeding season)	> 95%
Percentage calves born alive (of cows confirmed pregnant)	> 93%

Note that these figures apply to intensively managed dairy and beef herds in temperate climates. Comparisons should only be made between herds kept in the same or similar regions.

2.2.2 Economic aspects

There are three main components of economic loss due to fertility problems:
- losses due to incorrectly timed or ineffective AI
- extended calving intervals
- culling for reasons of reproductive failure of animals with high genetic potential

Losses due to incorrectly timed AI
Endocrine disorders affecting reproductive performance in cattle often manifest themselves in the irregularity of the oestrous cycle, inadequate signs of heat or delayed ovulation. The result is likely to be the incorrect timing of artificial insemination, which can also be due to poor management. Repeat inseminations increase the costs of service and are wasteful of semen.

Extended calving interval
Longer calving intervals result in a longer lactation and a longer dry period. The total loss increases with the length of the calving interval (see Table 3). Extended calving interval is a direct result of increased calving to conception interval and is expressed in the number of so-called 'days open'. It has been a commonly recognised fact that an increased calving to conception interval results in losses which can be expressed in reduced overall milk production (see Table.3).

Table 3 Estimated losses associated with days open in dairy herds

Source: Esslemont and Kossaibati, 2002

Lactation	Loss nett per day in milk litres
Medium milk yield - 6.000 L/lactation (305d)	
1	10.88L
5	15.03L
Average	13.72L
High milk yield of 10.000 L/lactation (305d)	
1	16.97L
5	21.18L
Average	19.87L

Culling for reasons of reproductive failure

Nowadays, the annual replacement rate can reach up to 34% in large commercial dairy operations in the US, and nearly as high in many larger dairies throughout the world, with fertility failure as one of the principal reasons.

The losses caused by premature culling due to infertility depend on the age and the production level of the cow culled (Fig 1). These losses represent the missed future income from that cow. They are maximal for a high-yielding cow in her second lactation, and thereafter decrease with age and lower production level (Dijkhuizen et al., 1991)

When a valuable young cow is culled, it is not only her future milk production which is lost, but also her genetic potential as the source of replacement heifers.

Figure 1 Estimated cost of culling in the herd

Adapted from Source: Esslemont and Kossaibati 2002

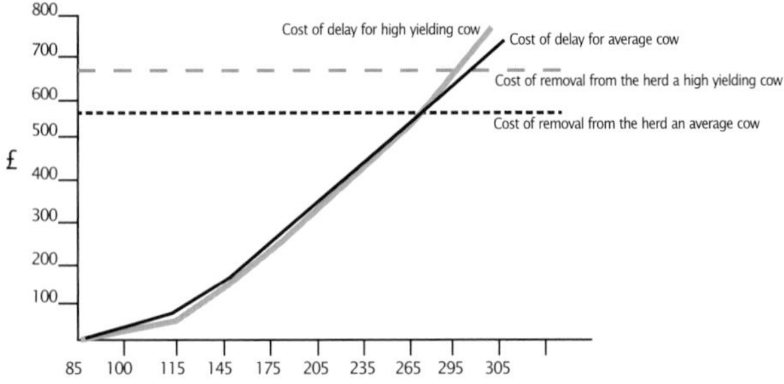

Moreover, with a high annual replacement rate, the age of the herd shifts towards an increasing proportion of first calving heifers. Above a certain threshold, this is unfavourable with respect both to milk production and also to reproductive efficiency, as first calvers are the group with the greatest frequency of post partum reproductive disorders.

2.2.3 Pregnancy diagnosis

Accurate and early diagnosis of pregnancy in both dairy and beef herds is essential for the maintenance of high levels of reproductive efficiency. It is required for the early identification of fertility problems at both individual animal and herd level.

Non-return to oestrus

If a cow is not observed in oestrus at around 3 weeks after service or insemination, she is generally assumed to be in calf. However, even if oestrus detection is good, not all of these cows will be pregnant. On the other hand, up to 7% of pregnant cows will show some signs of oestrus during pregnancy. Insemination of these animals may result in embryonic or foetal death.

Rectal palpation

Early pregnancy diagnosis (1-3 months) is based on a combination of the following: asymmetry of the uterine horns, lesser tone of the pregnant horn and fluctuant contents in the pregnant horn (later both horns), a palpable corpus luteum on the ovary on the same side as the pregnant horn, membrane slip and appreciation of an amniotic vesicle. In the later stages of pregnancy (>3 months), the cervix is located anterior to the pelvic rim and the uterus cannot be easily retracted. The uterus is flaccid and placentomes, and sometimes the foetus, are palpable. The median uterine artery increases in diameter and fremitus can be detected. See Table 4.

Table 4 Positive signs of pregnancy at rectal palpation

Stage of pregnancy	Membrane slip	Amniotic Vesicle	Foetus	Placentomes	Fremitus A.uterine media	
					Ipsilateral	contralateral
30 days	±	+				
45 days	+	+				
60 days	+	+				
75 days	+	+		+		
90 days	+		+	+		
105 days			+	+	+	
4 months			+	+	+	
5 months			+	+	+	+
6 months				+	+	+
7 months			+	+	+	+

The advantage of rectal palpation is that it provides an immediate answer and the non-pregnant cow be treated early. It requires minimum equipment and few personnel, if good handling facilities are available. A skilled practitioner can detect pregnancy in cattle as early as day 35.

Common reasons for errors in rectal palpation include failure to retract the uterus, abnormal uterine contents (pyometra or mucometra) and incorrect service dates. There is contradictory information regarding the possible risk to the embryo/foetus of palpation per rectum. Early or inappropriate palpation of the amniotic vesicle may damage the embryo and cause embryonic mortality. Nonetheless, a recent publication by Romano et al. (2007) indicated that pregnancy diagnosis by rectal palpation between days 34 and 41 of pregnancy, using the so-called 'membrane slip' technique did not affect embryonic/foetal viability.

Regardless of the advantages of the rectal palpation, pregnancy diagnosis by this method provides no information about foetal development (deformities, vitality etc.) and in the case of non-pregnancy, there is a relatively long period before insemination can be safely repeated.

Progesterone assay

The progesterone secreted by a functional corpus luteum between 18 and 24 days after service or insemination is an early indication of pregnancy. It can be assayed in milk or plasma. The optimum time for the assay is 24 days after service or AI, eliminating the problem of long oestrus intervals which might lead to a false positive diagnosis.

The sensitivity (i.e. accuracy in detecting pregnancy) of the cow-side milk progesterone (EIA) test was 93.1% in a study by Pieterse et al. (1989). However, its specificity (i.e. accuracy in detecting non-pregnancy) was only 39.3%, which meant that there was a rather large number of animals diagnosed as pregnant, which were in fact not pregnant. The most common reasons for error are pyometra/persistent corpus luteum, short oestrus intervals, cystic ovarian disease (luteal cysts) and the incorrect handling of the samples and test kit, as well as early embryonic mortality.

This indicates that relying on progesterone measurement on its own is unsatisfactory, and pregnancy must be confirmed by rectal palpation at 40 or so days after breeding. However, if a series of samples is collected between the day of insemination and days 21 and 24, the accuracy of early diagnosis of non-pregnancy approaches 95 to 100%. Thus milk progesterone tests could be used for the early identification of cows that have not conceived, allowing for their re-introduction into the breeding program.

Ultrasound examination

The use of transrectal ultrasonography to assess pregnancy status early in gestation is among the most practical applications of ultrasound for dairy cattle reproduction (Tab. 5). Early identification of non-pregnant cows following natural or artificial insemination improves reproductive efficiency and pregnancy rate by reducing the interval between AI services and increasing AI service rate. Real time (B-mode) ultrasound is a reliable and relatively simple method of diagnosing pregnancy. Under most farm conditions, pregnancy can be rapidly and accurately diagnosed using ultrasound as early as 26 days post AI.

Using ultrasound scanning techniques, an accuracy of over 99% can be achieved, enabling fertility problems to be identified rapidly. Generally, two factors affect the speed at which ultrasound examinations can be conducted on a dairy farm: operator proficiency and the availability and restraint of animals. When both factors are optimized, the speed of ultrasonography can approach that of rectal palpation, while exceeding the latter in the amount of information gathered from each animal. The main advantage of scanning is that it can give an accurate diagnosis earlier than rectal palpation.

Table 5 Day of first detection of ultrasonographically identifiable characterstics of the bovine conceptus.

Characteristic	First day detected	
	Mean	Range
Embryo proper	20.3	19 to 24
Heartbeat	20.9	19 to 24
Allantois	23.2	22 to 25
Spinal cord	29.1	26 to 33
Forelimb buds	29.1	28 to 31
Amnion	29.5	28 to 33
Eye orbit	30.2	29 to 33
Hindlimb buds	31.2	30 to 33
Placentomes	35.2	33 to 38
Split hooves	44.6	42 to 49
Foetal movement	44.8	42 to 50
Ribs	52.8	51 to 55

Adapted from Curran et al., 1986

Because pregnancy can be identified earlier using ultrasound than by rectal palpation, the rate of pregnancy loss detected is often higher. Of cows diagnosed pregnant at 28 days after AI, 10 to 16% experience early embryonic loss by 56 days (Mee et al., 1994; Vasconcelos et al., 1997). Therefore, cows diagnosed pregnant at 28 days after AI, using ultrasound, should be submitted to a subsequent examination at around 60 days, after which the rate of embryonic loss will be much less (Vasconcelos et al., 1997).

Identification of twin pregnancies

With transrectal ultrasonography, cows carrying twins can be accurately identified by 40 to 55 days post breeding. When conducting an early examination to identify twins, the entire length of both uterine horns must be carefully scanned to ensure that an embryo is not missed. Depending on the type of cow (dairy, beef or dual purpose) several management scenarios can be considered once twins have been identified, including abortion and rebreeding, or continued management until parturition. Although approaches to twin pregnancies are limited under field conditions, identifying cows carrying twins is always beneficial, so that extra care can be provided at calving.

Identification of foetal gender

Transrectal ultrasound can be used to determine the sex of bovine foetuses by evaluating the morphology and location of the genital tubercle; it is reliable and accurate from day 55 to 60 of gestation (Fricke 2002). A much greater level of proficiency and experience is required for determinating the sex of the foetus than that required for early pregnancy diagnosis or examination of ovarian structures. It must be stressed that, although it has its attractions, foetal sex determination should only be included in reproduction management, if the information generated can be put to good use from a managerial viewpoint. Knowing the percentage of cows carrying female foetuses can be of value in dairy operations, when replacement heifers are selected from within the herd. When the expected number of replacements does not match the requirement, plans can be made for the purchase of followers from another supplier. On the other hand, sexing the foetus can also be used effectively producing dairy bull calves of a specific parentage for sale to insemination centres and others.

Early pregnancy diagnosis based on the detection of pregnancy specific molecules

During the last ten years, techniques have been developed for early pregnanacy diagnosis in cattle based on the detection of pregnancy specific proteins.

PAGs

Pregnancy-associated glycoproteins (PAGs) are known under a variety of names, including pregnancy-specific protein B (PSPB). They constitute a large family of glycoproteins expressed in the outer epithelial cell layer (chorion/trophectoderm) of the placenta of eutherian species. The PAG molecules belong to a group of proteolytic enzymes known as aspartic proteinases (AP). Several closely related PAG molecules have been identified between early blastocyst development and parturition (Sousa et al., 2006). Pregnancy-specific protein-B was the first such protein to be identified in cattle (Butler et al., 1982) and was later found to have the same N-terminal AA sequence as pregnancy-associated glycoprotein (Xie et al., 1991; Lynch et al., 1992). Both pregnancy specific protein-B and PAG have subsequently been reclassified as boPAG-1.

Mean PAGs concentrations in cattle increase from 15 to 35 days of gestation. However, the variation between cows in serum PAG levels, limits their use as a reliable indicator of pregnancy until about 26 to 30 days of gestation (Humblot, 2001).

There are several different diagnostic approaches, employing either radioimmunoassay (RIA) (Haugejorden et al., 2006; Lopez-Gatius et al., 2007; Ayad et al., 2009) or variations of the enzyme-linked immunosorbent assay (ELISA) (Green et al., 2005; Silva et al., 2007; Friedrich and Holtz 2009). Several laboratories at universities or scientific institutes use the PAG-based assays for pregnancy diagnosis for experimental purposes, and some offer the tests to practitioners on a commercial basis.

An ELISA test for PSPB (BioPRYN™, BioTracking, Moscow, ID, USA) is available in the US, Canada, Australia and Hungary. The assay is performed on serum samples by licensed laboratories and is recommended for pregnancy detection from day 30 after insemination in dairy and beef cows, and from day 28 in heifers. In general, the data available so far indicate that this type of test is of great diagnostic value when performed from 30 days after insemination. It must be stressed that because PAG molecules persist for a long time in the circulation after calving, only cows served more than 60 days after calving should be included in any PAG-based assays.

ECF/EPF

Early pregnancy factor (EPF) was first identified in pregnant mice (Morton et al., 1987) and later in sheep and cattle (Nancarrow et al., 1981) by using the rosette inhibition test.

Early pregnancy factor was demonstrated to have specific growth regulatory and immunomodulatory properties and is required for the successful establishment of pregnancy and the proliferation of both normal and neoplastic cells in vivo and in vitro (Cavanagh, 1996). Significant differences in rosette inhibition titre were observed between pregnant and non-pregnant cows on days 13 to 16 and 25 post AI (Sakonju et al., 1993) suggesting that measurement of EPF activity could be used as a method of early pregnancy diagnosis. Several publications have reported conflicting results from trials assessing the accuracy of ECF/EPF-based laboratory tests, mainly indicating the low specificity of the assays when used in the early post breeding period (Cordoba et al., 2001; Ambrose et al., 2007)

Recently, a new early pregnancy test has become commercially available for use in cattle. The Early Conception Factor (ECF) test (Concepto Diagnostics, Knoxville, TN) is reported to detect a pregnancy-associated glycoprotein within 48 hours of conception. However, encouraging data are only limited, not enough to allow this test to be recommended on a wide scale in the field.

2.2.4 Oestrus and oestrus detection

Reproductive performance is a major factor affecting the production and economic efficiency of dairy and beef herds. For herds using artificial insemination, heat detection rate and calving rate are two major determinants of the compactness of the calving season and ultimately of the calving-to-calving interval. Insufficient and/or inaccurate oestrus detection leads to delayed insemination, reduced conception rates and thus extended calving intervals (Table 6).

Oestrus

Oestrus is the complex of physiological and behavioural signs occurring just before ovulation. The length of oestrus varies from 4 to 24 hours. The signs of oestrus are: standing when mounted; swollen vulva; hyperaemic vaginal mucosa; clear and elastic mucous vaginal discharge; ruffled tailhead, possibly with minor skin lesions; restlessness; group formation; chin rubbing; flehmen; licking, pushing, fighting, mounting other animals; lordosis; and possibly reduced feed intake and/or milk yield.

Oestrus signs, especially when several animals are in (pro-) oestrus simultaneously, are often misinterpreted. Of all the signs the standing reflex (standing when mounted) is a truly reliable indication of oestrus. The cow is then said to be in 'standing heat'.

Table 6 Accuracy of visual heat detection in relation to the number of observations per day.

Frequency of observation	Efficacy
Once a day	60%
Twice a day	80%
Three times a day	90%
Four times a day	95-100%

Heat detection aids

There are several aids to facilitate oestrus detection.

Heat mount detectors

Heat mount detectors are glued on the mid-line of the back of the cow, just in front of the tail-head. A 'triggered' detector indicates that the animal has been mounted. Experimental evaluation has produced conflicting results. Loss of the detector, poor performance in cold weather and a high proportion of false positives when animals are housed close together, have all been reported to account for this.
Recent technological advances have allowed heat-mount detection devices to become more sophisticated. Some detectors now flash to indicate how many times the cow has been mounted

and how much time has elapsed since it was first mounted. However, perhaps the most sophisticated detector comprises a pressure sensitive battery-operated radio transmitter. When activated, the transmitter emits a radio-signal which is picked up by a receiver. The signal is then digitalised and stored on computer together with the date and time, duration of each mount and the cow's identity. This has been widely used in the US.

Tail paint, a strip of brightly-coloured paint (20 cm long and 5 cm wide) lightly applied to the midline area in front of the tail head which will be rubbed by mounting cows, should last for at least 4 weeks unless rubbed. It appears to improve the efficiency of oestrus detection, though cubicle housing and high cattle density increase the number of false positives.

Teasers

Teaser animals, i.e. vasectomised bulls or testosterone-treated cull cows, will mount a cow in heat and thus attract the attention of the herdsman. They may be equipped with a chin ball marker or a raddle. Aggressive behaviour, and the development of favouritism (ignoring cows in heat other than favourites), are disadvantages of this system. Moreover, vasectomised bulls may be vectors of venereal diseases.

Pedometers

Cattle in heat walk at least twice as much as they do before and after heat. Thus, measuring the distance walked using pedometers can identify bulling cattle. However, the significant difference in normal walking activity between cows means that it is not possible to set a reliable general threshold over which cows are likely to be in oestrus. Comparisons can only be made for an individual cow. This requires computerisation and greatly increases the costs. Nevertheless, combining heat checks and pedometer detection is a highly efficient and accurate method of detection.

TV surveillance

This method involves camera surveillance and recording of the behaviour of cows in a confined area. It requires careful evaluation of a day's recordings and relies on the subjective interpretation of animals' behaviour.

Measurement of electrical resistance of vaginal mucus - Draminsky method
Changes in the electrical resistance of vaginal mucus are measured with a so-called Draminsky apparatus equipped with an intravaginal probe.
The method requires good records of results in individual animals from previous heats and at least two readings from the current heat, to be reliable. A single reading may be misleading (standard values are provided, but there is considerable individual variation).

2.2.5 Timing of insemination

Fertilization of the ovum occurs in the oviduct at the junction of the isthmus and ampulla. The life span of the ovum is around 12-18 hours and its viability decreases with time. About 8 hours after service, sufficient numbers of spermatozoa have reached the isthmus of the oviduct. Capacitation of the spermatozoa is required for fertilization and is characterised by their hypermotility and completed acrosome reaction. The optimal time at which insemination should take place relative to ovulation (insemination–ovulation interval = IOI) depends mainly on the fertile lifespan of spermatozoa and on the viable lifespan of the oocyte in the female reproductive tract.
Spermatozoa also have a limited lifespan, therefore if insemination takes place too early, the sperm cells will die before they can fertilize the ovum. Conversely, when insemination is delayed too long, the ovum will have lost its capacity to be fertilized.

Ovulation normally occurs between 10 and 15 hours after the end of oestrus. The optimum time for insemination is therefore towards the end of oestrus (see Table 7). Under practical conditions, cows are not observed continuously, so the end of oestrus is not apparent. Because of the limited lifespan of both ovum and sperm there is a 'window' of about 12 hours during which optimal conception rates are achieved.
A study by Roelofs et al. (2006) showed that the IOI with a high probability of fertilization is quite long (between 36 and 12 hours before ovulation). However, the IOI in which this fertilized oocyte has a high probability of developing into a good embryo is shorter (24–12 hours before ovulation).

Table 7 Optimum time of insemination in relation to oestrus

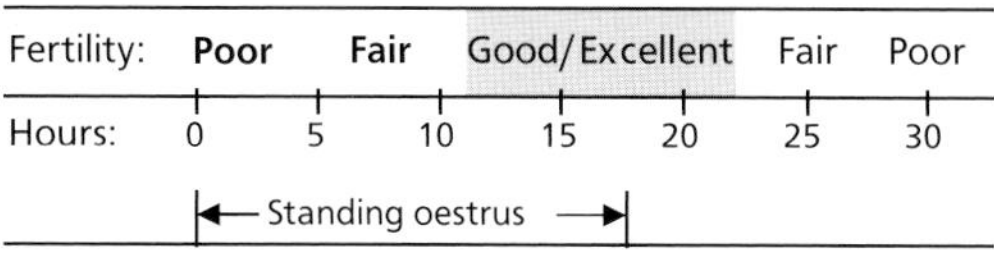

Fertility:	Poor	Fair	Good/Excellent		Fair	Poor
Hours:	0	5	10	15	20	25	30

|←Standing oestrus→| (0 to approx. 18 hours)

For practical purposes it is best to use the AM/PM rule: all cows seen in oestrus during the morning are inseminated during the afternoon. Cows still in heat the next morning are re-inseminated. Cows observed in oestrus during the afternoon or evening, are inseminated the following morning. This represents, in fact, a compromise between ensuring the best chance of fertilization and obtaining an embryo of optimal quality and developmental potential (Fig 2). In other words, early insemination gives good prospects for an embryo of high quality, but at a lower fertilization rate (decreased sperm survival due to "waiting" for the oocyte). On the other hand, late insemination makes a high fertilization rate possible (a lot of fresh sperm) but due to ageing of the oocyte which ovulated much earlier, there is a risk of low embryo quality (Saacke 2008).

Figure 2 Calculated pregnancy in relation to the insemination time (adapted from Saacke 2008)

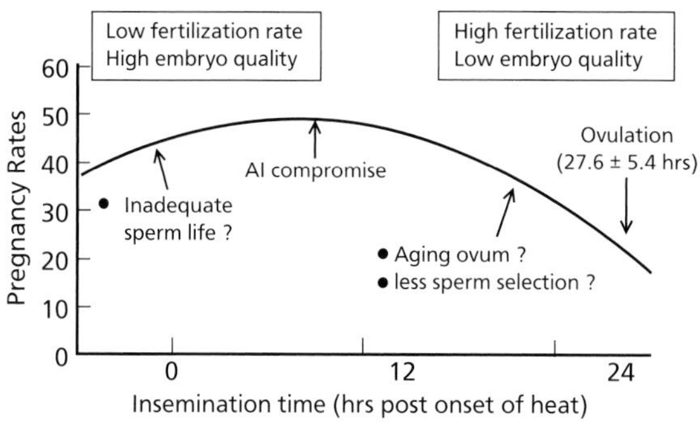

2.3 Control of oestrus

2.3.1 Reasons for oestrus control

The oestrous cycle can be regulated pharmacologically to induce or control the time of oestrus and ovulation.

Generally the main reasons for oestrus control in cattle can be grouped as follows:
- management of anoestrus/acyclia in both beef and dairy herds
- induction of oestrus within a predetermined time-window to facilitate oestrus detection and for management purposes (availability of AI technician, seasonal breeding)
- tight synchronization of oestrus in donors and recipients involved in embryo transfer
- treatment of certain disorders such as suboestrus, persistent corpus luteum, cystic ovarian disease

Planning and cost-effectiveness of oestrus management programs
There are several factors to be considered when making a decision about introducing planned oestrus management into a cattle herd, and especially when a pharmacological system needs to be chosen. Prior reproductive performance is very important when assessing which system is likely to be of best advantage to a given farm. The type of animals, age structure of the herd and the level of productivity should be carefully analysed. Human resources, the level of education/skills of the farm staff, and their work environment must all be taken into account also. This is especially important if a complex regime is to be implemented, as compliance in the accuracy and timing of the administration of products will have a decisive effect on the efficacy of the program.

It should be always borne in mind that the costs of any oestrus management program must be weighed not only against the possible improvement of pregnancy rates and reduction in days open, but also against the reduced labour costs of oestrus detection. Visual heat detection is more labour intensive, and thus more cost-sensitive than a synchronization program. The cost-effectiveness should be calculated for each individual herd when assessing the advantages of introducing systematic breeding programs.

Certain aspects of oestrus management need to be highlighted separately for beef and dairy herds.

Beef cattle
Beef herds are often managed extensively and on a group basis. Oestrus detection is therefore a much less intensive activity and less accurate than in dairy herds. The presence of a sucking calf and seasonal influences can depress or block cyclical activity in beef cattle. For these reasons many beef cows do not show signs of oestrus during the 40-60 days post partum when they should be served again.

Most beef herds are restricted to a specific breeding period. Cows that have not resumed ovarian activity in time, and therefore failed to conceive, will generally be culled.

In beef herds, AI has several advantages over natural service:
- Fewer bulls need to be kept.
- It allows the use of high quality semen, from progeny tested bulls, thus increasing the breeding value of the herd.
- More uniform calf production.

In beef herds, oestrus detection is often the limiting factor for the successful use of AI. Oestrus control and synchronization can offer a solution. The use of a progestagen/PMSG system at the start of the natural breeding period stimulates and synchronizes ovarian activity. It thus advances and compacts the calving period compared to reliance upon natural service.

The advantages of such a system are considerable:
- Close supervision during the shortened calving period which reduces calf losses due to dystocia.
- If weaned on a fixed date, calves will be older and heavier by sale time.
- A short calving period will improve herd fertility for the following season.
- Calves can be sold in batches of similar age and of consistent quality, which increases their value.
- It enables and/or facilitates the use of AI and allows more rational semen management.

Dairy cattle
In dairy herds which practise year-round calving, cows must be managed individually and more intensively than beef cattle. With a target of one calf per cow per year, the interval between calving and conception is limited to about 85 days during which involution of the uterus must take place, ovarian activity must be resumed and oestrus detected. Generally about 25% of dairy cows have not been observed in oestrus before day 40 post partum.

Oestrus control is used in dairy cattle for the following indications:
- to induce oestrus and ovulation in cows with post partum anoestrus in order to shorten the interval between calving and first insemination.
- to synchronize donor and recipient cows for embryo transfer
- to synchronize oestrus in groups of animals to improve oestrus detection or to reduce the time required for oestrus detection.
- to control a herd's calving period.

For many dairy farms the failure to observe oestrus efficiently significantly limits their reproductive performance. Increased levels of production, coupled with increased herd size, have influenced the way in which dairy farms manage reproduction, which has stimulated the development of oestrus synchronization programs that allow artificial insemination at pre-determined times without the need for oestrus detection.

For a more in-depth economic analysis see De Vries (2006) and Olynk et al. (2007, 2008).

2.3.2 Methods of oestrus control

The critical requirements for any effective system to control the oestrus cycle are a predictable and high frequency of oestrus and ovulation response during a specified 12-24h period, followed by a high pregnancy rate to a single pre-programmed AI after treatment.
Due to changing requirements of the ovarian follicles for gonadotrophin support during their development, it is difficult to develop one simple exogenous hormone treatment to stimulate the predictable emergence of a new wave in any animal treated, irrespective of the stage of the follicle wave at time of treatment.
All pharmacological methods of oestrus management should be regarded as useful tools whose main objective is increase the efficiency of breeding in the herds, improve breeding organization or correct some organisational deficiency. In some cases, oestrus management systems can be used as a treatment for certain reproductive disorders such as 'silent heat' or cystic ovarian disease.
Pharmacological methods for oestrus management should, however, never be perceived as replacing the proper nutrition and appropriate management of breeding cattle.

In cattle with active ovaries, the oestrous cycle can be manipulated in three ways:
- by the use of prostaglandins, to induce early regression of the corpus luteum.
- by the sequential use of prostaglandins and GnRH analogues to obtain synchronized follicular development after an induced luteolysis.
- by the use of progestagens that act as an 'artificial' corpus luteum.

In animals in anoestrus (failing to ovulate), systems should be employed that allow for the induction of follicular growth and ovulation followed by a luteal phase of physiological duration:
- progestagen-based systems usually combined with GnRH and/or PMSG/eCG
- stimulation of ovarian activity with GnRH followed by an Ovsynch-type protocol

Prostaglandins

Between day 6 and day 16 of the cycle (the period of natural prostaglandin $F_{2\alpha}$ release) an injection of prostaglandin (Estrumate®) will induce regression of the corpus luteum ending the luteal phase. A new follicular phase begins and the animal will come into oestrus and ovulate. The fertility at the induced oestrus is similar to that of a natural oestrus. For the synchronization of a group of cyclic animals, likely all to be in different and unknown stages of the cycle, one injection is not sufficient. A second injection should be given 11-14 days later, because, by then, all animals should have a functional corpus luteum.

Despite rapid luteolysis the interval to onset of oestrus after treatment with $PGF_{2\alpha}$ is variable and dependent on the stage of the animal's follicular development when treated (Fig 3). Animals with a functional dominant follicle are in oestrus within 2-3 days because the dominant follicle ovulates at the time of induced luteolysis (Fig 4). However animals at the pre-dominance phase of the wave will require 2-4 days to form a dominant follicle and hence have a longer and more variable interval to the onset of oestrus.

Figure 3 Interval from PGF injection to ovulation in cattle

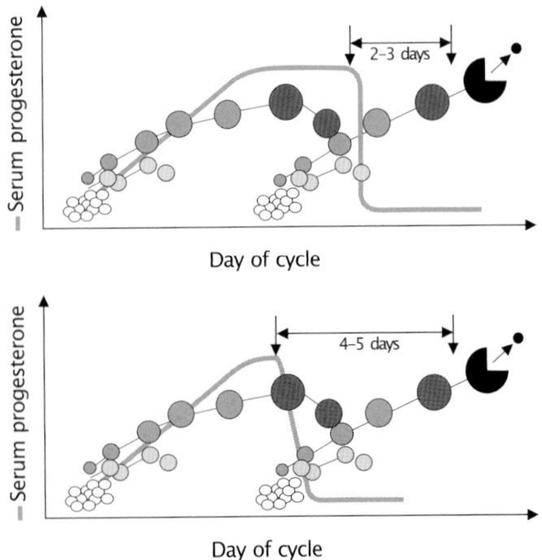

Figure 4 Distribution of oestrus in cows treated with PGF

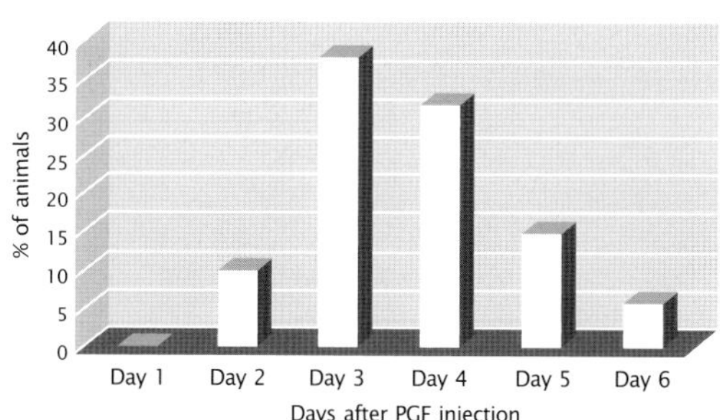

Insemination at an observed oestrus will give the best conception rates and is recommended for adult dairy cows in particular. Heifers show a more synchronous response and fixed time insemination at 72 and 96 hours can be used in cycling beef and dairy heifers. Because prostaglandins act on the corpus luteum, they can only be effective in cycling cattle.

Prostaglandins can be used in several different ways for oestrus control depending on the intentions of the herdsman, the type of animal and the conditions on the farm. An overview adapted from Cavalieri et al. (2006) outlines the most frequently used systems (Fig. 5).

Figure 5 Various systems of oestrus management with prostaglandins

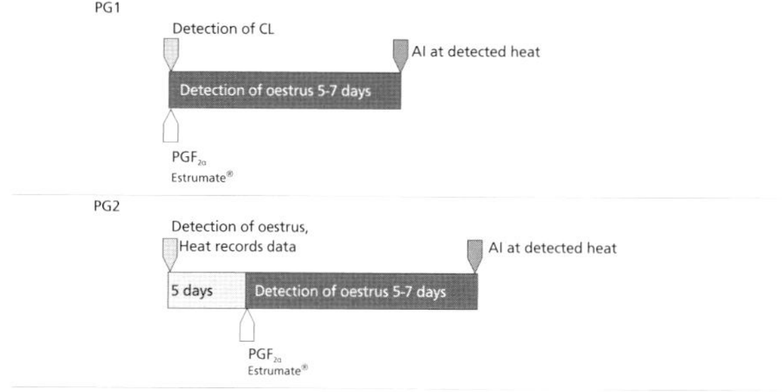

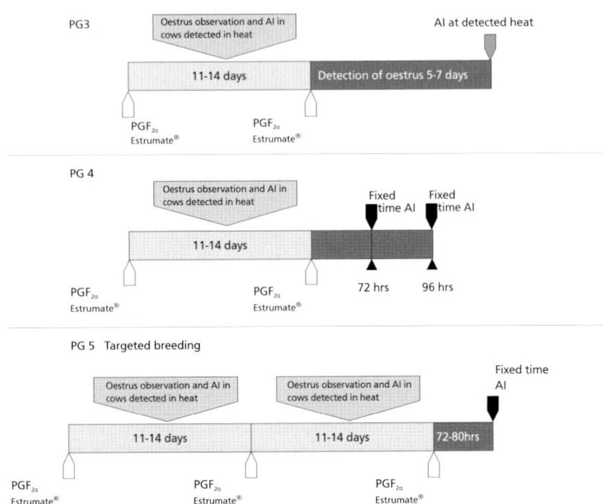

Multiple dose protocols are usually designed to synchronize oestrus in whole herds with the onset of oestrus expected in most cows within 7 days of treatment. Some single dose systems have also been developed with the aim of reducing the cost of treatment, but these offer far less flexibility than multidose protocols. They rely on the strategic administration of $PGF_{2\alpha}$ to cows in which luteolysis is most likely to occur after treatment, and then require oestrus detection over a longer period and/or detection of a corpus luteum to ensure a high rate of response to treatment.

A so-called Targeted Breeding programme was developed in order to improve reproductive efficiency in large dairy herds (Nebel and Jobst 1998). In this system cows are systematically treated on the same day of the week, to facilitate treatment and AI on weekdays. Animals receive a prostaglandin injection at 14-day intervals and are inseminated at the observed oestrus.

Cows not detected in oestrus after a third prostaglandin treatment, are inseminated at a fixed time 72-80 hours after the last $PGF_{2\alpha}$ injection.
These types of program using sequential PGF treatment were demonstrated to have a beneficial effect in herds with a high prevalence of post partum uterine infections. Prostaglandins promote uterine contractions, and are postulated to have a positive effect on the activity of endometrial immune cells. Moreover, with this approach, each consecutive luteal phase is shortened and thus the immunosuppressive influence of progesterone reduced. Some experts, however, argue that this may carry with it some risk for the future fertility of treated cows. If the treatment is initiated soon after the first post partum ovulation and continued without interruption for several cycles the treated cows practically never have a chance to experience a complete luteal phase. This may result in lower fertility due to a limited exposure to progesterone.

Application in beef cows.
Due to a high incidence of post partum anoestrus in beef cows, prostaglandins are not considered to be the method of choice for oestrus management in this class of animal. Should this method be used in spite of this, it is essential to ensure that the cows are cycling and in appropriate body condition.

Prostaglandins and GnRH analogues
A programme sometimes known as Ovsynch (Fig 6) is primarily indicated for dairy cows and involves two injections of a GnRH analogue separated by a single administration of $PGF_{2\alpha}$ (Pursley et al., 1995). Because, in the field, synchronization is likely to be used in cows which might be at any stage of the oestrous cycle, combining GnRH with prostaglandin leads to a greater homogeneity of ovarian follicular status at the time of the induction of luteolysis. As a result, the precision with which oestrus can be predicted after prostaglandin-induced luteolysis and the synchrony of the LH surge are both improved, which allows the synchronization of both follicular development and regression of the corpus luteum.

Figure 6 The Ovsynch protocol

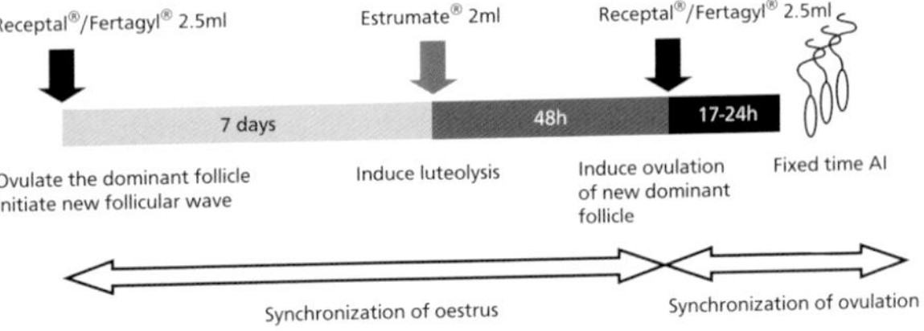

The first administration of GnRH is given at a random stage of the oestrous cycle and causes either ovulation or luteinization of a dominant follicle, if present, in about 85% of cows (Pursley et al., 1995). The administration of prostaglandin causes regression of any accessory corpus luteum or luteinized follicle induced by the GnRH or indeed of any corpus luteum present following an earlier spontaneous ovulation (Fig 7). In cows in which the fate of the current follicle wave was altered, a new dominant follicle should be present on the ovary by the time of the second GnRH treatment. Cows receiving GnRH at the pre-dominance phase of their follicular wave cycle should not have their follicular wave altered and would also be expected to have a dominant follicle present at the time of the second GnRH treatment. The ovulatory response in dairy cattle has been tightly synchronized, and occurs approximately 26-32 hours after the second GnRH injection. Thus a timed insemination at 17-24 hours after GnRH should result in a high probability of successful conception (Peters et al., 1999).

Figure 7 Follicular dynamics in cows treated with the Ovsynch protocol

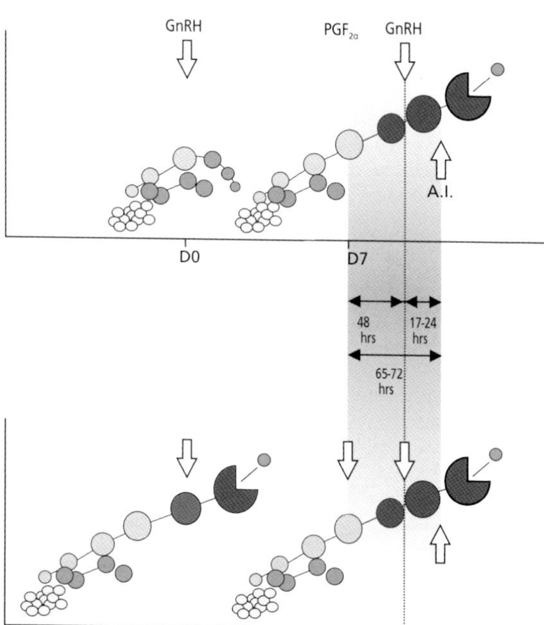

Ovsynch facilitates the precise scheduling of the first post partum AI, while improving reproductive performance during the early post partum period, with much saving of labour due to elimination of the need for oestrus detection.

Coleman et al. (1991) and Twagiramungu et al. (1992) reported that the fertility rate of cows synchronized with GnRH and $PGF_{2\alpha}$ varied between 35 and 65% and was similar to that of control animals inseminated at a first observed oestrus.

Efficacy of the Ovsynch protocol

The ability of GnRH-$PGF_{2\alpha}$ based protocols to synchronize oestrus and ovulation effectively is dependent on the stage of follicular development at the time of the initial GnRH injection. Fertility obtained with the Ovsynch protocol is greatest when cows ovulate to the first GnRH injection.

Vasconcelos et al. (1999) evaluated the influence of the day of the oestrous cycle on which the Ovsynch is initiated and resulting pregnancy rates in lactating dairy cows (Table 8).

Table 8 Efficacy of oestrus induction in Ovsynch protocol initiated on different days of the oestrous cycle. Vasconcelos et al. (1999)

Day of oestrous cycle	1st GnRH injection Ovulation	2nd GnRH injection Ovulation
1-4	23%	94%
5-9	96%	89%
10-16	54%	85%
17-21	77%	81%
Overall	64%	87%

From that study it can be concluded that the conception rates should be greatest when the Ovsynch protocol is initiated between days 1 and 12 of the oestrous cycle. Monitoring of the cow's oestrous cycle to select the most promising time to initiate the Ovsynch protocol is, however, impractical and, in a way, acts against the whole idea of this system as being practicable regardless of the cow's stage of the cycle.

Several studies conducted during the past few years compared pregnancy rates obtained with the use of the Ovsynch protocol and other oestrus management programmes such as the use of prostaglandins (Pursley et al., 1997; de la Sota et al., 1998; Keister et al., 1998; Stevenson et al., 1999,2000; Cartmill 2001), progestagens (Gaery et al., 1998; Williams et al., 2002) and various Ovsynch programme modifications (Bartolome et al., 2002; Pancarci et al., 2002) and natural breeding (Cordoba and Fricke 2001).

A meta-analysis performed by Rabiee et al. (2005) compared the results reported in numerous trials with the use of the Ovsynch protocol, natural breeding, single, double or triple prostaglandin injection, Select Synch, Heat Synch and modified Ovsynch. These authors concluded that pregnancy rates for Ovsynch programmes did not differ significantly from those obtained with natural breeding. Moreover the likelihood of conception and pregnancy did not differ significantly between the Ovsynch group and cows treated with prostaglandins. Comparison of the probability of pregnancy in cows treated with Ovsynch, Heat Synch and Select Synch did not differ significantly.

Modifications of the Ovsynch protocol (Fig 8)

Both ovulatory response to GnRH injection and luteal function following induction of ovulation with GnRH are dependent on the size of ovarian follicles at the time when GnRH is administered. Pre-synchronization and other modifications of the classical Ovsynch protocol are thought to increase the probability that ovulation will be induced by the first injection of GnRH and that luteolysis and a synchronized ovulation will ensue after the administration of prostaglandin and GnRH.

Figure 8 Examples of modifications to the Ovsynch protocol

Adapted from Cavalieri et al. (2006)

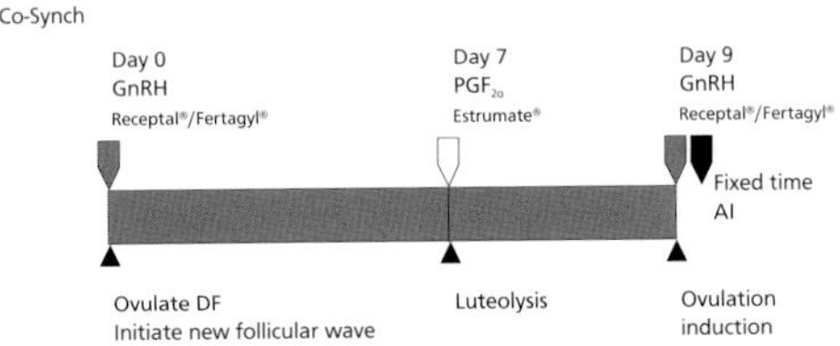

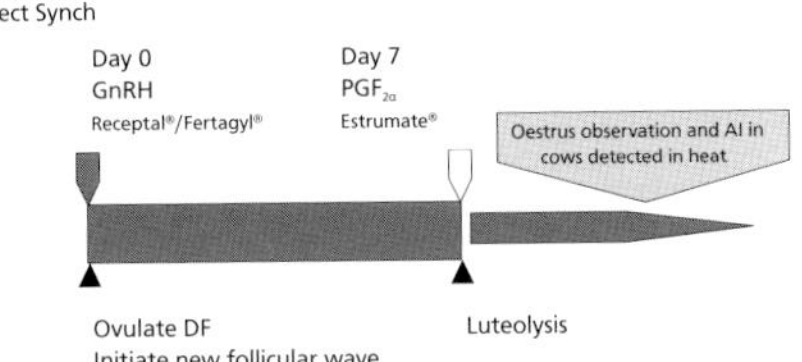

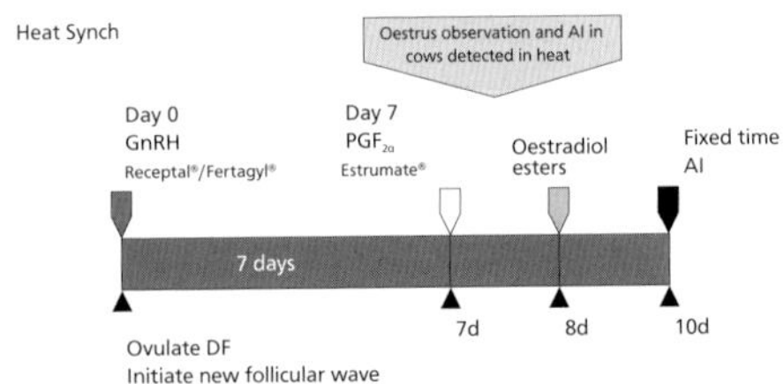

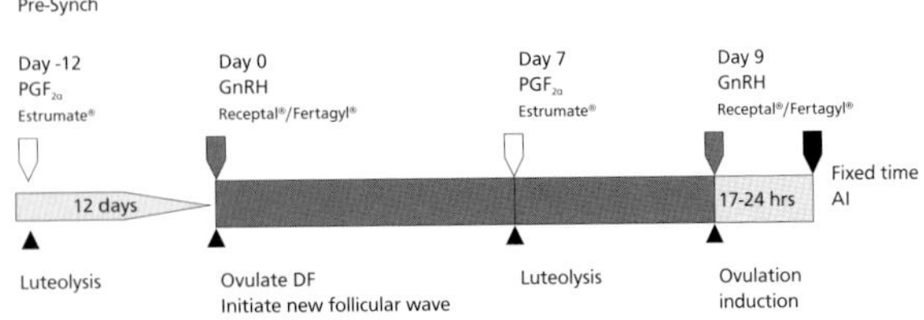

One of the simplest modifications of the classical Ovsynch system is the so-called Co-Synch protocol, the difference being that both the second injection of GnRH and AI are performed at the same time i.e. 48 hours after the treatment with prostaglandin (Small et al., 2000).
Although most research using the Co-Synch protocol has focused on a 48 hour interval between prostaglandin injection and GnRH+AI, intervals to oestrus following the treatment indicate that a 60-64 hour interval post PGF (as used in Ovsynch), would more closely match the appropriate insemination timing for beef (Geary et al., 2000; Stevenson et al., 2000; DeJarnette et al., 2001a) and dairy (DeJarnette et al., 2001b)
Reported results have been comparable with, or only slightly lower than, those obtained with the Ovsynch while the need to handle the animals is reduced (DeJarnette et al., 2003). Nonetheless, a stochastic analysis published by Olynk et al. (2009) indicated that risk-averse managers are willing to incur additional labour costs of breeding using Ovsynch and thus avoid the potential risk of a reduction in conception rate associated with Co-Synch.

Various pre-synchronization systems have also been proposed in order to unify the ovarian dynamics even further in cows ultimately subjected to a classical Ovsynch protocol (Fig 9). This provides the best chance of ensuring the majority of cows included in the final Ovsynch will have LH-responsive dominant follicles at the time of the first GnRH injection.
A pre-synchronization protocol prior to implementation of the Ovsynch protocol was developed by giving two injections of PGF, 14 days apart, with the second injection given 12 days prior to the first GnRH of the Ovsynch protocol. The Pre-synch-Ovsynch protocol increased pregnancy rates by 18% (25% to 43%) in lactating cyclic cows as reported by Moreira et al. (2001).
It should be stressed that prostaglandin-based pre-synchronization protocols can increase the efficacy of insemination after the final Ovsynch only in cyclic cows, as only these animals are capable of responding to the pre-synchronizing luteolysis.

Figure 9 Follicular dynamics in cows subjected to PGF-based Pre-Synch protocols

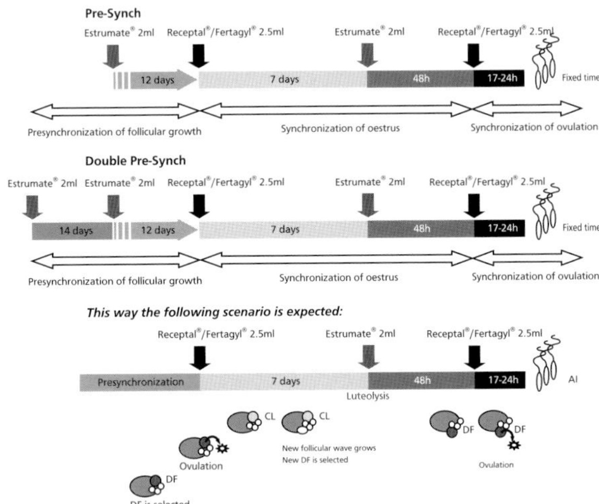

Post partum pre-synchronization with GnRH can also be undertaken at 7 days before the actual Ovsynch protocol. This approach also has the advantage of being potentially effective in both cyclic and anoestrus cows (Thompson et al., 1999; Stevenson et al., 2000) and this has been demonstrated to be advantageous in heifers also (Stevenson et al., 2008).

The combination of prostaglandin and GnRH as a pre-synchronization treatment preceeding the classical Ovsynch or Co-Synch protocol was also tried with variable success, usually resulting, nonetheless, in some improvement in pregnancy rates to the final Ovsynch AI (DeJarnette et al., 2003).

Heat Synch protocol, more widely used in the US, involves replacement of the second GnRH injection with oestradiol esters (Geary et al., 2000; Stevenson et al., 2004). Enthusiasts of this system indicate that oestradiol synchronizes the ovulation of the dominant follicle more tightly and increases the behavioural expression of oestrus in treated cows. With the growing concern for the use of oestrogens in food-producing animals, and practically no possibility of using them in Europe, the application of this system is limited geographically. Moreover, although the majority of studies involving the use of Heat Synch originate from the US, it should be stressed that at present there are no oestradiol-containing products licensed for use in dairy cattle on the US market.

Injections of hCG or implants containing a potent GnRH agonist, deslorelin, have also been used to replace the second GnRH injection in the Ovsynch protocol to induce ovulation. The use of hCG was associated with comparable results and similar pregnancy rates as per AI to GnRH (De Rensis et al., 2002), but implementation of a protocol with deslorelin resulted in prolonged interovulatory intervals (Bartolome et al., 2004) due to the desensitisation of the hypothalamus (Padula et al., 2002; 2005) and reduced pregnancy rates when a higher dose of deslorelin was used (Santos et al., 2004).
The use of hCG in place of the second GnRH injection during the classical Ovsynch protocol seems to be particularly promising. The effectiveness of hCG in inducing ovulation and the formation of a functional CL has been described by several authors (Rajamehendran et al., 1992; Schmitt et al., 1996s, 1996b). In the classic Ovsynch protocol, hCG is given to synchronize and induce ovulation (De Rensis et al., 2002).
Preliminary data provided in recent publications encourage the expectation that in high yielding dairy cows, and herds exposed to heat stress, this approach can provide a clear advantage over the GnRH-only based Ovsynch. De Rensis et al. (2008) submitted groups of lactating dairy cows to a classical Ovsynch protocol (GPG) and an hCG-Ovsynch (GPH) during late spring and summer. Mean plasma progesterone levels were higher in the GPH group than in the GPG group on days 3, 6 and 9 post insemination. The findings of this study indicate that the use of hCG to induce ovulation in a timed artificial insemination protocol increases plasma progesterone levels and improves fertility in dairy cows during the warmer months of the year. An abstract from Schmitz et al. (2008) presented at the 16th ICAR conference reported similar positive effects of the replacement of the second GnRH injection in a classical Co-Synch program with hCG, in dairy cows.

The beneficial results of the hCG injection in the Ovsynch-type programs can be attributed mainly to the luteotrophic action of hCG and its prolonged activity. It has been argued for some time that the induction of ovulation with hCG may lead to the formation of a corpus luteum with a greater steroidogenic capacity (Schmitt et al., 1996a,b). Moreover, human chorionic gonadotrophin treatment in sheep and cows has been linked to increased numbers of large luteal cells and a concomitant reduction in the number of small luteal cells, accompanied by increased plasma progesterone concentrations.

The Ovsynch protocol and the dose of GnRH

First fundamental studies on the use of GnRH in Ovsynch-type systems, and to induce ovulation, had been performed with the use of 8mcg of the potent GnRH analogue, buserelin. Many later studies have involved the use of gonadorelin, but at a dose of only 100mcg. This dose of GnRH is the norm in the US and has proved of considerable interest in many other countries, as it offers the possibility of reducing the cost of treatment.

But the reduced dose of gonadorelin would represent a substantial reduction in biological potency because buserelin was estimated to be between 40 and 200 times more potent than gonadorelin (Chenault et al., 1990). Since then, many authors have questioned the efficacy of a reduced gonadorelin dose to induce ovulation, especially in complex Ovsynch-type synchronization systems, in which the induction of ovulation in a high percentage of cows determines both the precision of the synchronization and its efficacy. Smaller doses of gonadorelin (25mcg and 100mcg) were shown to be only partially effective (100mcg) or incapable (25mcg) of ovulating a luteal phase dominant follicle (Mihm et al., 1998).The synchronized incidence of ovulation was only 68% in cycling cows as reported by Cartmill et al. (2001), when a 100mcg gonadorelin dose was used in the Ovsynch protocol. At the same time, Vasconcelos et al. (1999) and Fricke et al. (1998) showed comparable results, in terms of rates of induction of ovulation, when low and standard doses of gonadorelin were used.

However, some recent studies have indicated that many of the ovulations induced with the lower gonadorelin dose may not result in normal corpus luteum formation. This, in turn, would have a clearly detrimental effect on the subsequent maintenance of pregnancy and pregnancy rates, in treated cows. Cordoba

and Fricke (2002) and Shephard (2002) reported an increased incidence of short cycles in cows treated with the Ovsynch protocol using doses of 50mg or 100mcg of gonadorelin, indicative of a shortened luteal phase and failure of conception. These short cycles occurred in both cycling and anoestrus cows. This would indicate that the abnormal corpus luteum formation was most likely to be associated with the injection of the lower dose of GnRH having limited effectiveness on follicle atresia, ovulation and the development of the corpus luteum.
A very recent study reported by Colazo et al. (2009) tested the effect of three doses of GnRH (gonadorelin; 50mcg, 100mcg and 250mcg) on LH release in ovariectomized cows. The mean plasma LH concentration was affected by the GnRH dose in cows given 250mcg gonadorelin which released more pituitary LH than those given either 50 or 100mcg. Cows given 250mcg also had a longer-lasting LH surge than those given 50mcg of GnRH.

Progestagens
Progestagen treatments, such as Crestar®, mimic the luteal phase of the cycle. To obtain a normally fertile oestrus, the duration of treatment has been set at 10 -12 days.

A feature of all current progestagen-based systems is the administration of oestradiol at the start of the treatment to:
- shorten the life span of the corpus luteum
- terminate the existing wave and induce the emergence of a new follicle.

This second function of oestradiol esters used in conjunction with progestagens is especially important, as all progesterone/progestagen-releasing systems create subluteal levels of progesterone in the circulation of treated cows. These levels are sufficient to create a negative feedback and prevent a preovulatory LH surge, ovulation and heat. However, they are not able to block the LH release completely, and a small pulsatile secretion is maintained, allowing the persistence of a dominant follicle should it be present on the ovary at the start of treatment. It has been known that when the duration of dominance of the ovulatory follicle exceeds 4 days (persistent dominant follicle) there is a progressive decline in fertility which has been attributed to a reduction in oocyte competence and an increase in embryonic loss (Fig 10; Diskin et al., 2002).

Figure 10 Estimation of pregnancy rate as duration of dominance of the pre-ovulatory follicle increases (Diskin et al., 2002)

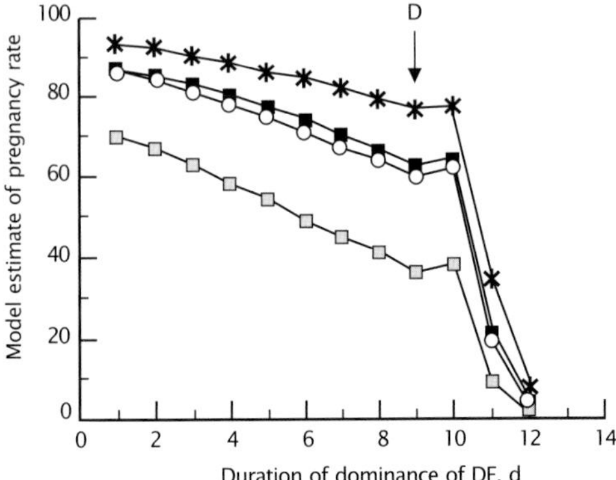

Exogenous oestradiol, administered with progesterone, suppresses the formation of, or decreases the diameter of, the dominant follicle, when administered before or during the emergence of the wave, presumably due to suppression of FSH and perhaps LH. When follicle selection has occurred, this treatment results in a decrease in dominant follicle diameter without consistently changing the timing of the emergence of the next wave (Fig 11). Treatment of cows classified as in anovulatory anoestrus with low doses of progestagens for 6-8 days rarely induces the formation of persistent dominant follicles, as would be expected in cows that are cycling without the presence of a functional corpus luteum (McDougal et al., 2004). Cerri et al. (2009) found that treatment of high-yielding cyclic Holstein cows which had had a progesterone-releasing intravaginal device (CIDR®) inserted, resulted in subluteal concentrations of progesterone, but in anoestrus high-yielders this treatment increased the induction of oestrous cycles with no effect on fertility at the first insemination.

Figure 11 Follicular dynamics in cows treated with oestradiol at the start of progestagen-based oestrus synchronization program

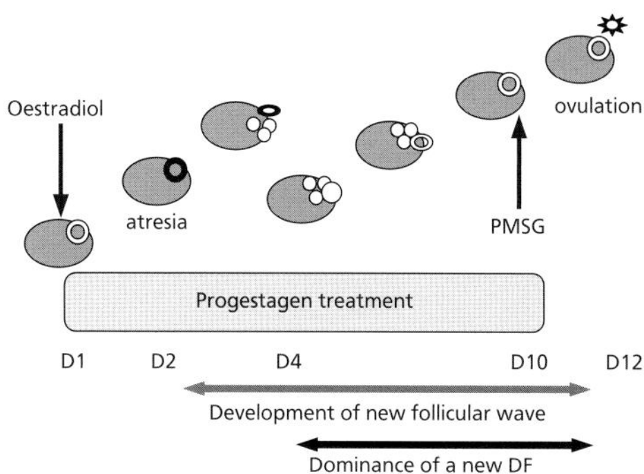

The use of oestradiol at the beginning of a progesterone synchronization treatment, even when the duration of treatment is extended to 12 days, does not always guarantee that corpus luteum regression is complete in all animals at the time of, or 24h after, progesterone withdrawal. Consequently, it is highly recommended that $PGF_{2\alpha}$ be administered at, or, before progesterone withdrawal, to ensure corpus luteum regression in those animals not responding to oestradiol.

One of the advantages of progestagen-based treatments such as Crestar® is that they are capable of initiating oestrous cycles in anoestrus cows. In non-cyclic cows, the progestagen sensitises the hypothalamo-pituitary-gonadal axis and facilitates a normal lifespan of the corpus luteum. The administration of PMSG when the progestagen is removed, further stimulates follicular maturation and ovulation. The success rate of Crestar® and other progestagen-based methods in the treatment of anoestrus can be variable (50-70%) depending on the post partum interval at the time of treatment, the body condition of the cow and other underlying causes of anoestrus. Nonetheless, Crestar® and other progestagen-based systems should be seen as the method of choice in managing oestrus in beef cows, as they allow for compact breeding early in the season with a high percentage of cows conceiving at the first synchronized oestrus. This, in turn, facilitates the rapid representation of cows for AI that have not conceived during the first oestrus, and allows of a tighter calving season. Oestrus and ovulation, after treatment with progestagens, occur earlier and with more precise timing than when following prostaglandin injection. For Crestar® a single, fixed time insemination is recommended (Table 9).

Table 9 Use of Crestar® in different production systems of heifers and cows

Type of animals	Day 0	48h before implant removal	Day 9-10	Artificial insemination
Beef heifers	Crestar® implant and injection	x	Implant removal injection of 400-600IU PMSG (Folligon®)	48h after implant removal
Dairy heifers	Crestar® implant and injection	x	Implant removal	48h after implant removal
Beef cows	Crestar® implant and injection	x	Implant removal injection of 500-700IU PMSG (Folligon®)	56h after implant removal
Dairy cows	Crestar® implant and injection	Prostaglandin injection (Estrumate®)	Implant removal injection of 300-400IU PMSG (Folligon®)	56h after implant removal

In recent studies, systems have been proposed in which the injection of oestradiol was replaced by GnRH administration at the start of the treatment (Thompson et al., 1999; Stevenson et al., 2000; Garcia et al., 2004). This change is clearly associated with the ban on the use of oestradiol esters in food-producing animals in Europe (Lane et al., 2008). Moreover, the restrictions within the EU have wider implications, beyond the European Union borders. For example, they have forced changes in both New Zealand and Australia. In New Zealand, oestradiol benzoate use is effectively banned for all veterinary indications, while in Australia there is a voluntary agreement not to use oestradiol benzoate in lactating dairy cows.

The mechanism of action used in systems combining GnRH and progestagens is slightly different to that of the oestradiol-progestagen based ones, because GnRH induces ovulation of the dominant follicle and the creation of an additional corpus luteum (Fig 12) (Cavalieri et al., 2006).

Figure 12 Follicular dynamics in cows treated with GnRH at the start of progestagen-based oestrus synchronization program

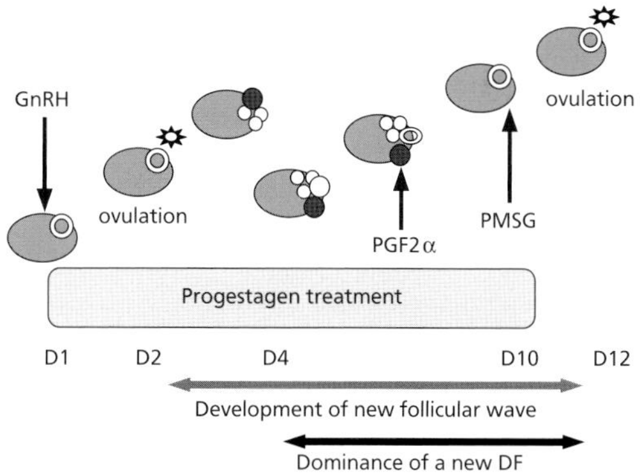

If this system is to be adopted, there are certain important aspects to be considered.
By replacing oestradiol with GnRH, additional benefits can be expected such as stimulation of follicular growth (especially important in anovulatory cows) and the creation of an additional corpus luteum, which increases the concentrations of progesterone and has a positive effect on fertility at the induced oestrus. As the administration of GnRH is going to induce formation of an additional corpus luteum in a considerable percentage of cows, and no pro-luteolytic factor is included (oestradiol in the traditional system), it is necessary to administer a $PGF_{2\alpha}$ analogue to all treated animals, preferably 48h before the removal of the progesterone source (Fig 13).

Figure 13 Example of a progestagen-based oestrus synchronization program with administration of GnRH at the start of the treatment

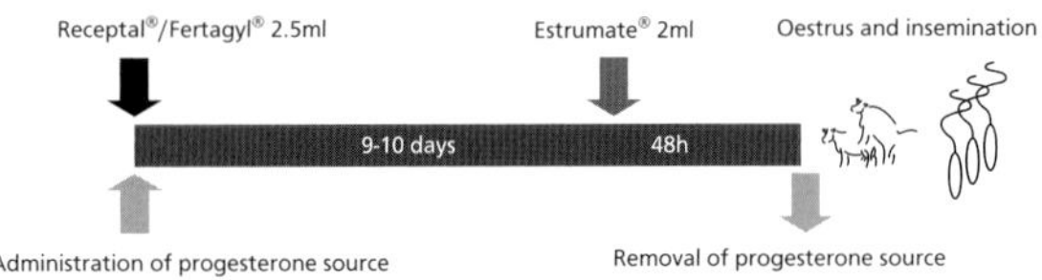

This approach has also found application in an increasingly popular combination of progestagen/progesterone with the complete classical Ovsynch protocol. Such programs include insertion of a progesterone relasing device (e.g. PRID® progesterone releasing intravaginal device) at the time of the first GnRH injection of the Ovsynch protocol. The device is then removed and a prostaglandin injection administered , followed by the second GnRH dose 48h later. This system has been shown to increase the efficacy of the classical Ovsynch in dairy herds (El-Zarkouny et al., 2004; Ambrose et al., 2005; Stevenson et al., 2006) but it may also be effective in beef cows.

Undoubtedly the supplementation of progesterone during the development of the follicular wave and the future ovulatory follicle should have an obvious beneficial effect on the quality of the oocyte, and also reduce the occurrence of shortened luteal phases after insemination when used in the treatment of anoestrus cows. Melendez et al. (2006) showed that cows subjected to the Ovsynch program and supplemented with exogenous progesterone had higher pregnancy rates and concentrations of progesterone after AI than those subjected to the Ovsynch protocol which received no additional progesterone.

Re-synchronization of oestrus in cows returning to oestrus
Various strategies have been used to re-synchronize returns to oestrus in previously synchronized cows, in order to increase the number of cows re-inseminated in a timely manner. These include the use of progesterone-releasing devices or the enrolment of previously inseminated cows in Ovsynch-type protocols.

When the timing of re-synchronization is to be considered the appropriate systems can be generally divided as follows:

1. *Blind recruitment*
   Re-synchronization begins before the non-pregnant cows of an inseminated group have been identified. These systems are based on the use of GnRH in inseminated animals, which is a licensed indication for some GnRH analogues in many countries. GnRH is usually administered on day 23-24 post AI and followed 7 days later by an ultrasound examination (Chebel et al., 2003;). Cows identified as non-pregnant then receive a $PGF_{2\alpha}$ injection and can continue with the complete Ovsynch protocol. Thus re-insemination takes place approximately 32 days after the previous AI. Although the period before re-insemination is significantly shorter than in the targeted approach, use of these systems results in many cows which are already pregnant being treated unnecessarily.
2. *Targeted recruitment*
   The re-synchronization program begins as soon as the non-pregnant cows in a group have been identified. These systems are based on the early use of ultrasound pregnancy diagnosis (days 27-28 post AI) or early pregnancy tests (see section 2.2.3). Non-pregnant cows receive a $PGF_{2\alpha}$ injection and can be inseminated at the next observed heat or enrolled into a pre-synchronized Ovsynch (Bartolome et al., 2005a,b,c). Thus re-insemination can take place approximately 30-31 days after the previous AI (with prostaglandin induced oestrus and AI at observed heat) or even 49 days after (if the full pre-synchronized Ovsynch is used).

Although the time between insemination and the identification of empty cows and re-insemination is longer than with the blind recruitment approach, the targeted system means that only non-pregnant animals are treated, which is more economical, and complies with recommendations for the prudent use of medication.

Various other combinations of progestagens and oestradiol have also been used with variable results (Galvao et al.,2007; Calavalieri et al., 2008). Moreover, possible adverse effects of oestradiol used post AI, on the function of the corpus luteum require further investigation.

2.3.3 Factors affecting fertility of inseminated cows

In dairy cattle, fertilization rates are similar in lactating and non-lactating cows averaging 76.2% (ranging from 55.3 to 87.8%) and 78.1% (ranging from 58.0 to 98.0%), respectively (Santos et al., 2004). In beef cattle the rate averages 75.0%, with a range from 60 to 100%.
Humblot (2001) showed that fertilization failure and early embryonic loss were responsible for 20-45% of pregnancy failures, late embryonic loss/foetal loss for 8-17.5%, and late abortion for 1-4%. Two sources of pregnancy failure exist in addition to breeding, fertilization failure and pregnancy loss.
This means that factors contributing to losses after insemination can be grouped as follows:

1. Factors contributing to fertilization failure:
   a. unfavourable endocrine environment causing impaired follicular growth and poor oocyte quality
      - heat stress
      - negative energy balance
      - infection with BVDV and IBRV
   b. ovulation delay and/or failure
      - heat stress
      - negative energy balance
   c. factors affecting the quality of spermatozoa
      - factors affecting spermatogenesis: infections with BVDV, IBRV, *Brucella spp.*, heat stress, fever
      - factors affecting the survival of sperm before deposition in the female reproductive tract:
      semen preservation technique, semen management
2. Factors affecting early embryonic development, pregnancy recognition and implantation
   a. impaired early luteal function
      - high metabolic rate in dairy cows
      - infections with BVDV and IBRV
      - lack of progesterone priming in the first post-anoestrus cycles
      - luteotoxic factors causing precocious luteolysis: mycotoxins, bacterial toxins associated with mastitis
   b. impaired function of endometrium and unfavourable uterine environment
      - increased levels of plasma urea nitrogen
      - subclinical endometritis

3. Factors causing late embryonic/foetal death
   a. infectious factors directly detrimental to the foetus or impairing the function of the placenta
      - viral infections: BVDV, IBRV,
      - bacterial infections: *Brucella spp., Chlamydia spp.,*
      - protozoan infections: Neospora caninum, Trichomonas spp.
   b. non-infectious factors directly detrimental to the foetus or impairing the function of the placenta
      - mycotoxins,
      - certain substances such as: PVP, lead etc.

2.3.3.1 Delayed ovulation

Variations in the duration of oestrus, and problems with oestrus detection, may lead to the inappropriate timing of insemination and poor success rates. On the other hand, in high-yielders, both delayed ovulation and follicular atresia can contribute to the failure of conception. They are responsible for a high proportion of the so-called 'asymptomatic' failures to conceive observed during the spring months.

Ovulation takes place about 30 hours after the onset of oestrus, that is, after the end of behavioural oestrus. Various factors can, however, influence the actual time of ovulation in relation to the oestradiol peak (maximal oestrus signs). As mentioned in other chapters, compromised luteal function due to metabolic deficiencies and excessive metabolic rate, or the effects of high ambient temperature (heat stress) can lead to a delay in ovulation. Delayed ovulation after oestrus minimizes the chances of successful fertilization in cows.

With the relatively short survival time of frozen semen, the success of AI is very much dependent on the proper timing of insemination relative to the time of ovulation. The fertilization rate of the oocyte decreases significantly 8 to 12 hours post ovulation, and insemination 25 to 40 hours before ovulation is associated with a significant reduction in conception rates.

Moreover, prolonged follicular dominance is associated with compromised oocyte competence and increased embryonic loss (Diskin et al., 2004).

In a recent study published by Bloch et al. (2006) the endocrine profile of cows with different oestrus-to-ovulation intervals was investigated. The results indicated the existence of an association between preovulatory reduced oestradiol concentrations and a small and delayed preovulatory LH surge, on the one hand, and an extended oestrus-to-ovulation interval, on the other (Fig 14).

Figure 14 Concentrations of plasma preovulatory LH surges in cows with various oestrus-to-ovulation intervals (Adapted from Bloch et al., 2006)

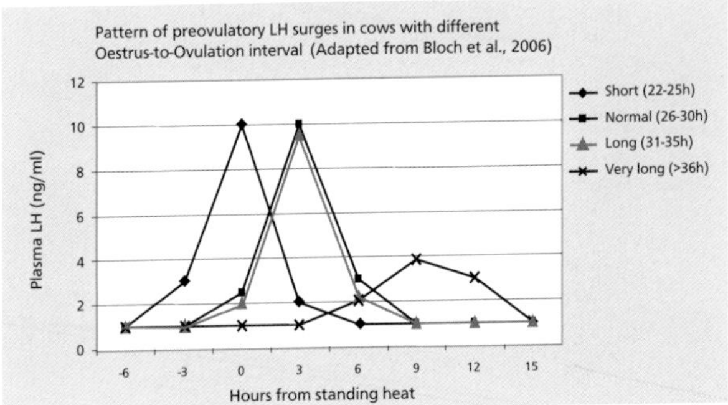

Moreover, this study found lower post ovulation progesterone concentrations during the mid-luteal phase in animals with a long or very long oestrus-to-ovulation interval as compared to those with a short or normal interval. This provides important clues about the possible contribution of delayed ovulation and prolonged oestrus-to-ovulation interval to early embryonic losses caused by an inadequate early progesterone pattern.

2.3.3.2 Inadequate uterine environment

Other factors which limit fertility in the dairy herd include the accumulation of toxic concentrations of urea and nitrogen in cows fed high levels of crude protein in the face of an inadequate energy supply. As the amino-acids are degraded, the concentrations of both ammonia and urea in the circulation increase. This, in turn, is believed to lead to unfavourable changes in the pH of the endometrium, which can impair implantation. In addition, it has been postulated that increased concentrations of nitrogen and urea, in both the blood stream and the endometrial fluid, might affect the embryo's viability and its capacity for further development. The greatest changes in the uterine environment occur during the mid-luteal phase, which is a critical period for early embryo development that ultimately determines long-term embryo survival. Recent work by Rhoads et al. (2006) revealed that high plasma urea nitrogen concentrations in lactating dairy cows reduce the viability of the embryo through effects exerted on the oocyte and embryo before its recovery from the uterus 7 days after insemination.

There is limited information, in cattle, about the possible effect of subclinical endometritis and the irreversible morphological changes in the endometrium caused by a prolonged inflammatory process on the success of implantation. The data available in mares, however, (see chapter on Equine Reproduction) clearly indicate that such changes can have a negative effect on the recognition of pregnancy and impair the implantation process, leading to early embryonic losses. Moreover Hill and Gilbert (2008) found reduced quality of bovine embryos cultured in media conditioned by exposure to an inflamed endometrium. This can indicate altered embryo quality as a mechanism for early embryonic failure in cows with subclinical endometritis

2.3.3.3 Importance of early luteal function in pregnancy recognition and maintenance

It has been established for many years that the concentration of progesterone during early pregnancy has a marked effect on the outcome of insemination.

As reviewed recently in Robinson et al. (2008) the formation of a functional corpus luteum and the post-ovulatory rise in progesterone are of critical importance for the developing embryo. Peripheral progesterone concentrations begin to increase by about day 4 after ovulation and reach maximal levels by day 8-10. It is this rapid decline in oestradiol concentrations and the subsequent rise in progesterone that ensures the timely control of both oviductal and endometrial functions supporting the survival and development of the embryo. Progesterone receptor levels are maximal in both endometrial glands and the sub-epithelial stroma from day 4 to 10 post ovulation. These endometrial glands synthesize, secrete and transport a complex of amino acids, glucose, transport proteins and growth factors called histotroph. Histotroph is an essential source of nutrients and regulatory molecules for the developing blastocyst in the pre-attachment period.

Numerous studies have revealed lower concentrations of progesterone in milk (Lamming et al., 1989; Mann et al., 1995) and plasma (Mann et al., 1995, 1996; Buttler et al., 1996; Mann et al., 2001) in cows that fail to maintain pregnancy (Fig. 15).

Figure 15 Progesterone profiles after AI in cows confirmed later as pregnant or non-pregnant (Adapted from Mann et al., 1999)

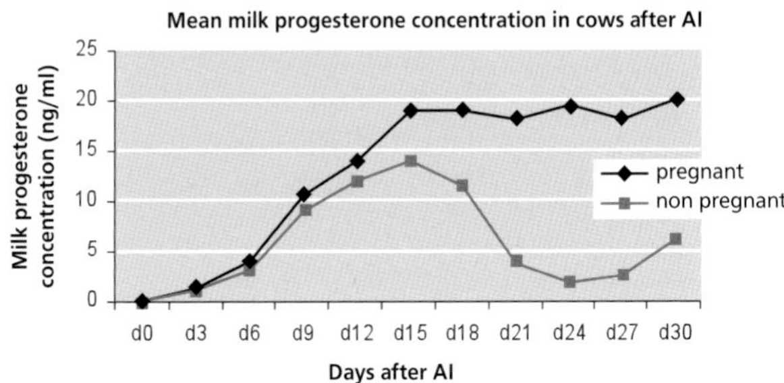

Embryos from cows with higher progesterone concentrations showed more advanced development as early as 5 days post ovulation (Green et al., 2005).

It is well established that fertility and milk production are negatively associated in dairy cows. Lopez et al. (2005) indicated that high-yielding cows have lower circulating concentrations of progesterone than low-yielders, which may possibly be associated with their higher metabolic rate and consequently higher rate of progesterone catabolism (Wiltbank et al., 2006).

Several studies of pregnancy recognition and maintenance in cattle have revealed that these two groups of factors are closely connected, as the sufficient developmental potential of the embryo is a prerequisite for continued luteal function in cattle. In the study by Mann et al. (2001), it was demonstrated that the degree of embryo development was closely related to the maternal progesterone environment. In this study, even a single day's delay in the post ovulatory rise in progesterone concentrations was shown to reduce significantly the subsequent development of the embryo.

Poor progesterone support of the developing embryo clearly can affect its ability to synthesize and secrete interferon-τ, a widely recognised embryonic signal for the maternal recognition of pregnancy in ruminants (Mann et al., 1999). The elongation of the blastocyst initiates interferon-τ production, which is detectable in uterine flushes from day 12 to day 25 post ovulation. Cows with poorly developed embryos on day 16 after the first insemination that produced little or no interferon-τ, exhibited a delayed increase in progesterone concentration after ovulation and had a lower luteal phase plateau than did cows with well-developed embryos.

2.3.3.4 Influence of high ambient temperatures on reproductive efficiency in cattle

Heat stress is perceived to be a major factor contributing to the low fertility of dairy cows inseminated in the late summer months. The reduced conception rate during the hot season can vary between 20-30% compared to the winter months (Wolfenson et al., 2000; Rensis et al., 2003).
The substantial rise in milk yields in recent years has further aggravated the summer infertility syndrome, as the high level of productivity increases the cows' metabolic rate and metabolic heat production. The upper limit of ambient temperature at which lactating dairy cows can maintain a stable body temperature (upper critical temperature) is as low as 25-27°C. The problem of heat stress is thus not confined to tropical regions of the world, and imposes a considerable cost on the dairy industry.

There is a proven carry-over effect of the summer heat stress on fertility in the autumn months (Wolfenson et al., 1997; 2002). This negative effect on reproduction persists over the first one or two months of autumn even though the cows are no longer exposed to the heat stress (Fig. 16). It is thought to be a result of the summer heat stress effect exerted on antral follicles, which will develop into dominant follicles 40-50 days later (Roth et al., 2000; 2001a; Wolfenson et al., 2002).

Figure 16 Seasonal variation in 90-day non-return rate in Holstein cows in South Georgia and Florida in various milk yield groups (adapted from Wolferson et al., 1997)

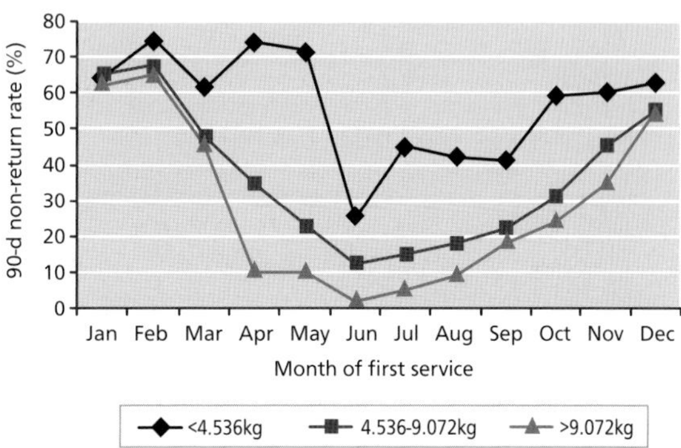

Mechanisms of the negative impact of heat stress on reproductive function in cattle

The detrimental effect of high ambient temperatures on reproductive processes in dairy cattle has been well documented and includes:

- Negative effect on reproductive behaviour patterns
- Impaired endocrine interactions
- Changed follicular development pattern
- Decreased quality of oocytes and embryos
- Negative effect on the nutritional status and energy balance

Effect of heat stress on reproductive behaviour patterns
Under the influence of heat stress, the duration and intensity of oestrus are reduced with a clear decrease in motor activity and other manifestations of oestrus such as mounting. Nobel et al (1997) found that Holstein cows during the summer have 4.5 mounts per oestrus versus 8.6 per oestrus in winter.
Higher incidence of silent heat and anoestrus is therefore one of the most common observations in cows exposed to high ambient temperatures.

Influence of heat stress on endocrine environment and follicular development pattern

The mechanisms by which heat stress influences the function of the hypothalamic-hypophyseal-ovarian axis remain incompletely understood. The secretion of FSH from the pituitary gland appears not to be impaired in animals exposed to high ambient temperatures. In contrast, a clear reduction in both the frequency and amplitude of the LH pulse release has been observed in heat stressed cows. It can therefore be concluded that in high ambient temperatures, the dominant follicle develops in a low LH environment which results in reduced oestradiol secretion. This, in turn, leads to the poor expression of oestrus and reduced fertility (Rensis et al., 2003). In addition, the reduction in the LH pulse (frequency and amplitude) leads to a prolonged follicular dominance, delayed ovulation and formation of persistent dominant follicles which are associated with a markedly reduced quality of oocytes and reduced pregnancy rates (Diskin et al., 2002; Bridges et al., 2005). Alterations in the steroidogenic capacity of the follicles carry over to their final development, causing reduced adrostenedione production by thecal cells and low oestradiol concentration in follicular fluid collected from the dominant follicles.

The development of a greater number of larger follicles with lower oestradiol production probably also leads to an increased rate of double ovulations and twin calving (Wolfenson et al., 2000).

Low circulating progesterone concentrations in cows have been associated with compromised reproductive function and reduced pregnancy rates (Butler et al., 1996; Lamming et al., 1989; Mann et al., 1995; 2001). There is much debate on whether insufficient progesterone secretion by the corpus luteum could be a possible cause of low fertility in cattle exposed to heat stress. Recent work published by Wolfenson et al. (2002) analysed progesterone production, in vitro, by theca and granulosa cells obtained from cows in cool and hot seasons, as well as progesterone concentrations in the general circulation. This study demonstrated that under chronic summer stress conditions, progesterone production was markedly reduced, especially by luteinized theca cells. The results indicated a 25% decrease in plasma concentrations of progesterone in cows in summer, compared to those in winter. The authors postulated that heat stress-induced damage to follicular function was carried over to the subsequent corpus luteum. In a recently published study, Kornmatitsuk et al. (2008) found a higher percentage of abnormal luteal activity in the cows during the hot season, with delayed luteal activity and anovulation being the most frequently reported features.

Influence of heat stress on the quality and development of embryos
The formation of gametes and the development of early embryonic stages have been shown to be highly temperature sensitive.
Heat stress causes hyperthermia of the scrotum and testes which can lead to poorer morphological and functional semen quality. Hansen (1997) reported deterioration of bull fertility caused by heat stress during the summer months. Heat stress has less severe effects on semen quality of zebu bulls than on bulls of the European breeds, a phenomenon associated not only with the generally more efficient thermoregulation observed in zebu cattle but also specific adaptations that enhance the local cooling of blood entering the testis (Brito et al., 2004).

Heat stress through delayed ovulation and follicular persistence can lead to the ovulation of aged, poor quality oocytes which are associated with low fertilization rate and embryonic mortality (Sartori et al., 2000; Al-Katanani et al., 2001; Roth et al., 2001). Aroyo et al. (2007) demonstrated that cleavage to the two- and four-cell stages following chemical activation was delayed in bovine oocytes collected during the hot season, as compared with the oocytes harvested during the cool months. As the timing of the initial cleavage is considered to have a major and long-lasting effect on the subsequent embryonic development potential, this may explain the inferior developmental competence of the embryos in cows exposed to high ambient temperatures.
High temperature has a negative effect on pre-attachment embryos (Ryan et al., 1993; Ealy et al., 1993), but the embryos' resistance to these effects increases as they develop (Ealy et al., 1993; Sartori et al., 2002, Hansen et al., 2001).
A recent study by Garcia-Ispierto et al. (2006) indicated that heat stress can compromise the success of gestation dur-

ing the peri-implantation period to the extent that a high temperature-humidity index during days 21-30 of gestation can be considered to be a risk factor for early foetal loss.

Marked differences were noted in the magnitude of effects of high temperatures on the developmental potential and quality of oocytes and embryos between *bos taurus* and *bos indicus*. Higher resistance to heat stress of embryos derived from *bos indicus* cows was demonstrated by Paula-Lopes et al. (2003) and Hernandez-Ceron et al. (2004) and summarised by Hansen (2004).

Heat stress compromises the uterine environment with decreased blood flow to the uterus and increased uterine temperature, which can lead to implantation failure and embryonic mortality. These effects are thought to be associated with the production of heat-shock proteins by the endometrium during the stressful period and reduced production of interferon-tau by the conceptus. Moreover heat stress can affect endometrial prostaglandin secretion, leading to premature luteolysis and embryo loss. Malayer and Hansen (1990) also found clear differences between Brahman and Holstein cows in endometrial responses to culture at elevated temperatures.

However, it should be recognised that although the resistance of *bos indicus* to the effects of high ambient temparatures is greater than that of *bos taurus* breeds, it is not without limits. As a recent study by Torres-Junior et al. (2008) indicated, long-term exposure of *bos indicus* cattle to heat stress has a delayed deleterious effect on the ovarian follicular dynamics and oocyte competence.

Negative effect on the nutritional status and energy balance

It is very clear that the negative effects of heat stress on reproduction can be the result of both direct action on reproductive function and embryonic development, but also of indirect influences mediated through changes in energy balance. In heat stressed dairy cows, a reduction in dry matter intake is often observed which prolongs the period of negative energy balance and negatively influences the plasma concentrations of insulin, IGF-I and glucose (Jonsson et al., 1997; Ronchi et al., 2001). This leads to poor follicular development, low expression of heat and poor quality oocytes.

Moreover, a recent study by Kornmatitsuk et al. (2008) recorded a decrease in the mean body condition score at 5 weeks post calving in cows during the hot season, which was clearly associated with a reduced feed intake by the affected animals. In the same experiment, a higher frequency of abnormal luteal activity was observed in the cows during the high temperature period with delayed luteal cyclicity and anovulation being the most common atypical features of ovarian function.

2.3.4. Improvement of conception rate at and after AI

The challenge to improve the reproductive performance of lactating dairy cattle requires an understanding of the biochemical and physiological principles controlling reproduction and lactation. This then needs to be integrated into nutritional, production and reproduction management systems to optimise the fertility of the herd.
Pharmacological attempts to improve fertility in inseminated cattle have concentrated on three areas so far:

- timely induction of ovulation
- prevention of early embryonic loss through increasing progesterone concentrations in the general circulation or prevention of precocious luteolysis (see chapter on early embryonic mortality)
- minimising the reproductive effects of heat stress

Prevention of delayed ovulation - to ensure timely ovulation in relation to service
One of the methods of obtaining satisfactory conception rates is to ensure that ovulation occurs within 7-18 hours of AI. One possible method is by the administration of GnRH around the time of service. Depending on the size and maturity of the dominant follicle, preovulatory LH surge and ovulation usually occur within 24 hours of GnRH injection, which is similar to the time between the onset of oestrus and ovulation (Fig 17).

Figure 17 Influence of GnRH (buserelin, Receptal®) administration on the peripheral LH concentrations in cows (adapted from Kaim et al., 2003)

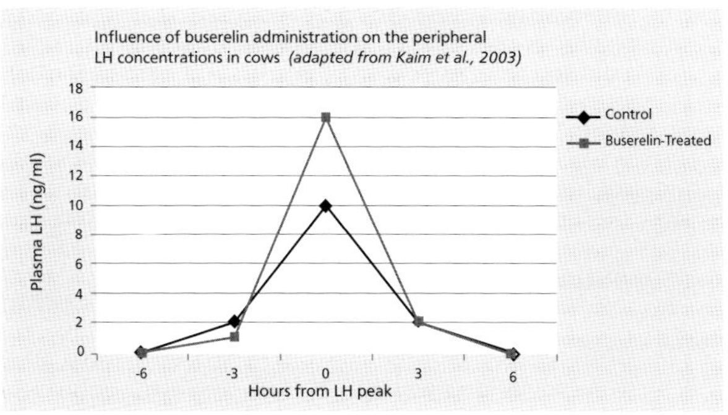

It is postulated that the administration of GnRH analogues at the time of insemination may modify the function or characteristics of pre-ovulatory ovarian follicles and the secretory capacity of the developing corpus luteum (Mee et al., 1993). Results reported by these authors suggest that GnRH may have served to enhance or alter theca-lutein or granulosa-lutein differentiation in the pre- or post-ovulatory follicle, or developing corpus luteum, and may have acted on the developing corpus luteum to promote the conversion of small to large luteal cells, thereby increasing the progesterone secretion.

Timing of the GnRH treatment

Bearing in mind the chronological relationship between endogenous LH release, the duration of heat, and ovulation, as well as the survival time of sperm and oocyte, it is best to use GnRH at the time of AI, or up to 6 hours beforehand (Rosenberger et al., 1991). Numerous trials have shown that GnRH injection early in oestrus, followed by AI within 5-10 hours produces the best results, both in terms of the timing of ovulation and improved pregnancy rate. In practice, however, GnRH is usually administered at the same time as AI with very satisfactory results.

Results of the treatment
Rosenberger et al. (1991) evaluated the effect of GnRH injection during oestrus (10mcg Receptal®, Intervet; /250mcg Fertagyl®, Intervet) on plasma LH and conception, in relation to the timing of the treatment and insemination. In groups suffering from low conception rates following the first post partum AI, treatment with GnRH improved the insemination results. It was suggested that GnRH treatment could reduce the variation in the timing of ovulation or prevent ovulation failure. Several earlier studies demonstrated that treatment with GnRH at the time of insemination in repeat breeders improved pregnancy rates (Stevenson et al., 1988, 1989; Lee et al., 1983; Phatak et al., 1986; Kharche et al., 2007).

The study by Morgan and Lean (1993) presented an extensive analysis of the possible effect of treatment with GnRH at the time of insemination on conception rate in cattle. The article compared results from numerous previous studies in which GnRH or GnRH analogues had been used at AI, and submitted them to meta-analysis.
There was a significant increase in the likelihood of pregnancy in cows treated with a GnRH analogue at the first post partum insemination, at the second service after calving and in repeat breeder cows treated at the time of insemination. Repeat breeders responded better to the treatment than the other groups, which supports the hypothesis that a proportion of repeat breeders have failed to conceive beforehand because of a failure in the timing or the magnitude of GnRH, LH or FSH surge at oestrus.
Heuwieser et al. (1994), in a large study involving 2,437 dairy cows, analysed the relationship between the administration of GnRH, body condition score and fertility. Conception rate improved when GnRH was administered at the first breeding post partum in cows with a body condition score below 3.0, regardless of their parity.
Ullah et al. (1996) evaluated the effect of GnRH administration in lactating Holstein cows exposed to heat stress, and found that treatment with GnRH at oestrus improved the fertility results in comparison with an untreated group. A study reported by Kaim et al. (2003) involving the administration of buserelin (Receptal®), indicated that the use of GnRH eliminated differences

in conception rates for cows inseminated early or late relative to the onset of oestrus, and increased the efficacy of insemination in cows suffering from post partum reproductive disorders. The authors of this study concluded that the administration of GnRH at the onset of oestrus increased LH surges, prevented delayed ovulation, and may have increased subsequent progesterone concentrations. Treatment with buserelin in this trial increased conception in primiparous cows during the summer, and in cows with lower body condition scores.

Support of luteal function and prevention of precocious luteolysis
Several attempts have been made in high-yielding cows to prevent early embryonic loss, especially in those exposed to heat stress, and embryo transfer recipients.

Several methods have been tried to increase conception rates by increasing plasma progesterone concentrations during the luteal phase. This can be achieved by inducing the formation of accessory corpora lutea, which can be obtained by hCG treatment for an average of 4-6 days after insemination (Binelli et al., 2001). Apart from the initiation of additional corpora lutea, this treatment is believed to provide further LH support to the corpus luteum verum, which results from the ovulation of the dominant follicle.
Santos et al. (2001) administered hCG on day 5 after AI in high yielding dairy cows and noted that the treatment induced the formation of accessory corpora lutea, enhanced plasma progesterone concentrations and improved conception rates, when evaluated on days 28, 45 and 90, especially in cows which were losing body condition in the month following AI. Similarly Breuel et al. (1989); Sianangama et al. (1992); Rajamahedran and Sianangama (1992) reported a significant increase in pregnancy rates with the administration of hCG at 7 days post AI. Keneda et al. (1981) and Kerbler et al. (1997) achieved improvements in pregnancy rate with the administration of hCG at a dose of 1500 i.u. after AI.

Early embryonic losses which contribute to the low success rate of embryo transfer are the particular focus of attention, especially in view of the relatively high cost of the procedure.
The following factors were suggested as contributing to early embryonic losses following embryo transfer:

- transfer of an embryo of morphologically poor quality
- inadequate synchronization of oestrus between donors and recipients
- heat stress
- subclinical endometritis
- poor nutritional status of the recipient
- luteal insufficiency in recipients

The administration of progesterone, hCG and GnRH have been used to prevent the early loss of transferred embryos caused by luteal insufficiency, and with the general aim of improving the pregnancy rate following embryo transfer.

On day 5 of the oestrous cycle, granulosa cells of the dominant follicle contain LH receptors, so that hCG will induce ovulation and the formation of an accessory corpus luteum. Therefore administration of hCG 5 days after AI has the potential to increase progesterone secretion during early pregnancy. The positive effect of hCG on conception rates is mediated by reducing early embryonic losses. In addition, most of the benefit of hCG treatment was observed in lactating dairy cows that were losing body condition during the breeding period. Since high yielders have a greater metabolism of progesterone (Wiltbank et al., 2006) they are more likely to be responsive to hCG treatment.
Human chorionic gonadotrophin is usually administered at a dose of 1500 i.u. on the day of embryo transfer. It was shown that the administration of hCG at this time directly supports the development and function of the corpus luteum resulting from ovulation, but also induces the ovulation/luteinization of receptive follicles of the first wave of the subsequent follicular development. This results in the formation of induced corpora lutea, an increase in progesterone levels and a reduction of oestradiol concentration. Small et al. (2002) evaluated the influence of hCG (Chorulon®, Intervet; 2500 i.u./cow) administration on day 7 in embryo transfer recipients and

inseminated cows. They found that treatment with hCG at the time of embryo transfer, 7 days after AI, improved timed-AI pregnancy rates in cows carrying twins and first calving heifers. The authors postulated that treatment with hCG at 7 days post AI may be used to improve pregnancy rates in metabolically stressed cows and first-calving heifers.
Nishigai et al. (2002) administered hCG 6 days after oestrus in embryo transfer recipients. The trial results showed that the administration of hCG (1500 i.u./cow) 6 days after oestrus improved the pregnancy rate for non-surgical frozen embryo transfer 7 days after oestrus, by enhancing luteal function and depressing oestradiol secretion. A recent study reported by Chagas e Silva et al. (2008) evaluated the influence of hCG administration on the day of embryo transfer in high yielding dairy cows in a highly discriminative set-up (the transfer of bisected embryos). The treatment with 1500iu of hCG enhanced the survival of low viability embryos (half-embryos) and increased progesterone concentrations associated with the formation of an additional corpus luteum.

Although the rationale for the administration of GnRH and hCG on the day of embryo transfer is the same, few studies have reported positive results in terms of improvements in pregnancy rates in embryo recipients after treatment with GnRH. Ellington et al. (1991) evaluated the effect of the administration of buserelin at the time of embryo transfer and at 4 to 7 days after transfer, but found no significant improvement in pregnancy rates in comparison with the untreated controls.

Prevention of precocious luteolysis

A number of recent studies have been devoted to the analysis of the effect of GnRH treatment in mid-cycle (usually 11-14 days post insemination) on embryo survival and the resulting pregnancy rate. GnRH treatment aims at enhancing embryo survival by suppressing the luteolytic mechanism that ensues if there is no maternal recognition of pregnancy. Depending on the stage of follicular development, treatment with GnRH analogues during the luteal phase causes luteinization or ovulation of the existing responsive luteal phase follicles, which continue to grow after the ovulation of the dominant follicle of the previous cycle. Thus, not only is progesterone secretion increased, but also oestradiol concentrations are reduced as follicular turnover reduces oestradiol production. It results in a failure to upregulate the oxytocin receptors and hence blocks $PGF_{2\alpha}$ secretion. This thesis was confirmed in a study reported by Matsui et al. (2008), who found that oestradiol secretion by a dominant follicle from the first follicular wave after insemination had a negative effect on conception rate.

Mann et al. (1995) concluded that GnRH attenuated the luteolytic signal, allowing embryos more time to develop their antiluteolytic ability. Depending on the stage of follicular development, treatment with GnRH analogues during the luteal phase causes advanced atresia, luteinization or ovulation followed by luteinization of the responding follicle. Administration of GnRH between 11 and 13 days after service produced a marked increase in pregnancy rates (MacMillan et al., 1986; Mee et al., 1990; Peters et al., 1992; Stevenson et al., 1990; Ryan et al., 1994). Peters (2000) summarised the results of various studies analysing the effects of GnRH injections between days 11 and 13 of the oestrous cycle on pregnancy rates in cows, and noted a wide variation both in respect of the experimental design and the degree of improvement in pregnancy rates obtained. This analysis suggested that in certain circumstances GnRH treatment after insemination may produce significant benefits.

This thesis was further supported in a study reported by Sterry et al. (2006) who found that treatment with GnRH 5 days after fixed time insemination in dairy cows improved the pregnancy rate per insemination for non-cycling, but not for cycling, cows.

Lopez-Gatius et al. (2006) demonstrated that GnRH treatment at the time of insemination, and 12 days later, increases the conception rate in high yielding dairy cows during the warm season. Although less effective than double dosing, undoubted benefits were obtained following a single GnRH treatment at insemination.

Similar beneficial effects of the post insemination treatment with GnRH were found by Bech-Sabat et al. (2009) in certain target groups of cows.

On the other hand, two experiments reported by Franco et al. (2006a,b) failed to show any significant improvement in pregnancy rate in cows treated with GnRH after AI or embryo transfer. These results highlight the fact that treatment with GnRH post insemination may be of considerable value in certain groups of cows but, due to the complex aetiology of embryonic loss in cattle, will not always bring consistent improvement in pregnancy rates.

Several recent publications have reported on the use of non-steroidal anti-inflammatory drugs (NSAIDs) such as flunixin meglumine during the post insemination period in dairy cows. This approach is based on the ability of NSAIDs to interfere with the synthesis of various pro-inflammatory molecules from arachidonic acid, including prostaglandins. Thus the precocious synthesis of $PGF_{2\alpha}$ can be inhibited in cows the development of whose embryos are delayed and/or which produce inadequate amounts of INT-τ. Guzeloglu et al. (2007) described an increase in pregnancy rate in heifers treated with flunixin meglumine on days 15 and 16 post insemination, as compared with untreated animals. Similarly, Merril et al. (2007) found that treatment of inseminated cows with flunixin meglumine increased pregnancy rates, irrespective of whether they were subjected to transportation stress or not. By contrast, the administration of flunixin meglumine 11-16 days post AI in beef cows did not result in improvement in pregnancy rate (Lucacin 2008). Ketoprofen used in the same experimental design by Guzeloglu et al. (2008) did not bring any significant improvement in pregnancy rates as compared to an untreated control group.
If confirmed in further trials, this approach may become particularly attractive in situations in which precocious luteolysis is thought to be the main reason for early embryonic loss. At present, however, such treatment, although promising, should be considered cautiously, as the controlled studies are limited and registration conditions of products containing NSAIDs generally do not include the treatment of dairy cows after AI for improving fertility.

Strategies to decrease the negative impact of heat stress on reproduction in dairy cattle

Measures aimed at reducing the negative impact of heat stress on reproduction in dairy herds should always include reducing the exposure of cows to heat as well as any biotechnical or pharmaceutical approaches aimed directly at fertility improvement.

The possible options include:

- Changes in production system
- Selection of heat resistant breeds (*bos indicus* and crosses)
- Embryo transfer
- Hormone therapy

Changes in the production system

The most direct and most frequently adopted measures include temperature and humidity control by means of water sprinklers, fans, shades or overhead sprays. Younas et al. (1993) demonstrated that cooling and fanning brought a tendency towards more pre-ovulatory LH surges and a higher oestrus response rate, but needed to be initiated several weeks before the planned breeding to produce significant reproductive improvements. Their findings were confirmed by Bucklin et al. (1991) and Armstrong (1994). In a study by Morton et al. (2007) a clear reduction in conception rate was observed when cows were exposed to high temperatures from the day of service to 6 days after service, and for a week before breeding. High temperature exposure for between 3 and 5 weeks before insemination was also associated with reduced conception rates. Thus, management interventions aimed at ameliorating the effects of heat on conception rates should be implemented at least 5 weeks before anticipated service and should continue until at least 1 week after service.

In another study, Roth et al. (2001b) found that a period of two to three oestrous cycles is required for recovery from damage caused by heat to follicles and the appearance of competent oocytes.

Some benefits were also observed with dietary supplementation with minerals, vitamin E and β-carotene, especially when combined with cooling and fanning of the cows and pharmacological oestrus management. Arechiga et al. (1998) reported that timed AI in combination with β-carotene supplementation improved pregnancy rates during periods of heat stress in dairy cows. Supplementation with selenium and vitamin E was found by Arechiga et al. (1998) to have a beneficial effect on fertility in cows in a hot environment. On the other hand, Ealy et al. (1994) reported that cooling improved pregnancy rates slightly in heat stressed cows, but supplementation with vitamin E had no obvious positive effect on pregnancy rates.

Selection of heat resistant breeds

It is now well established that *bos indicus* has a greater resistance to the indirect harmful effects of heat stress on production and reproduction.

Under heat stress conditions, zebu cattle exhibit less severe reductions in feed intake, growth rate and milk yield. Thus, in hot zones, in spite of their low milk production and relatively slow growth rate, *bos indicus* breeds are the best choice for extensive meat and milk production, though not, of course, for intensive dairy operations.

Embryo transfer

Embryo transfer using embryos produced in vitro or embryos derived from donors not exposed to high ambient temperatures has been employed with encouraging results as a means of reducing the adverse effects of heat stress on fertility (Drost et al., 1999; Rutledge 2001; Al Katanani et al., 2002).

Such encouragement should be viewed with caution, however, since an uncompromised embryo transferred into a recipient suffering the effects of heat stress does not avoid the negative effects on the endocrine balance and the uterine environment.

Moreover embryo transfer is not often an economically or technically viable option for many countries in the high temperature zones.

Hormone therapy

Hormone therapy does not address the cause of the harmful effects of heat stress, but can alleviate some of its direct effects on the endocrine balance and thereby help to reduce its negative influence on reproductive performance in cattle, during the summer and early autumn months.

Hormone therapy should never be relied upon as the only measure to combat heat stress. The obvious management measures should be also implemented, preferably before any pharmacological intervention.

The following strategies can be adopted to improve reproductive results during periods of heat stress:

- Oestrus synchronization for timed AI
- GnRH administration at oestrus
- GnRH or hCG administration post AI

Oestrus synchronization for a fixed time AI

The negative effects of heat stress on the reproductive pattern in dairy cows include the poor expression of oestrus behaviour and the tendency for oestrus to be obvious only during the night. This markedly reduces the efficiency of heat detection and leads to a reduction in the number of inseminations and an increase in the proportion of inseminations that fail to result in pregnancy due to the wrong timing of AI. The pharmacological management of oestrus aimed at fixed time insemination, removing the need for oestrus detection, improves submission rates and consequently improves overall pregnancy rates. However, the various systems for inducing and synchronizing oestrus should always be combined with other measures such as cooling or spraying to reduce the direct influence of high temperature.

The preferred methods for oestrus management in heat stressed dairy cattle involve so-called Ovsynch-type protocols. In these systems, any responsive follicle is caused to ovulate by the injection of GnRH or hCG followed by a luteolytic dose of $PGF_{2\alpha}$ after 7 days and, 47 hours later, a second dose of GnRH or hCG which induces the ovulation of a new dominant follicle. The results of recent studies suggest that the principal benefit of these approaches is induction of ovulation and removing the need for heat detection during the summer months. Some authors suggest that the treatment with GnRH or hCG at oestrus can also contribute to the creation of normal and fully functional corpora lutea associated with good fertility (Rensis et al., 2003, 2008).

De la Sota et al. (1998) evaluated the effects of Ovsynch synchronization and timed insemination during summer heat stress in lactating dairy cattle. They found that the Ovsynch programme improved the reproductive performance in the treated group.
Pregnancy rates were higher for the timed inseminated cows (Ovsynch group-13.9%±2.6 versus Control group 4.8%±2.5) as was the overall pregnancy rate by 120 days post partum (Ovsynch-27%±3.6 versus Controls-16.5%±3.5). The authors also reported a reduction in the number of days open for cows conceiving by 120 days post partum in the treated group (Ovsynch -77.6±3.8 versus Controls – 90.0±4.2) as well as in the interval to first service (Ovsynch-58.7±2.1 versus Controls-91.0±1.9).
Moreover an economic evaluation of the programme applied to the first service of the summer months revealed an increase in the net income per cow.

In a recent publication, De Rensis (2008) reported that the use of hCG in place of the second GnRH injection in a classical Ovsynch protocol increased plasma progesterone levels, and improved fertility, in dairy cows during the warmer months of the year.

The pharmacological management of oestrus brings further benefits when combined with other measures, such as vitamin and mineral supplementation. Arechiga et al. (1998) evaluated the effect of timed insemination and supplemental β-carotene on the reproductive performance and milk yield of dairy cows under heat stress. Using the Ovsynch protocol, this group found that the pregnancy rate at first AI was similar among the treated and untreated group in both hot and cooler months. However, during the hot months, the percentage of cows pregnant by 90 days post partum was greater in those treated under the Ovsynch protocol with fixed time insemination, than in the cows inseminated at an observed heat (16.5% versus 9.8% and 34.% versus 14.3%). These authors came to the conclusion that timed AI can improve pregnancy rates during periods of heat stress, while supplementation with β-carotene may increase pregnancy rates and can increase milk yield, for cows in the summer.

Fertility in post partum dairy cows in winter and summer following oestrus synchronization with GPG (GnRH+$PGF_{2\alpha}$+GnRH) or CPC (hCG+$PGF_{2\alpha}$+hCG) protocols was analysed by Rensis et al. (2002). Oestrus management with either of these systems improved pregnancy rates, which approached the results obtained in untreated animals during the winter. Moreover oestrus synchronization reduced the calving to conception interval in both summer and winter.
The benefits of oestrus management with Ovsynch-type protocols in dairy cows exposed to heat stress were also confirmed by Almier et al. (2002) and Cartmil et al. (1999).

Administration of GnRH at the time of artificial insemination
The administration of GnRH during the early stages of oestrus is believed to induce an enhanced LH surge and to improve the synchronization of the intervals between oestrus, LH surge, ovulation and insemination. Moreover, induction of ovulation, with the administration of GnRH at oestrus, allows for a reduction in the incidence of delayed ovulation and prolonged follicular dominance associated with the effects of heat stress.

Treatment of lactating cows with GnRH at the time of oestrus detection during late summer increased their conception rate from 18% to 29% (Ullah et al., 1996).
As some authors suggest, improvements in fertility after treatment with GnRH or hCG at AI, apart from ensuring the timely ovulation of better quality oocytes, can be due to improved luteal function, and consequently higher concentrations of progesterone during the first 30 days after AI. In the study reported by Ullah et al. (1996) the mean progesterone concentrations were higher for cows treated

with GnRH at oestrus than for the controls. Moreover, at the second pregnancy diagnosis after 45 days, a significant reduction in pregnancy rates was observed for the control cows, in comparison with the results of the early diagnosis, except for those cows given GnRH at oestrus, which suggested better embryonic survival in treated cows. The authors thus concluded that GnRH treatment at AI enhanced the secretion of luteal progesterone and improved embryo survival in heat stressed cattle (Ullah et al., 1996).

This thesis was further supported by the results of Kaim et al. (2001) who found an increase of approximately 16.6% over that of untreated controls in the pregnancy rate of lactating cows injected with a GnRH analogue (buserelin, Receptal®) at the first signs of standing heat during the summer and autumn months, in Israel. Moreover, in the trials reported by Kaim et al. (2001), treatment with GnRH at oestrus significantly improved conception rates in cows with low body condition scores at AI, and in those with high body condition scores during the summer. The effect of the treatment was especially obvious in cows with low body condition scores, as treatment with GnRH at oestrus significantly improved their conception rates in both summer and winter. Interestingly enough, these authors also found that treatment with GnRH at oestrus more than doubled the conception rates in cows which had experienced post partum reproductive disorders.

Administration of GnRH or hCG after artificial insemination

Few studies have specifically addressed the use of luteotrophic hormones to obtain an endocrine environment more conductive to embryo development and conceptus survival in heat stressed cattle.

Treatment with GnRH or hCG after insemination is believed to lead to elimination of the first wave dominant follicle of the luteal phase, and in this way to decrease the concentration of oestradiol and prevent the initiation of a luteolytic cascade.

Moreover, ovulation of early luteal phase follicles also leads to the creation of accessory corpora lutea, and consequently to the increase in progesterone concentration, which has been associated with higher pregnancy rates (Butler et al., 1996; Lamming et al., 1989; Mann et al., 1995; 2001; Lopez-Gatius et al., 2006).

Although administration of both hCG (at 4-6 days) and GnRH (at 11-12 days) after insemination are well established approaches to improving pregnancy rates in dairy cattle, there are only limited studies of supplemental hCG and GnRH administration post breeding in heat stressed cattle.
The effect of GnRH administration post insemination on serum progesterone and pregnancy rates in dairy cattle exposed to mild heat stress was evaluated by Willard et al. (2003). These workers reported that treatment with GnRH, at either 5 or 11 days after insemination, induced a more dynamic rise in progesterone levels which reached higher values between 8 and 15 days later, when compared with untreated cows. Untreated controls tended to have lower pregnancy rates than those treated with GnRH (5 or 11 days post AI) with the greatest improvement being obtained after the later treatment.

Bearing in mind the positive effects of hCG administration at 4-6 days post AI, and in embryo transfer recipients (Greve et al., 1982; Kaneda et al., 1981; Lewis et al., 1990; Nishigai et al., 2001, 2002; Santos et al., 2001; Sianangama et al., 1992) and GnRH injection at 11-12 days post AI (Peters et al., 2000) the possibilities of implementing such treatment as a means of reducing the harmful effects of heat stress on reproduction in dairy cattle, need further investigation.

2.4 Reproductive disorders

Infertility can be a serious problem, especially in high-yielding dairy cows. During the post partum period, there must be a rapid and uneventful involution of the uterus and early resumption of normal ovarian activity, followed by an accurately detected oestrus with a high conception rate. At the same time, the cow is being asked to produce large amounts of milk while in the early post partum negative energy balance. It is not surprising that fertility problems are common. To achieve and maintain good herd fertility requires their early diagnosis and treatment.

The reproductive problems of the individual cow can be divided into the following groups:
- Retained placenta
- Uterine infections
- Anoestrus
- Cystic Ovarian Disease (COD)
- Embryonic mortality
- Repeat breeders
- Abortion

All of these will be discussed in the following chapters, starting with the physiological aspects of the post partum period.

2.4.1 Physiological aspects of the post partum period

Uterine involution
It generally takes 3 weeks for the uterus to return to its normal non-pregnant size. The time required for complete physiological involution (including regeneration of the epithelium of the endometrium) varies from 40 to 50 days.
Endogenous levels of prostaglandin $F_{2\alpha}$ metabolites are elevated during the first 7 to 23 days after calving, which supports rapid uterine involution.
Uterine involution involves physical shrinkage, necrosis and shedding of caruncles, and the regeneration of the endometrium. Following the loss of the allanto-chorion, necrosis of the uterine caruncles takes place, which are normally separated and shed by 12 days after parturition. The separation of the caruncles contributes significantly to the rapid reduction in weight of the involuting postpartum uterus from 13 kg at parturition to about 1 kg 3 weeks later. Lochia is formed from the caruncles and the remains of foetal fluids and blood from the ruptured umbilicus, leading to a noticeable loss of fluid and tissue debris during the first 7 to 10 days after calving. The volume can vary from 500 ml in primipara to 1000-2000 ml in pluripara.

Although the correlation between uterine involution and ovarian activity in the early post partum period has not yet been completely elucidated, there is strong evidence that such a correlation exists and that it can influence subsequent fertility. The early resumption of normal ovarian activity is known to hasten uterine involution. Moreover, the marked increase in uterine tone, and reduction in the size of the uterus from day 10 to 14 post partum which occurs in normal cows, usually coincides with the onset of the first oestrus and oestrogen production. At the same time, oestrogens are known to exert a beneficial effect on the uterine defence mechanisms and the contraction of uterine smooth muscle fibres (Hussain 1989). On the other hand, the influence of uterine involution on the resumption of ovarian activity is mainly based on the massive post partum release of $PGF_{2\alpha}$ by the endometrium (Kindahl et al., 1992). It was concluded that in cows with a normal puerperium, and in those in which the duration of the post partum release of prostaglandin is extended, uterine involution was completed more quickly, and the first ovulation (followed by a luteal phase of normal duration) occurred earlier. In cows with an abnormal puerperium, characterised by prolonged uterine involution, the resumption of ovarian activity was markedly delayed.

Ovarian activity

It has been clearly shown that during the post partum anovulatory period a distinct pattern of follicular activity can be observed in most cows. Their ovaries are characterised by several small to medium-sized follicles, leading to the recruitment of a first dominant follicle within a considerably short time after parturition (Opsomer et al., 1996). However the interval between calving and first ovulation in commercial cattle herds varies greatly depending on the breed, nutrition, milk yield, season and the presence of a sucking calf.

In milked dairy cows, medium follicles are detectable by day 5 post partum with the first dominant follicle ovulating between days 15 and 27 post partum. The majority of dairy cows should have resumed cyclic activity by day 40 post partum. Under farm conditions, however, many of them are not observed in oestrus.

In suckled beef cows, the first ovulation occurs later, with considerable variation both within and between herds. Short cycles (luteal phase <10 days) are frequently found during the post partum period. In suckled beef cows, medium follicles are present by day 5 to 7 post partum while the dominant follicles are detectable by day 10 to 21 post partum. These dominant follicles, however, fail to undergo their final maturation and ovulation due to the absence of appropriate LH pulses, and become atretic. The absence of LH pulses in the early post calving period is associated with the depletion of LH stores in the anterior pituitary gland and is independent of suckling (Yavas and Walton 2000). After the replenishment of LH stores between days 15 and 30 post calving, the absence of LH pulses becomes suckling dependent. The stimuli generated by suckling suppress pulsatile LH release by inhibiting GnRH secretion from the hypothalamus. Ovarian oestrogens modulate this inhibitory effect. Suckling increases the sensitivity of the hypothalamus to the negative feedback effect of ovarian oestrogens, suppressing LH release from the pituitary gland (Yavas and Walton 2000). The pulsatile LH release recovers around days 25 to 32 post partum and cows start cycling again between days 29 and 67 post partum.

Complications of the post partum period
Slow recovery of reproductive competence during the post partum period is a major limitation to the success of subsequent reproduction management programmes

2.4.2 Retained placenta

The release of foetal membranes (placenta) post partum is a physiological process that involves the loss of foeto-maternal adherence, combined with contractions of the myometrium.
The separation of foetal membranes is based on a complex immunological process. Maternal immunological recognition of foetal MHC (major histocompatibility complex) class I proteins expressed by trophoblast cells, triggers an immune/inflammatory response that contributes to placental separation at parturition (Davies et al., 2004).

Normally the placenta is expelled within 6-8 hours of calving. A placenta which has not been shed by 24 hours after calving is often referred to as 'retained' placenta or retained foetal membranes. The incidence of retained placenta varies from 4.0- 16.1%, but can be much higher in problem herds.

Failure of placental detachment appears to be largely due to an inability of the immune system to successfully degrade the placentomes at the end of pregnancy. Davies et al. (2004) presented evidence from various published works that indicate impaired function of the immune processes leading to the failure of timely separation of foetal membranes in cattle. Bovine placentomes from cows with normal placental separation contain a chemotactic factor for leukocytes which is lacking in placentomes from cows with retained placenta. Leukocytes and neutrophils of cows with retained placenta are less reactive to chemotactic stimuli than in cows with normal placental separation

It is important to recognise that the lack of uterine contractility to expel the placenta plays little or no role in the occurrence of retained foetal membranes (Eiler, 1997); cows with retained placenta have normal to increased uterine activity in the days after calving (Frazer, 2005).

There is a clear association between cows' metabolic status and their ability to expel their foetal membranes. Cows in a more profoundly negative energy balance pre partum are 80% more likely to have retained placenta, and those with lower circulating vitamin E are also at greater risk of this condition (LeBlanc et al., 2004; LeBlanc 2008).

Retention of the foetal membranes is a common disorder that has a detrimental effect on the reproductive efficiency of the cows, predisposing them to uterine infections later in the post partum period and affecting the resumption of ovarian activity after calving.

It is estimated that pregnancy rate in affected cows is reduced by approximately 15% compared with unaffected cows, but it is likely that impaired reproductive performance only occurs if placental retention leads to the development of metritis or endometritis.

Although it has been established that several genetic, nutritional, immunological and pathological factors influence the separation of the bovine placenta, the aetiology of retained placenta is not fully understood.

The manual removal of the placenta can traumatise the uterus and delay the return to normal reproductive status (Bolinder et al., 1988). It appears to be better to allow the placenta to separate of its own accord, or to withdraw it gently from the uterus 7-10 days post calving.
The aim of therapy should be to prevent the adverse effects of post partum endometritis. Local therapy with various forms of intra-uterine antibiotics is well-established yet brings limited benefits. Moreover, the results of some trials indicate that treatment of retained foetal membranes with parenteral antibiotics, but without intra-uterine manipulation and treatment, can be as effective as conventional treatment, including detachment and local antibiotic treatment (Drilrich et al., 2001). Several studies indicate that approximately 50–80% of cows with untreated retained placenta have a temperature >39.5°C on at least 1 day within 10 days of parturition (Drillich et al., 2003, 2006). It is not clear, however, if all these require systemic antibiotic treatment. This was confirmed in a later study in febrile cows (Drilrich et al., 2006) in which neither intra-uterine antibiotics, nor manual removal of foetal membranes, alone or in combination, reduced the percentage of cows needing therapy, or improved the reproductive parameters in the current lactation, when compared with systemic antibiotic treatment alone. Systemic treatment alone was effective, assessed on elevated rectal temperature, and reduced the use of antibiotics compared with therapies that included intra- uterine antibiosis.

One of the pharmacological approaches to the prevention and treatment of retained foetal membranes is the administration of prostaglandins immediately after calving (Stevens et al., 1995). The efficacy of this approach is difficult to assess because of the scarcity of controlled trials. Drugs that increase uterine motility - oxytocin, ergot derivatives, calcium - have shown, at best, a limited benefit.
The reduced incidence of placental retention when vitamin E and selenium were administered, alone or in combination, suggests that oxidative stress has a part to play in the aetiology of the disorder (Campbell et al., 1998; Gupta et al., 2005). To date, therefore, prevention remains limited to general guidance on hygiene at calving, adequate nutrition (Ca, Se, Vit E, etc.) and the control of infectious disease.

Whichever therapeutic approach is selected, the body temperature and clinical appearance of cows with retained placenta must be monitored, as typically 25–50% of affected cows develop metritis.

2.4.3 Uterine infections

Uterine bacterial infections are important because they disrupt not only the function of the uterus, but also the ovary, and the higher control centres in the hypothalamus and pituitary. Due both to the uterine bacterial infection itself, as well as through the associated immune response, the animal's health and fertility are compromised. For the veterinary practitioner, therefore, the accurate diagnosis and adequate treatment of uterine disease is a key component of all reproduction management programmes.

Typically, 25–40% of animals have clinical metritis in the first 2 weeks after calving, which persists in up to 20% of animals as clinical endometritis. Numerous factors, either directly associated with the function of the reproductive tract and the general health of the cow, or indirectly with management conditions, are known to predispose cows to uterine infections (Table 10).

Table 10 Risk factors for the establishment of uterine bacterial disease in cattle

Adapted from Sheldon and Dobson (2004)

Risk factors for the establishment of uterine bacterial disease in cattle
Uterine damage - Stillbirth, twins, dystocia, caesarean section operation - Retained placenta - Delayed uterine involution
Metabolic conditions - Milk fever, ketosis and left displaced abomasum
Balance between pathogenicity and immunity - Disruption of neutrophil function - Type of bacterial flora in the uterine lumen - Progesterone or glucocorticoid administration; early formation of corpus luteum - Level of hygiene of the environment, cows or calving boxes may be less important

Definition

For many years, both research scientists and veterinary practitioners have identified a need for a clear set of definitions to describe various uterine conditions. One of the most popular classifications separated acute endometritis (vaginal discharge, enlarged uterus and clinical disease) occurring up to 14 days post partum from subacute-chronic endometritis (limited vaginal discharge, absence of clinical signs) occurring after 14 days post partum.

Recently, Sheldon et al. (2006; 2008) proposed clear clinical definitions which allowed most important uterine problems to be described and differentiated.

Puerperal metritis

An acute systemic disease caused by a bacterial infection of the uterus taking place usually within the first 10 days post partum. Clinical signs include a fetid, brown, watery uterine discharge and usually pyrexia. In severe cases, reduced milk yield, dullness, inappetance, elevated heart rate and apparent dehydratation may also be present.

Puerperal metritis is often associated with retained placenta, dystocia, stillbirth or twin pregnancy. It is proposed that animals with an abnormally enlarged uterus and a purulent uterine discharge detectable in the vagina within the first 21 days post partum, but not clinically ill, should be classified as having clinical endometritis.

Clinical endometritis

Clinical endometritis is characterised by the presence of purulent (>50% pus) or mucopurulent (approx. 50% pus and 50% mucus) uterine exudate in the vagina, 21 or more days post partum, not accompanied by systemic signs.

Subclinical endometritis

Endometrial inflammation of the uterus usually determined by cytology, in the absence of purulent material in the vagina. It is proposed to define a cow with subclinical endometritis by the presence of >18% neutrophils in uterine cytology samples collected 21-33 days post partum or >10% neutrophils at 34-47 days, in the absence of clinical endometritis.

The prevalence of subclinical endometritis reported in various studies ranges from 19 to 90% depending on the diagnostic method employed and the timing of the post partum examination. Affected cows show a significant reduction in their reproductive performance (Lincke et al., 2007).

Immunological aspects of uterine diseases in cattle

Bacteria from the environment contaminate the uterine lumen of most post partum cows. The elimination of this contamination is dependent on uterine involution, regeneration of the endometrium and the uterine defence mechanisms.

The immune system of the cow's uterus is active during pregnancy, playing an important role in maintaining pregnancy, supporting foetal growth and preventing infection.

The innate defence system is principally responsible for combating bacterial contamination of the uterus by a range of anatomical, physiological, phagocytic and inflammatory mechanisms. Neutrophils are the earliest and most important phagocytic cell to be recruited from the peripheral circulation to the uterine lumen in the case of bacterial infection.

Hormonal changes and alterations in immune responsiveness during the peri-parturient period have been associated with increased susceptibility to infections of the uterus, udder and other tissues. Following normal delivery, the phagocytic capacity of bovine neutrophils in the peripheral circulation remains high throughout the period around parturition, but the bactericidal capacity and oxidative burst activity of neutrophils is slightly impaired during parturition itself (Singh et al., 2008). These activities are enhanced one week after parturition, which favours the spontaneous resolution of uterine infections.

During the pre-partum period there is a rise in cortisol levels, which leads to peripheral leucocytosis. This is followed by peripheral leucopaenia during the first week post partum, which is thought to be due to the migration of neutrophils towards the uterine lumen immediately after calving.

There is now compelling evidence that both metritis and endometritis are associated with reduced feed intake, a more pronounced negative energy balance, and reduced immune function, and these differences are measurable from 2 weeks before calving, i.e. 3–7 weeks before the conditions are diagnosed (Le Blanc 2008)

Zerbe et al. (2000) demonstrated that metabolic disease, and especially an increased blood level of liver triacilglycerols were associated with reduced cytotoxic activity in neutrophils obtained from both the general circulation and the uterine wall, most probably predisposing the cows to uterine disease.

Role of progesterone, oestradiol and prostaglandins
The post partum endocrine environment has a profound effect on the uterine immune response. It is generally accepted that a high progesterone environment suppresses cervical mucus production, myometrial contractility, uterine gland secretion and the phagocytic activity of uterine neutrophils. It has been shown and summarised by Lewis (2003) that luteal phase concentrations of progesterone suppress the immune response, making the uterus more susceptible to bacterial infection. As Lewis concludes from the numerous trials reported, susceptibility to uterine infections is associated with increased progesterone concentrations, reduced $PGF_{2\alpha}$ production and reduced lymphocyte proliferation in vitro.

Uterine immune function appears to improve under the influence of oestrogens. It is unclear, however, whether oestradiol causes an absolute increase in phagocytic and bactericidal activity of the endometrial immune cells, or whether the observed enhancements are simply relative to the situation which occurs under progesterone dominance (Le Blanc 2008). Sheldon et al. (2004) found that administration of oestradiol into the lumen of the previously gravid uterine horn did not enhance the elimination of post partum uterine bacterial infection.

The physiological role of $PGF_{2\alpha}$ in the first month post partum is unclear, but it might help to promote uterine contractility and so contribute to uterine involution. From the immunological point of view, $PGF_{2\alpha}$ is pro-inflammatory stimulating the production of cytokines that enhance phagocytosis and lymphocyte function. If produced in significant concentrations, $PGF_{2\alpha}$ can enhance uterine immune defences by mitigating the immunosuppressive effects of progesterone.

Bacteriology of uterine infections

Acute endometritis is characterised by the presence of Coliforms, Gram-negative anaerobes, *Arcanobacterium pyogenes* and other bacteria (including peptostreptococci) each with a similar frequency. Endotoxins and lipo-polysaccharides excreted by coliform bacteria are among the most important virulence factors leading to complications in cases of dystocia and retained placenta in cattle. These endotoxins have a direct cytotoxic effect, which probably favours the establishment of infections with *A.pyogenes*. Zerbe et al. (2001) showed that prolonged contact between fragments or solubles of *E.coli* and *A.pyogenes* and bovine neutrophils resulted in a functional depression of these cells. A similar effect was obtained with neutrophils exposed to uterine secretions from cows infected with *A.pyogenes* and *E.coli* (Zerbe et al., 2002). Thus it can be concluded that a high level of contamination of the endometrium with *E.coli* during the early post partum period has a negative effect on the function of endometrial immune defence mechanisms and facilitates the persistence of uterine infections.

In cows with subacute/chronic endometritis the bacteria most commonly isolated from the uterus are *Arcanobacterium pyogenes* and Gram-negative anaerobes. This opportunistic, Gram-positive facultative anaerobe is commonly present in mixed culture with a wide variety of organisms, but most often with the anaerobes *Fusobacterium necrophorum* and *Prevotella melaninogenicus, E. coli* or *Streptococcus spp.*

There appears to be a synergism between *Arcanobacterium pyogenes* and Gramnegative anaerobes. *Bacteroides melanogenicus* and *B. fragilis* produce and release certain substances which can impair the phagocytosis of bacteria by immune cells. *F.necrophorum* has been shown to produce leucotoxins, which exert their cytotoxic effect on phagocytic immune cells. *A. pyogenes* is capable of releasing growth-factor-like substances stimulating multiplication of *F.necrophorum*.

Recent in vitro studies (Donofrio et al., 2007) have suggested that bovine herpesvirus-4 might play a role in endometritis.

Effects of uterine health on fertility

The negative influence of uterine bacterial infections is associated with both the presence of the bacteria and their toxins, and also the damage caused by the inflammatory process taking place in response to the infection. The presence of *A.pyogenes* or anaerobic bacteria lead to reduced fertility. It is extremely important to realise that endometritis causes infertility at the time of the infection and subfertility even after the successful resolution of the disease. It is estimated that in cows with endometritis the conception rate is approximately 20% lower, and calving interval 30 days longer, resulting in 3% more animals culled for reasons of reproductive failure (LeBlanc et al., 2002).

The subfertility associated with uterine infections also involves disruption of ovarian function. Opsomer et al. (2000) suggested that uterine damage disrupts the luteolytic mechanism causing the prolonged luteal phase. These epidemiological studies also indicated that uterine infection leads to delayed ovulation. Moreover Sheldon et al. (2002) showed that ovarian function is disturbed in cattle with greater bacterial contamination after parturition, which is manifested by a slower growth rate of, and oestradiol production by, the first post partum dominant follicle.
As well as the effects on fertility, uterine infections contribute to lower milk yields, particularly if associated with retained placenta (Esslemont and Kossaibati 2002; Sheldon et al., 2004).

Data on the prevalence of endometritis in dairy herds vary, ranging from 7.5-8.9% to over 40% (Gilbert et al., 2006). However later research by these authors found the prevalence of cytologically diagnosed endometritis to be 37%-74% between 40 and 60 days post partum. Regardless of the mechanisms underlying the subfertility caused by uterine infections, it is important for veterinary practitioners to diagnose and treat uterine disease promptly and effectively.

Diagnosis of uterine infections
Generally speaking, the diagnostic protocol for assessing uterine health in cattle follows that of a detailed clinical examination, supported by additional laboratory investigation of samples collected during this process (Tab. 11). Data regarding the animal's reproductive history, although not providing a definite diagnosis, is of considerable value, both in assessing the likely causative factors and the duration of the disease process, as well as in deciding on treatment options (e.g. distinguishing between cyclic and non-cyclic cows when selecting the most appropriate treatment).

Table 11 Diagnostic steps in the assessment of uterine health in cattle

Phase of diagnostic process	Information obtained
Reproductive history	Time elapsed since calving Service history since calving Recent treatments (general and/or focused on reproductive tract)
General clinical examination	**General appearance of the animal:** posture, alertness, mobility Presence of vaginal discharge, presence of dried exudate in the perineal region and legs Position of the tail (elevated tail base, held to one side) Body temperature
Detailed clinical examination of the reproductive tract	**Palpation of vaginal walls and visual examination of the vaginal discharge:** presence of discharge in the vagina, presence of lesions in the vaginal walls. Character of the vaginal discharge: colour, smell, consistency **Rectal palpation:** position and size of the cervix and the uterus, uterine tone, presence of fluid in the uterine cavity, presence of corpus luteum and other structures on the ovary **Vaginoscopy:** external cervical orifice: degree of closure, presence, character and volume of discharge; vaginal mucosa. **Transrectal ultrasound examination of the reproductive tract:** Uterus: position, size, thickness of the uterine wall, presence of fluid in the uterine lumen Ovaries: presence of corpus luteum, other ovarian structures
Laboratory tests	**Cytology:** evaluation of the presence and type of cells in the endometrial smear (percentage of PMNs) **Microbiological culture of uterine discharge:** type of bacteria and their sensitivity to antibiotics **Endometrial biopsy:** histological evaluation of biopsy samples of endometrium: presence and degree of inflammation, degree of morphological changes in endometrium.

Diagnosis of metritis within the first 10 days post partum is relatively easy. It is associated with pyrexia, fetid pus within the uterine lumen and vagina and discharging from the vulva, with delayed uterine involution. Care however should be taken when assessing the tract for the early diagnosis of metritis, in view of the physiological process of uterine involution. The presence of abundant red-brown lochia is normal in the first 2 weeks post partum. Additionally, fever of 1–2 days duration is common in the first week after calving, and is not well correlated with uterine infection (Sheldon et al., 2004a).

Endometritis, expecially when subclinical, may be more difficult to diagnose. In a study undertaken by Intervet, only 51% of the cows with subacute/chronic endometritis showed any externally visible vaginal discharge.

Rectal palpation allows for a general estimation of size, contents and position of the uterus. Detection of fluid accumulation is possible if considerable amounts of exudate have accumulated in the uterine lumen, but no information can be gained about the character of this fluid or the condition of the uterine wall.

The use of transrectal ultrasonography allows a more objective measurement of the diameter of the uterine horns and cervix, and the appreciation of the presence of mucus and pus within the uterine lumen.

Vaginoscopy can be performed using autoclavable plastic, metal or disposable foil-lined cardboard vaginoscopes, which allow inspection of the contents of the vagina. It is a rapid and simple technique, but because a positive diagnosis is based on the presence of cervical exudate, it tends to underestimate the proportion of cows with uterine pathology. Vaginoscopy is a far superior diagnostic technique to transrectal palpation of the uterus for the detection of endometritis, but is underutilised by veterinary practitioners mainly because they overestimate the time and effort needed, and the cost of the equipment.

The definitive diagnosis of endometritis is made on the basis of the histological examination of endometrial biopsy samples, which are also useful for assessing subsequent fertility (Bonnet et al., 1993). However, this technique is costly, time-consuming and not easily accessible under field conditions. Moreover, there is some evidence that collecting biopsy samples can have a negative effect on fertility.

Cytology of the uterine contents provides very valuable information, allowing the diagnosis of subclinical cases (Gilbert et al., 2004; Kasimanickam et al., 2004, Sheldon et al., 2004b, 2006, 2008). Polymorphonuclear neutrophils (PMNs) are the predominant inflammatory cell type found in accumulations of intrauterine fluid and the determination of the relative proportion of PMNs has been shown to be predictive of reproductive performance in the post partum cow.
The samples can be collected using either a protected cotton swab inserted into the uterus, by uterine lavage or with a small device called a cytobrush.
A recent study by Barlund et al. (2008) compared the accuracy of endometritis diagnosis by vaginoscopy, ultrasonographic assessment of uterine fluid volume, ultrasonographic assessment of endometrial thickness, endometrial cytology collected by cytobrush and endometrial cytology following uterine lavage. The cytological examination of samples collected by the cytobrush was found to be the most reliable method of diagnosing endometritis in cattle.

Neither of these methods is widely used in the field, and the diagnosis of uterine disease usually depends entirely on clinical examination.

The most accurate method for the diagnosis of endometritis in clinical conditions is examination of the vagina for the presence of pus. The use of vaginoscopy is therefore highly recommended or, alternatively, the vagina can be explored manually, withdrawing the cervical mucus for examination. The advantage of the latter method is that it is cheap, quick, and allows vaginal lacerations and the odour of any vaginal discharge to be detected (Sheldon et al., 2006). The procedure involves cleaninig of the vulva using a dry paper towel and the insertion of a clean, lubricated and gloved hand through the vulva into the vagina followed by the withdrawal of the mucoid contents of the vagina for examination. Manual vaginal examination does not cause uterine bacterial contamination, provoke an acute-phase protein response, or affect uterine horn diameter

Also, a new device called Metricheck (Metricheck®, Simcro, New Zealand) which consists of a stainless steel rod with a rubber hemisphere can be used to retrieve the vaginal contents.
Some important points should be taken into account when using this simple and very effective device:

- The tool should be cleaned and disinfected before use in each animal (which requires a sufficient number of devices to be available for routine post partum examinations in larger herds).
- The perineum must be cleaned to avoid the introduction of faecal material into the vagina.
- The animals need to be restrained to ensure the security and comfort of both animal and operator.

The assessment of endometritis is made on the basis of the uterine status and the characteristics of the vaginal mucus. A mucus scoring system is widely adopted to indicate the degree of the inflammation process (Table 12).

Table 12 Clinical Endometritis Score (Sheldon and Dobson 2004).

The vaginal mucus is scored for character and odour according to the following descriptions. The sum of the two scores gives the endometritis score.

Description	Score
Mucus character	
Clear or translucent mucus	0
Clear or translucent mucus containing flecks of white pus	1
< 50ml exudate containing < 50% white or cream pus	2
> 50ml exudate containing > 50% white, cream or bloody pus	3
Mucus odour	
No unpleasant odour	0
Fetid odour	3

Currently accepted general guidelines in the treatment of uterine infections in cattle

In the therapy of acute puerperal metritis, there are three main objectives to be addressed: elimination of the bacterial infection, treatment of the general clinical signs of toxaemia and supportive measures aimed at sustaining the animal's homeostasis and minimising the damage caused by the inflammatory process and toxaemia. Antibacterial treatment should employ antibiotics with a broad spectrum of activity (especially against *E.coli*). Intrauterine products can be used, but the fact that many affected cows have an elevated body temperature prompts practitioners to select parenteral antibiosis. Moreover, as affected cattle have moderate to severe illness, there is usually little dispute that cows with metritis require systemic antibiotic treatment. Injectable preparations of cephalosporins such as ceftiofur are currently in common use (Sheldon et al., 2004d; Drillich et al., 2006).

Animal welfare and evidence of a destructive nature of the inflammatory process to the endometrium motivates many practitioners to add non-steroidal anti-inflammatory drugs (NSAIDs) to their standard treatment of acute metritis. Although there is, so far, little evidence that this practice has any beneficial effect on reproductive efficiency, reduction in body temperature and improved clinical appearance have been demonstrated (Drillich et al., 2007). Whenever a decision is made to include NSAIDs in the therapy of metritis it should be borne in mind that these products inhibit the production of endogenous prostaglandins from arachidonic acid, and can thus lead to impaired uterine involution. In such cases, exogenous $PGF_{2\alpha}$ should always be administered.

The possible benefits of the routine inclusion of prostaglandins in the treatment of uterine infections in the early post partum period remain disputed. There is little evidence to support the use of $PGF_{2\alpha}$ before 3 weeks post partum (LeBlanc 2008), though many practitioners report highly satisfactory results.

The antibiotic chosen to treat endometritis must be able to eliminate the bacterial infection whilst remaining active in the anaerobic uterine environment. What is more, it should lead to minimal drug residues in milk or meat.

Metricure® has been developed especially for this indication and meets these requirements, treated cows having been shown to eliminate the uterine bacterial contamination, leading to improved reproductive performance (Kasimanickam et al. 2005; LeBlanc et al., 2002; McDougall et al., 2001).

In a study in New Zealand, reported by McDougall et al. (2001), intrauterine treatment with Metricure® improved reproductive performance of dairy cattle, especially those with a history of retained placenta, stillbirth or a vulval discharge.

One of the important features of this product is its ability to provide adequate concentrations of the active, cephapirin, not only in the uterine lumen but also in the endometrium (Table 13). This allows for an effective elimination of the bacteria from endometrial crypts.

Table 13 Concentrations of cephapirin in endometrium and plasma at 4, 8, 24 and 72 hours after administration of Metricure (Data source: Intervet product file)

Hours after administration of Metricure	4h	8h	24h	72h
Concentration of cephapirin in endometrium (mcg/g)	9.62 (>38MIC)	23.08 (>92 MIC)	4.9 (>19 MIC)	0.8 (>3MIC)
Concentration of cephapirin in plasma (mcg/g)	0.06	0.02	<0.01	<0.01

MIC90 for A. pyogenes = 0.25 mcg/ml
Detection limit – 0.01mcg/ml

Antibiotic treatments which have led to the rapid and effective elimination of uterine infections with *A.pyogenes* have been associated with improved reproductive performance in treated cows. Cephapirin was found to be very effective against the major uterine pathogens involved in endometritis in cattle (Sheldon et al., 2004d).

It is extremely important to ensure that any intrauterine treatment used for the treatment of uterine infection has no irritatant effect and does not impair the function of the endometrial defence mechanisms. Few antibacterial substances have actually been examined in controlled studies in this respect. Cephapirin, at clinical dose rates, has been demonstrated to have no negative effect on neutrophil function or on their ability to eliminate the bacteria (Dosogne et al., 1998).

Sometimes the chronic/subacute condition is only spotted when small flecks of pus are detected in the vaginal mucus or on the end of an insemination pipette. It is not uncommon for these flecks to appear in the vaginal mucus some 2-3 hours after AI, because the manual examination of the uterus and cervix allows small amounts of exudate to find their way out of the uterine lumen. In such cases the cow may still be inseminated, and given intra-uterine treatment the day after AI (e.g. a single dose of Metricure®). The embryo will remain protected in the oviduct, only arriving in the treated uterus on around day 5.
When treating uterine infections during the later post partum period (>21 days post calving) the strategy should be based on the severity of clinical signs and ovarian activity (Fig 18).

Figure 18 proposed decision tree in the therapy of endometritis in cattle

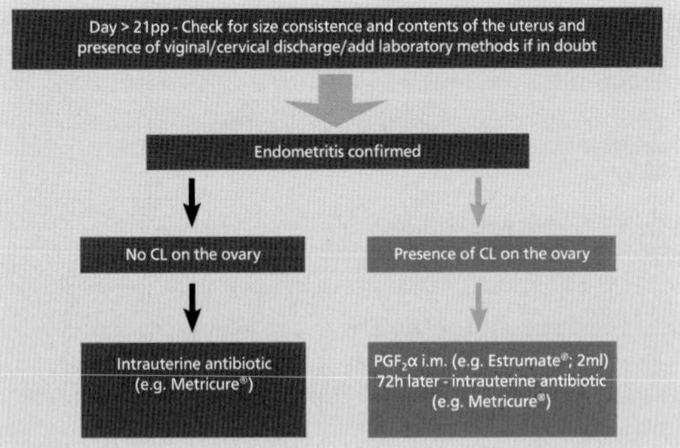

In cases of endometritis in which a corpus luteum is present, the treatment of choice is a combination of prostaglandin injection and intra-uterine antibiotics. The induced luteolysis eliminates the immunosuppressive effect of progesterone and improves uterine tonicity. The intra-uterine administration of broad spectrum antibiotics not only eliminates the bacterial contamination responsible for the inflammatory process, but also avoids some bacteria remaining in the uterine lumen and multiplying during the next luteal phase, with a consequent recrudescence of the endometritis (Lewis 2004).

Routine use of prostaglandins in treatment and prevention of uterine disorders

Prostaglandins have been used for decades as a treatment of both metritis and endometritis, as well as a form of prophylaxis when administered routinely post partum. As is well known, exogenous $PGF_{2\alpha}$ induces luteolysis, which reduces circulating progesterone levels, eliminating its immunosuppressive effect and permitting the uterus to rid itself of infections (Murray et al., 1990; Lewis 1997; Heuwieser et al., 2000). The results of clinical trials of $PGF_{2\alpha}$ for the treatment of clinical endometritis in the absence of an active corpus luteum are inconsistent (Sheldon and Noakes 1998; LeBlanc et al., 2002; Mejia Lacau-Mengido 2005). Lewis (2004) suggests, however, that even the administration of prostaglandins in endometritis without an active corpus luteum being present, can bring certain advantages through a direct beneficial effect of $PGF_{2\alpha}$ on the function of the uterine immune defences.

As already mentioned, a combination of prostaglandin and intrauterine antibiotics seems to provide the best possible solution for eliminating infection and preventing a relapse during subsequent luteal phases (Lewis 2004; Kasimanickam et al., 2005; Sheldon et al., in 2006, LeBlanc 2008).

However, there has been much controversy over the claimed value of the routine use of prostaglandins in the early post partum period, in the absence of a functional corpus luteum. There are conflicting reports of the efficacy of exogenous prostaglandins in increasing the rate of uterine involution, causing the evacuation of bacterial and debris from the uterus, consequently improving conception rates. Prostaglandin would be more consistently effective in these instances if it was administered when there is a corpus luteum present. In most post partum cows this would be at approximately 17-24 days post partum. Many practitioners believe that sequential luteolysis with exogenous prostaglandin treatment at specific times post partum results in exposing the uterine environment to normal concentrations of progesterone for shorter intervals, thereby reducing the susceptibility of the uterus to bacterial infection. Many published studies have failed to demonstrate a clearly measurable benefit of such a treatment (Burton and Lean 1995 (meta-analysis; Hendricks et al., 2005), while others have shown a reduction in uterine problems, and improved fertility (Etherington et al., 1994; Nakao et al., 1997; Fernandes et al., 2008a,b).

Pyometra can be regarded as a specific form of chronic endometritis, i.e. one featuring a persistent corpus luteum and closed cervix. During the progesterone-dominated phase, the uterus has a reduced resistance to infection:

- The pH is lower, which creates better conditions for the common uterine pathogens.
- The leucocyte activity is delayed and reduced.
- The uterine secretion has no detoxifying effect.

In cases of pyometra, prostaglandin $F_{2\alpha}$ release from the uterus is insufficient to cause luteolysis. Prostaglandin injections can, therefore, be used to treat this condition. The corpus luteum regresses, followed by the maturation of a new follicle. The uterine contractility increases, the cervix relaxes and the purulent material is expelled. The change in the hormone balance (increased oestrogen/decreased progesterone) stimulates the uterine self-defence mechanisms. It should be mentioned, however, that the result of the treatment is largely dependent on its timing, and treated cows should be closely monitored, as relapse is common. It is therefore strongly recommended that these animals receive a second prostaglandin injection after 12 to 14 days. Insemination can begin once the endometrium is restored , which usually takes 4 to 8 weeks. Intra-uterine antibiotic therapy (Metricure®) can be used, in addition.

In view of the destructive nature of pyometra, any intra-uterine infusion should be non-irritant to prevent even more destruction of the endometrium.

Vaginitis

In heifers, vaginitis is quite a common sequel to natural mating and usually requires no treatment. In adult cows, vaginitis may be due to environmental infection and can easily lead to endometritis. It is often difficult to differentiate between these two conditions. Non-pregnant animals are best treated as for endometritis. Prevention must be based on improving hygiene. A number of specific infections are accompanied by vaginitis and/or endometritis. See under abortion (Chapter 2.4.8).

2.4.4 Anoestrus

When a dairy cow is not observed in oestrus by 60 days post partum, whether actually cycling or not, the condition is defined as Post Partum Anoestrus (PPA).

Some definitions will prevent misunderstanding:

Anoestrus	The cow is not observed in oestrus either beause she has not come into oestrus (not cycling) or because oestrus was not detected (cycling).
True anoestrus	The cow does not come into oestrus because it has inactive ovaries.
Suboestrus	The cow has normal cyclic activity, but is not observed in oestrus due to weak or absent oestrus behaviour, or inadequate observation

Cyclic cows

Suboestrus

Suboestrus, or failure to observe oestrus, accounts for most reported post partum anoestrus. It includes animals showing normal oestrus behaviour, weak oestrus behaviour or none at all. Differentiation between these is practically impossible. Action must be based, firstly, on improving oestrus detection: knowing what to look for, observing for long enough, often enough, clear identification of individuals, good fertility records, and possibly the use of milk progesterone test kits. See under oestrus detection (2.2.4).

The control of oestrus and ovulation by the use of prostaglandins, gonadotrophin-releasing hormone or progestagens may ameliorate some of the problems of oestrus detection by defining the period in which the farmer can expect to observe oestrus. See under oestrus control (2.3).

Non-cyclic cows

True anoestrus

Resumption of cyclic activity after calving is influenced by nutrition, body condition, suckling, lactation, dystocia, breed, age, season, uterine pathology and concurrent disease. In most well managed dairy herds fewer than 10% of cows fail to ovulate by day 40 post partum. In beef cattle, this may be up to 60% due to the suppressive effect of suckling, nutrition, season etc. The duration of post partum anoestrus is not determined by the emergence of follicular waves, but rather by follicular deviation and/or the fate of the dominant follicle.

Benefiting from the use of ultrasonography and the growing knowledge of follicular dynamics in cattle, Wiltbank et al. (2002) proposed the following classification of anovulatory status:

1. *Anovulation with follicle growth up to the emergence stage.* In this form of anoestrus, cows exhibit very small follicles which grow only to the emergence phase and proceed no further. The authors speculate that this form of anoestrus is related to a relative deficiency in FSH release.
2. *Anovulation with follicle growth up to deviation phase.* In this form of anoestrus, follicular growth takes place and proceeds through emergence and deviation but does not continue to ovulation. It is a form of anoestrus frequently reported. It appears to occur in all cows during the prepubertal period, and commonly occurs in the post partum period in lactating dairy and suckling beef cows. The characteristic signs are small ovaries with no corpus luteum or follicles of ovulatory-size, even though they show continuing growth in a dynamic wave pattern up to the deviation phase. The underlying physiological problem is the inhibitory effect of oestradiol on GnRH/LH pulses that does not allow the growth to the final phase, or oestradiol production by the post-deviation dominant follicle.
3. *Anovulation with follicular deviation, growth, and the establishment of a dominant follicle, which fails to ovulate but becomes a persistent follicular structure.* Persistent follicular structures may become follicular cysts or they may luteinize (luteal cysts).
   For more details see in section 2.4.5.

2.4.4.1. Treatment of anoestrus in cattle

Improved knowledge of the physiological backround of various types of anovulatory conditions in cattle allows the use of more adequate and appropriate treatment approaches which address the underlying endocrine disorder.

Improvement in the energy status in dairy cows by providing optimal nutrition during the transition period and early lactation can reduce the anoestrus period associated with the lack of LH pulses. In beef cows, an improvement in energy status and/or reduction of the frequency with which the calves are allowed to suck can increase LH pulses and reduce the time to first ovulation. Hormonal treatment can be used to stimulate anovulatory cows, especially if combined with increased energy supplementation in dairy cows, and energy supplementation and/or reduced suckling frequency in beef cows.

In the anovulatory condition with follicular growth progressing only to the emergence stage (type 1), the possibilities for pharmacological treatment are rather limited. It is often found in cows at pasture, especially in *bos indicus* breeds reared in tropical zones. Such cows usually have poor quality feed and are exposed to very demanding climatic conditions. Field experience indicates that treatments with GnRH analogues usually have no effect, but FSH treatment can increase follicle growth. FSH-based products used routinely for the stimulation of multiple ovulation in oocyte/embryo donors in cattle are relatively expensive. Careful dosing with PMSG/eCG (e.g. Folligon®) could be used to stimulate further follicular growth in cows suffering from this type of anoestrus. It must be stressed that without radical improvement in the nutrition of the treated cows the prospects for success are rather low.

The type of anovulation with follicular growth up to deviation phase (type 2) is especially common in high-yielding dairy cows and in suckled beef cows of relatively good body condition. Regardless of any pharmacological intervention, improvement in energy status by the provision of optimal nutrition during the transition period, as well as during early lactation, should be considered as the primary means of reducing the period of anovulation caused by the lack of LH pulses. In addition, disease conditions should be minimised. Anovulatory lactating dairy cows can be effectively treated with a regular Ovsynch protocol as many such animals have follicles of a sufficient size and ovulatory capacity to respond to a pharmacologically stimulated LH surge. Beef cows, on the other hand, are preferably treated with progestagens combined with a temporary weaning of their calves. Vasconcelos et al. (2009) described a trial comparing the results of temporary weaning and the use of a progesterone-releasing device in anoestrus crossbred *bos indicus/bos taurus* cows. Their findings indicated that temporary weaning alone increased the incidence of oestrous behaviour, whereas the use of progesterone-releasing devices alone benefited conception. Combining the two improved pregnancy rate, with direct benefits on behavioural oestrus and conception.

Treatment of anovulatory conditions leading to the formation of a persistently dominant follicle or follicular cysts is discussed in section 2.4.5.

Use of progestagens in anoestrus cows

Treatment with progestagens/progesterone is now considered to be the preferred option for the induction of cyclicity and management of oestrus in anoestrus cattle, especially beef breeds (for reviews see: Yavas et al., 200a,b; Peter et al., 2009).

The use of progesterone or progestagens to treat anoestrus is beneficial because it initiates the oestrous cycle with ovulation, and facilitates the subsequent luteal phase of a normal length. The best results have so far been obtained with the use of progesterone or progestagens, such a norgestomet (Crestar®), combined with an injection of oestradiol at the start of treatment.

Injection of PMSG/eCG (Folligon®) may be used following a period of progesterone treatment, and forms an integral part of the Crestar® system to induce oestrus and ovulation in anovulatory anoestrus cows.

Using daily transrectal ultrasonography, Rhodes et al. (2000) demonstrated that anoestrus cows treated with small doses of progesterone did not develop persistent ovarian follicles such as those seen in cows treated after oestrous cycles had begun. Therefore it should be possible to obtain satisfactory results in this group of cows with progesterone or progestagen treatment alone.

Gonadotrophin-releasing hormone analogues may also be used at the start of progesterone treatment to cause the regression of the dominant follicle present and synchronize the emergence of a new cohort of follicles. This protocol has the additional effect of inducing ovulation and the formation of a corpus luteum in a majority of cows, resulting in elevated concentrations of progesterone in plasma compared, with cows not treated with GnRH (Xu et al., 2000a). To ensure the absence of luteal tissue following the removal of a progesterone-releasing device, prostaglandins are generally included in such protocols. Oestradiol has been used to stimulate ovulation and the expression of oestrus following progesterone treatment, especially in New Zealand, but with the recent ban on the application of this class of hormones the practice has had to be abandoned.

In suckled cows in deep anoestrus, temporary weaning (separating calf and dam for 48 hrs) at the time of progesterone/ progestagen removal, provides additional ovarian stimulation.

GnRH analogues in combination with prostaglandins

The capacity of GnRH analogues to induce ovulation during the postpartum anovulatory anoestrus period, allows for the use of programmes such as Ovsynch to treat anoestrus in cattle, providing that follicles responsive to LH stimulation are present on the ovaries. Use of this protocol, in conjunction with separating cow and calf, was compared with the use of norgestomet implants and injection of oestradiol valerate in anoestrus beef cows, and in cows which had resumed oestrous cycles. Pregnancy rates were similar in previously anoestrus cows treated with either protocol, and were equivalent to those obtained in cows that had resumed oestrous cycles before treatment with the Ovsynch protocol (Geary et al., 1998).

In anoestrus grazing dairy cows, use of an Ovsynch protocol resulted in similar conception rates to first insemination and in a median interval to conception compared with cows treated with CIDR® devices and oestradiol benzoate and inseminated at the observed oestrus (McDougall et al., 2001). However, the results

suggest that the Ovsynch protocol may be of benefit in treating anoestrus cows in situations in which oestrus detection is a problem, although pregnancy rates are lower than those obtained in cows that have resumed oestrous cycles (Cartmill et al., 2001).
Hormone treatment can effectively reduce the interval to first ovulation, and synchronize oestrus, across a variety of physiological states. However, response to treatment is not uniform either between herds or within herds, and appears to be dependent on those factors influencing the prevalence of anoestrus, such as age, body condition, and interval after calving. In post partum anoestrus cows with low body condition, both oestrus response rates and pregnancy rates are usually disappointing, regardless of the method used.

In view of the fact that uterine infections were shown to be associated with the delayed resumption of ovarian activity (Opsomer et al 2000; Sheldon et al., 2004a,b) anoestrus cows should always be checked for signs of endometritis.

Persistent Corpus Luteum/Pyometra.
Persistent corpora lutea are generally accompanied by a uterine disorder preventing the release of sufficient prostaglandin for luteolysis. As already mentioned, abnormal luteal activity, often associated with uterine infections, is commonly found in high-yielding dairy herds (Shrestha et al., 2004), especially during the warmer months of the year (Kornmatitsuk et al., 2008). Treatment consists primarily of the administration of exogenous prostaglandin to cause regression of the persistent corpus luteum. This can be combined with GnRH administration to cause ovulation of the dominant follicle from a new follicular wave, followed by insemination.

Cystic Ovarian Disease.
Anoestrus is a possible symptom of cystic ovarian disease. For more information, see under cystic ovarian disease (chapter 2.4.5 Cystic Ovarian Disease).

2.4.5 Cystic Ovarian Disease

Traditionally, cysts have been defined as anovulatory follicular structures (diameter, >25 mm) that persist for 10 or more days in the absence of a functional corpus luteum, and accompanied by abnormal oestrus behaviour (irregular oestrus intervals, nymphomania or anoestrus). However, recent data using ultrasonography, indicate that typically follicles ovulate when 17 mm in diameter, so follicles that persist at that diameter or greater may be considered to be 'cystic' (Vanholder et al., 2006a), which is the reason for the term Cystic Ovarian Follicles (COF) to be in common use, rather than ovarian cysts.

Ovarian follicular cysts are the most common reproductive disorder in dairy cows, developed by approximately 6-19% of this class of animal (Garverick 1997). In the early post partum period, the incidence is probably much higher, because about 60% of the cows that develop 'ovarian cysts' before the first ovulation, re-establish ovarian cycles spontaneously (Ijaz et al., 1987). The economic impact of cystic ovarian disease is a function of their impact on days open, and other associated costs. Each occurrence of ovarian follicular cysts has been estimated to add between 22 and 64 extra days open and cost US$137 in reduced milk production and veterinary expenses (Silvia et al., 2002).

Though no single cause can be blamed for cystic ovarian disease, high yield, season, stress, and negative energy balance are all considered to be predisposing factors. Post partum problems such as placental retention, milk fever and endometritis have been associated with an increased risk of cystic ovarian disease.
There is evidence to indicate the existence of a genetic background to cystic ovarian disease. Moreover, beside the existence of a genetic predisposition for COF, a genetic correlation between cysts and milk production traits has been established, indicating that continuing to select cows for production parameters will increase the incidence of COF. Nutritional factors include β-carotene deficiency and phyto-oestrogens.

Nutritional deficiencies (negative energy balance, NEB) are thought to be one of the most important factors contributing to the formation of cystic follicles during the early post partum period. Moreover, there seems to be a link between COF incidence and the magnitude and/or duration of the NEB (Vanholder et al., 2006a). Although elevated serum ketone concentrations increased the risk for the formation of cystic follicles in post partum dairy cows, they were not found to exert any negative effects on bovine follicle cells in vitro (Vanholder et al., 2006b). Therefore, ketone concentrations in the post partum dairy cow seem to be an indicator of the severity of the NEB, rather than a mediator of the negative effects of the NEB on reproduction at the ovarian level.

COF formation may result from functional disorders at both ovary/follicle and hypothalamus/pituitary levels. The most widely accepted hypothesis to explain the formation of a cystic follicle is the altered release of LH from the hypothalamus-pituitary: the pre-ovulatory LH surge is either absent, insufficient in magnitude, or occurs at the wrong time during the maturation of the dominant follicle.
It is believed that an altered feedback mechanism of oestrogens on the hypothalamus-pituitary can result in aberrant GnRH/LH release, ovulation failure and cyst formation. A GnRH/LH surge occurring prematurely during follicle growth, i.e. when no follicle capable of ovulation is present on the ovary, can render the hypothalamus unresponsive to the feedback effect of oestradiol, which results in the formation of a cystic follicle.
An altered feedback mechanism and GnRH/LH release may be attributed to factors interfering at the hypothalamic-pituitary level.
Based on this finding, Silvia et al. (2002) proposed a new model for the ethology of follicular cysts in cattle. Ovarian follicular cysts develop due to a lack of the pre-ovulatory LH surge that should take place in response to the pre-ovulatory rise in oestradiol. The primary cause lies in the hypothalamus, which fails to release a surge of GnRH in response to an oestradiol stimulus. Hypothalamic insensitivity to oestradiol may be induced by intermediate (subluteal) concentrations of circulating progesterone. If progesterone is administered at intermediate levels (0.5–2 ng/ml), it will block the LH surge, prevent ovulation,

and result in the formation of a follicle with a greater diameter and persistency than those of normal dominant follicles (Hatler et al., 2003). This concept has been proved with the discovery that treatment with low doses of progesterone, such as delivered by many progesterone-releasing devices used for oestrus synchronization, can lead to the formation of a persistent dominant follicle.
Primary dysfunction at the level of the follicle may disrupt the hypothalamic-pituitary-ovarian axis causing the formation of COF. Alterations in LH-receptor expression and content may cause anovulation of the follicle. Besides these, alterations in steroidogenesis by the dominant follicle may also be involved in cystic degeneration.

Macroscopically, cysts can appear as either follicular or luteal, but these are considered to be different forms of the same disorder. Luteal cysts are believed to develop in the presence of LH concentrations that are insufficient to induce ovulation, but capable of causing luteinization of the follicular walls. Luteal cysts are associated with anoestrus, but it is not possible to differentiate between follicular and luteal cysts on the basis of behaviour alone. Luteal cysts have a thicker wall which only few experienced clinicians seem able to detect by rectal palpation. A high progesterone level in milk or plasma is indicative of a luteal cyst. Care should be taken not to confuse luteal cysts with hollow corpora lutea, which are not pathological at all.

The clinical signs that accompany ovarian cysts can vary considerably. Anoestrus is most common, especially during the post partum period. Irregular oestrus intervals, nymphomania, relaxation of the broad pelvic ligaments and development of masculine physical traits are other signs of the presence of oestrogenically active follicular cysts, especially later in lactation. Luteal cysts are almost invariably associated with anoestrus.

Treatment of cystic ovarian follicles in cattle
In spite of a relatively high self-recovery rate, the development of ovarian cysts, untreated even when diagnosed, can extend the calving to conception interval by 64 days, leading to economic losses of $55 to $160 per lactation (Bartolome et al., 2005d).

The administration of GnRH (Receptal®, Fertagyl®; 5.0ml) is the treatment of choice. It acts by stimulating the pituitary gland to release LH and FSH. The induced LH surge leads to luteinization of the cystic follicle. Depending on the type of cyst, and possibly the dose of GnRH, some cystic follicles may be induced to ovulate. Moreover, the GnRH-induced increase in FSH concentration causes recruitment of a follicular wave that usually restores normal cyclicity. Following treatment, 60-80% of cows will come into oestrus between 18 and 23 days after injection.
It is essential to recognise that it is the stimulation of the normal follicular turnover and the induction of ovulation from a new follicular wave that produces the desired result, not the physical elimination of the cystic follicle. For this reason, manual rupture of the cyst often fails to restore cyclicity. Besides, the transrectal squashing of cysts carries a considerable risk of damaging the delicate ovarian tissues and inducing adhesions.

Since both follicular and luteal cysts respond similarly to this kind of treatment, differentiation is unnecessary, and authors generally agree that GnRH administration remains the best initial therapy for the majority of cows with cystic ovarian disease. Intravenous hCG (Chorulon®; 3000 IU) is another possibility. hCG is a gonadotrophin with strong LH activity. It has a half-life in cattle of nearly 2 days, and thus exerts a long-acting luteotrophic effect directly on the cyst, and is frequently reserved for recurrent cases.

Various studies have indicated that prior exposure of the effector cells of the ovarian follicle to sufficient levels of progesterone is essential for their sensitisation to further gonadotrophin stimulation. Therefore the use of progesterone or progestagens is a logical treatment for follicular cysts and has led to very encouraging results, either alone or in combination with GnRH (Calder et al., 1999; Todoroki et al., 2001; Ambrose et al., 2004).

In order to reduce the number of days open, and to reduce the incidence of cystic ovarian disease, a GnRH/prostaglandin-based system was proposed by White et al. (1996) and further tested by Lopez-Gatius et al. (2002). This regime can be used between

30 and 90 days post calving and involves the administration of GnRH (Receptal®, Fertagyl®) when the cyst is detected, followed 9 days later by $PGF_{2\alpha}$ (Estrumate®).
Once luteinization of the cyst has been initiated by the GnRH, luteal tissue is developed within 9 days of treatment. The resulting corpus luteum should then respond to the subsequent prostaglandin treatment, and a new oestrous cycle begins.

Alternatively a classic Ovsynch protocol can be used for the treatment of ovarian cysts in lactating dairy cows, as demonstrated by Bartolome et al. (2000), who reported that synchronization of ovulation and timed insemination with an Ovsynch protocol, resulted in pregnancy rates similar to those of oestrus synchronization and insemination at an induced oestrus within 7 days. Further studies by Bartolome et al., (2005), De Vries et al. (2006) and De Rensis et al. (2008) confirmed the suitability of the Ovsynch-type protocols for the treatment of cystic ovarian follicles in dairy cows.

Cows that have not come into oestrus within 23 days of GnRH or hCG treatment must be checked and treated if necessary. The same applies to animals that show signs of oestrus within 14 days, since this indicates that they failed to respond to the first injection.
Prevention of cystic ovarian disease can be approached by identifying and eliminating the contributory causes of the disease (periparturient stress, nutritional inadequacies and uterine infections). Furthermore, the administration of GnRH on day 14 post partum has been shown to reduce the incidence of ovarian cysts (Britt et al., 1977). Earlier administration is ineffective because the pituitary gland is not capable of releasing LH in response to GnRH before 12-14 days post partum.

Prostaglandin therapy is also used to treat cows with luteal-type cysts. However, the response and cure rate are dependent on the presence of luteal tissue and the accuracy of diagnosis that the cyst is indeed luteal. Because palpation has been reported as being inaccurate as a means of differentiating between luteal and follicular cysts, diagnosis is better based on plasma or milk progesterone concentrations or on the use of ultrasonography.

2.4.6 Embryonic mortality

The period from conception to day 45 of pregnancy is known as the embryonic stage. It is followed by the foetal stage that lasts until parturition. Embryonic mortality is regarded as one of the major causes of reproductive failure in cattle resulting in reduced pregnancy rates, slower genetic improvement and substantial financial losses to dairy and beef production.
Recent estimates indicated that the average value of a pregnancy was US $278 in high-yielding herds in the USA, whereas the cost of the loss of a pregnancy was substantially greater (De Vries, 2006).

It is generally accepted that the fertilization rate is in the order of 90% and that embryonic loss accounts for a 29-39% of losses after fertilization, most of them (estimated 70-80%) between days 8 and 16 after fertilization (Roche et al., 1981; Dunne et al., 2000; Diskin and Morris 2008).
With the advent of ultrasonography, accurate pregnancy diagnosis has been possible as early as 25 days after AI in cattle, thereby facilitating the study of embryonic mortality after the period of maternal recognition of pregnancy. The frequency of this late embryonic loss is estimated at approximately 7%. While the extent of late embryonic mortality is much lower than early mortality, it is nevertheless an important cause of serious economic loss. These losses can be especially severe in seasonally bred herds when cows which lose embryos towards the end of the breeding season will not be rebred, but culled because of reproductive failure.

Embryonic mortality refers to the losses which occur in the period between fertilization and the completion of the stage of differentiation at approximately day 42.
Early embryonic mortality, i.e. before day 15, does not affect the length of the cycle. When the embryo dies after this time, the cow returns to oestrus when the corpus luteum has regressed, and the cycle is thus lengthened. Embryonic mortality in the late embryonic phase (after day 35-45) may be diagnosable. Although in some cases the embryo and the membranes are

aborted, the remnants will frequently be resorbed. The corpus luteum may persist for a long time thus delaying the return to oestrus. Usually the only obvious sign is a return to oestrus behaviour as late as 35-50 days after insemination.

Some of the factors influencing embryonic mortality are:
- Inherent fertility of both the sire and the cow
- Embryonic chromosomal abnormalities
- Age of the cow
- Uterine abnormalities (e.g. endometritis)
- Damage to the embryo by rectal palpation (e.g. at pregnancy diagnosis)
- Diseases inducing fever
- Heat stress
- Delayed insemination (reduced fertility of the ovum)
- Insufficient luteal function

Mechanisms of pregnancy recognition in cattle
During the normal oestrous cycle, an efficient mechanism involving oxytocin and prostaglandin $F_{2\alpha}$ ensures prompt luteolysis of the corpus luteum and initiation of a new oestrous cycle. Oxytocin produced by the corpus luteum binds to the specific oxytocin receptors in the endometrium thus stimulating the release of $PGF_{2\alpha}$ from endometrial cells (Silvia et al., 1991; Wathes et al., 1995; Mann et al., 2001). Prostaglandin is released into the blood stream, reaches the ovary and causes regression of the corpus luteum. Increasing levels of oestrogens, produced by growing ovarian follicles, stimulate the expression of oxytocin receptors.

In order to sustain the corpus luteum and maintain pregnancy, an effective mechanism for pregnancy recognition has to take place. In other words, the developing embryo has to produce a specific signal to prevent luteolysis which would otherwise be triggered towards the end of the oestrous cycle. It has been demonstrated that early bovine and ovine embryos produce and release a specific pregnancy protein – interferon-τ (INF-τ) (Farin et al., 1989; Mann et al., 1999). The mechanism of luteolysis inhibition by INF-τ is now well established and involves inhibition of oxytocin receptors on the uterine luminal epithelium (Robinson et al., 1999) and induction of a prostaglandin synthesis inhibitor (Thatcher et al., 1995). In cattle, mRNA for interferon-τ is first detected in trophoectoderm, the principal site of its production, at approximately 12 days and reaches its maximum levels between days 15 and 16 (Farin et al., 1990). Interferon-τ can be detected in significant amounts first in the uterine flushings at 14-16 days coinciding with the start of the embryo elongation (Mann et al., 1998).

If retardation of embryonic development occurs, or if the growth of the embryo and the progress of the maternal oestrous cycle are not synchronous (e.g. due to delayed ovulation or late insemination), insufficient or delayed INF-τ production results, inhibition of luteolysis fails and the embryo is lost. The main reason for this impaired secretion of INT-τ by the embryos, resulting from fertilization of oocytes liberated through delayed ovulation, is supposed to be an ageing process in the oocyte associated with a prolonged period of follicular dominance. It has been argued that due to this extended period, and delayed ovulation, precocious maturation changes take place in the oocyte, which in turn reduce its fertilization and developmental capacity. Poor embryonic development is, in turn, associated with low interferon-τ production, failed inhibition of luteolysis and embryo loss (Mann et al., 1996, Mann et al., 1998). As mentioned in section 2.3.3, a close correlation exists between the early post insemination rise in progesterone concentrations, embryonic development and its production of INT-τ (Kerbler et al., 1997; Mann et al., 1999; 2001).
Figure 19 is a schematic representation of the interactions between the embryo and the cow during the early embryonic phase and pregnancy recognition.

Figure 19 Matenal-embryonic interactions preceeding pregnancy recognition in cattle

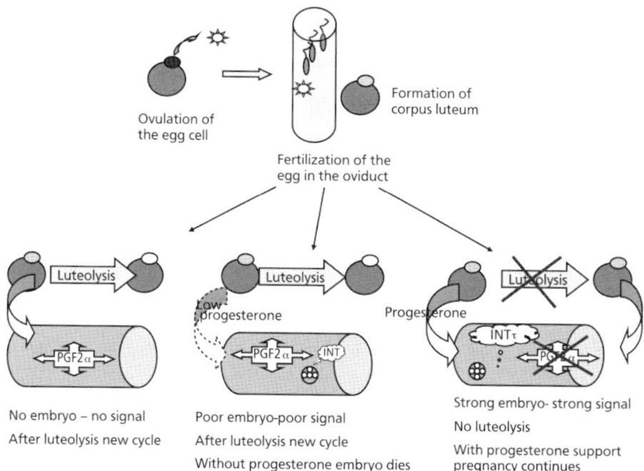

Pharmacological measures to prevent early embryonic mortality
At present the most popular strategies and pharmacological treatments aimed at the improvement of pregnancy rates in cattle can be classified into two groups:

1. Prevention of delayed ovulation
2. Support of early luteal function and prevention of precocious luteolysis

For the pharmacological measures to reduce the incidence of early embryonic mortality see chapter 2.3.4.

2.4.7 The repeat breeder cow

The repeat breeder cow is defined as a normally cyclic cow, with no clinical abnormalities, which has failed to conceive after at least two successive inseminations. In practice, some of these animals will have been inseminated at the wrong time. Others may have pathological changes in the bursa or oviduct that are difficult to palpate, or undiagnosed uterine infections.

The three other pathological conditions associated with repeat breeding are:
- Subclinical endometritis
- Delayed ovulation
- Insufficient corpus luteum function

See chapters 2.4.3; 2.3.4 for more information.

2.4.8 Abortion

Abortion in the cow is defined as foetal death and expulsion between day 45 and day 265 of pregnancy.
It is a significant cause of reproductive wastage and is of economic importance especially when there is large scale abortion in a herd. Moreover, some of the infectious causes of abortion in cattle represent an important zoonotic risk to humans.
An annual abortion rate up to 5% is considered to be normal. This figure excludes most abortions occurring during the second and third month of gestation as these often go undetected. An abortion rate in excess of 10% is considered to be an abortion storm. The diagnosis of the cause of abortion is difficult; unfortunately in only 20-30% of cases is a diagnosis made. Lack of suitable samples and poor sample quality are major reasons for this low success rate. One of important causes is that, in cattle, there is frequently a delay between the death of the foetus and its expulsion. Autolysis develops rapidly before expulsion and can severely affect the quality of the samples taken for diagnosis. Serology is often inappropriate. A whole range of infectious and non-infectious causes of abortion have been reported.
Non-infectious causes of abortion include physical causes, such as trauma, erroneous insemination of pregnant cows and

hyperthermia (also associated with pyrexia). Nutritional factors rarely cause abortion in cattle. An increase in abortion rate can be observed in herds suffering from severe vitamin A deficiency. Several plant toxins, and mycotoxin, can cause abortion as well as inorganic poisons such as nitrates/nitrites, lead or cadmium. Iatrogenic abortions are not common, but abortions induced by the administration of prostaglandins and glucocorticoids have been reported especially in herds with poor animal identification and inadequate treatment records, and when cows are misdiagnosed as being non-pregnant.

Infectious causes of abortion in cattle include a wide range of bacterial, viral and protozoan microorganisms (Anderson et al., 2007).

It is important to remember that some genetic and developmental abnormalities can cause foetal death and abortion in cattle. These include so-called complex vertebral malformation (CVM), dyschondroplasia (bulldog calves) and various chromosomal abnormalities.

The summary in Table 14 listing various abortion causes in cattle is, of necessity, incomplete.

Table 14 Differential diagnosis of abortion in cattle.

Non-infectious causes	Infectious causes
Genetic aberrations: Chromosomal abnormalities Phyto-teratogens: lupin senecio spp	**Viruses:** Bovine Herpes Virus 1 (BHV1) Bovine Herpes Virus 4 (BHV4) Bovine Virus Diarrhoea Virus (BVDV) Para-Influenza 3 Virus (PI-3) Parvo virus
Nutritional: Toxic plants Nitrate poisoning Phyto-oestrogens Iodine deficiency Vit. A deficiency Selenium deficiency Lead poisoning, Cadmium poisoning	**Bacteria:** Brucella abortus Campylobacter foetus Chlamydia psittaci Leptospira hardjo/pomona Listeria monocytogenes Staphylococci, Streptococci Salmonella dublin/typhimurium Pasteurella spp, E. coli etc.
Stress: Handling High ambient temperature Trauma Surgery Drying off Anxiety Vaccinations	**Protozoa:** Toxoplasma gondii Sarcocystis Neospora caninum Trichomonas foetus
Miscellaneous: Multiple pregnancy Insemination Corticosteroid therapy Prostaglandin therapy Allergy Dehydration	**Fungi:** Aspergillus spp. Mycoplasma spp.

Basic information on the diagnostic investigation of abortion in cattle

For a detailed investigation of possible causes of abortion with the best chance of identifying the causative agent (especially infectious) it is essential to collect the correct samples and the appropriate additional data. Ideally, the entire foetus and placenta should be submitted to the laboratory for anatomical, histopathological and microbiological evaluation, accompanied by a serum sample from the dam for serological testing. Farmers and veterinary practitioners should make every effort to include the placenta, as it is often in placental tissues that the evidence of certain infectious pathogens is found.

Formalin-fixed tissues for histopathological examination include foetal brain, lung, heart, liver, kidney, adrenals, spleen, thymus, lymph node, skeletal muscle, abomasum, small intestine, eyelid and placenta.

Serological evaluation of paired serum samples from an aborting cow may help determine if there had been exposure to an agent but cannot usually differentiate between vaccination and natural exposure (unless marker vaccines are used), or between recent and previous exposure to infection. Maternal serology is most useful when serum from unvaccinated animals is examined, when several animals from the herd are tested, and when each animal's history is provided.

Additional information should be provided including:

- *The aborting cow:* age, stage of production, duration of pregnancy, any general clinical signs preceeding the abortion, housing and maintenance details (housed or at pasture) vaccination status, any health-care measures performed within 1-2 weeks of abortion (especially administration of pharmaceutical preparations)
- *The herd:* average abortion level in the herd, recent increase in abortions, number of abortions to date, herd vaccination schedule, any recent herd-wide medication, feeding regime and feed changes, recent introductions into the herd

It must be remembered that there are zoonotic considerations associated with bovine abortion pathogens such as those causing Brucellosis, Leptospirosis, Listeriosis, Salmonellosis, etc. Appropriate precautions should be employed while sampling and shipping specimens.

Table 15 lists the main symptoms of the most important infectious causes of abortion with suggestions for the most relevant samples.

Table 15 Symptoms of the main infectious causes of abortion.

Infectious factor Common names	Abortion rate	Abortion timing	Recurrence of abortion	Foetal lesions	Samples
			Bacterial		
Brucella abortus Brucellosis Bang's disease Zoonosis	Up to 80% of unvaccinated animals infected in 1st or 2nd trimester	6-9 months Abortion or stillbirth 2 wk to 5 mo after infection	Majority abort only once	Placenta: retained, cotyledons necrotic, red-yellow,; area between thickened Calf: normal or autolytic with bronchopneumonia	placenta, foetus, or uterine discharge Diagnosis: maternal serology, IFAT for Abs in placenta, bacteria isolation
Campylobacter fetus venerealis Vibriosis	>10%	5-8 months	Uncommon, convalescent cows resistant to infection	Placenta: mild placentitis, hemorrhagic cotyledons and an edematous intercotyledonary area. Foetus: fresh or autolysed; mild fibrinous pleuritis, peritonitis, bronchopneumonia.	Placenta, foetal abomasal contents, vaginal flushing Diagnosis: microscopic detection, isolation
C fetus fetus C jejuni	Sporadic	4-9 months	Uncommon, convalescent cows resistant to infection	See above	See above
Leptospira interrogans serovars grippotyphosa pomona hardjo canicola icterohaemorrhagiae Zoonosis	5-40%	Last trimester Abortion 2-5 weeks after infection	Immunity to the serotype causing abortion but sensitive to other types	Placenta: diffuse placentitis with avascular, light tan cotyledons and edematous, yellowish intercotyledonary areas Foetus: autolysed	Placenta, foetus Diagnosis: IFAT for Abs or PCR testing for Leptospira
Arcanobacterium (Actinomyces) pyogenes	Sporadic	Any stage	Not known	Placenta: endometritis and diffuse placentitis, reddish brown to brown colour. Foetus: autolysed, fibrinous pericarditis, pleuritis, or peritonitis	Placenta, foetus Identification in bacterial culture from placenta or abomasal contents
Listeria monocytogenes Zoonosis	Usually sporadic but can reach 50%	Last trimester	May recur	Dam: fever, inappetance Placenta: retained Foetus: autolysed Fibrinous polyserositis and white necrotic foci in the liver and/or cotyledons	Placenta, foetus Identification in bacterial culture from placenta or abomasal contents

Infectious factor Common names	Abortion rate	Abortion timing	Recurrence of abortion	Foetal lesions	Samples
Fungal					
Aspergillus sp (60-80%) Mucor sp , Absidia , or Rhizopus sp	Usually sporadic but can reach 5-10%	4 months to term most common in winter	May recur	Placenta: severe, necrotising placentitis Cotyledons enlarged, necrotic, intercotyledonary area is thickened and leathery. Foetus: autolysed ~30% have gray ringworm-like skin lesions principally involving the head and shoulders	Foetus, placenta Diagnosis: isolation from the stomach contents, placenta, and skin lesions.
Protozoan					
Tritrichomonas (Trichomonas) foetus Trichomoniasis	Sporadic	first half of gestation	Animal gains immunity but probably not life-long	Placenta: retained, mild placentitis with hemorrhagic cotyledons and thickened intercotyledonary areas covered with flocculent exudates Foetus: no specific lesions	Placenta, foetus, vaginal/ uterine discharge Diagnosis: detection in abomasal contents, placental fluids, and uterine discharges
Neospora caninum Neosporosis	High in first gestation and when infection enters the naïve herd Up to 30% first outbreak Enzootic: 5-10%	Any stage, but most often 5-6 months	Decreases with parity but always possible	Placenta, foetus: no specific gross lesions, autolysed Microscopic: focal encephalitis with necrosis and nonsuppurative inflammation, hepatitis	Placenta, foetus (brain, heart, liver, body fluids), serum samples from the dam Diagnosis: detection of antigen in brain histology samples Immunochemistry in tissue samples Abs - PCR, ELISA
Viral					
Bovine Viral Diarrhoea Virus BVD-MD	Usually low	Complex pathology Abortion usually up to 4 months	Uncommon, immunity develops	Placenta: retained, no specific lesions Foetus: no specific lesions, autolysed, mummified	Placenta, foetus (preferred -spleen), dam and herdmates serum Diagnosis: isolation, immunologic staining, PCR, or detection of precolostral antibodies in aborted calves

Bovine Herpesvirus type I (BHV I) Infectious Bovine rhinotracheitis virus (IBRV) IBR IBR-IPV	5-60% in non vaccinated herds	Possibly any stage but most common from 4 months to term	Uncommon, immunity develops	In the majority of cases there are no gross lesions in the placenta or foetus Placenta: necrotizing vasculitis Foetus: autolysed, foci of necrosis in the liver	Placenta, foetus, serum samples from the dam Diagnosis: Immunochemistry in samples from kidney and adrenal glands, blood serology, PCR
Blue tongue virus Blue tongue	Usually low	Variable	Unlikely	No specific Foetus: autolysed	Placenta, foetus, serum samples from the dam Diagnosis: virus isolation
Epizootic Bovine Abortion Foothill Abortion etiologic agent has not been definitively determined, vector – tick Ornithodoros coriaceus	Can reach 75% Limited mainly to California in the US	Usually in the last trimester	Unlikely	Placenta: No specific Foetus: hepatomegaly, splenomegaly, and generalized lymphomegaly. Microscopically - marked lymphoid hyperplasia in the spleen and lymph nodes and granulomatous inflammation in most organs.	Anamnesis Diagnosis: elevated foetal Ig-G
Factors not typical for cattle or rarely occurring					
Chlamydophila abortus (Chlamydia psittaci serotype 1) enzootic abortion of ewes Zoonosis	Sporadic	Near the end of the last trimester	Unlikely	Placenta: placentitis, thickening and yellow-brown exudate adhered to the cotyledons and intercotyledonary areas. Foetus: fresh, minimal autolysis, pneumonia, hepatitis	Placenta, foetus Diagnosis: isolation from the placenta, lungs, and/or abomasal contents
Ureaplasma diversum	Usually sporadic, but outbreaks possible	Third trimester	Possible	Placenta: retained, intercotyledonary areas thickened, nonsuppurative placentitis Foetus: no gross lesions, pneumonia	Placenta, foetus Diagnosis: isolation from the placenta, lungs, and/or abomasal contents
Salmonella spp	Usually sporadic but can take form of an abortion storm	Any stage	Possible	Cows: clinically ill Placenta and foetus: autolysed and emphysematous.	Placenta, foetus Diagnosis: isolation from the abomasal contents and other tissues.
Other infectious factors that potentially can cause abortion in cattle: Parainfluenza 3 Virus (PI3V), Mycoplasma spp , Histophilus somni (Haemophilus somnus), Staphylococcus spp, Streptococcus spp, Pasteurella spp, E.coli, Toxoplasma gondii					

Neosporosis

Neospora caninum is a protozoan parasite, closely related to *Toxoplasma gondii*, that has emerged as a major cause of reproductive failure in cattle worldwide (Dubey 2003; Hall et al., 2005; Dubey et al., 2007).

Up to now, the dog and the coyote have been identified as definitive hosts for *Neospora caninum* (Dijkstra et al.,2001; Gondim et al., 2004) while a clinical form of neosporosis has been described in cattle, goats, sheep, deer and horses (Dubey 2003.).

Cattle appear to be the most important intermediate host for the parasite. The presence of neospora-specific antibodies has been demonstrated in numerous species, but the consequences of seropositivity remains unclear in many of them: sheep (Dubey et al., 1990), goats (Dubey et al., 1992), buffaloes (Fuij et al., 2001), foxes (Buxton et al., 1997), coyotes (Lindsay et al., 1996), racoons (Lindsay et al., 2001), dingoes (Barber et al., 1997), cervids (Tieman et al., 2005), llamas and alpacas (Wolf et al., 2005) and European bison (Cabay et al., 2005). In a recent publication by Sedlak and Bartova (2006) antibodies to *N. caninum* were found in 31 of 556 zoo animals (5.6%), representing 18 of 114 species tested: Eurasian wolf (*Canis lupus lupus*), Maned wolf, fennec, cheetah, jaguar, Eurasian lynx, Indian lion, fisher, blackbuck, European bison, lechwe, African buffalo, eland, sitatunga, Thorold's deer, Eastern elk, Vietnam sika deer, and Père David's deer.

The consequence of infection in pregnant cattle will depend on several factors, including the gestational age of the foetus at the time of infection and the immune status of the dam. The stage of pregnancy at which infection/parasitaemia occurs is an important determinant of the severity of disease. Neospora infection in the first trimester of pregnancy may have more severe consequences for the foetus than infection occurring in the final trimester (Innes 2007). Clinical consequences of infection during pregnancy may include abortion of the foetus, birth of a weak calf sometimes showing neurological signs or birth of a clinically healthy but persistently infected calf (Innes et al., 2005).

One of the most interesting, but also still poorly understood, aspects of abortion caused by neospora in cattle is the immunological relationship between the host, its developing foetus and the parasite. The immune system of a pregnant dam, regulated through cytokines, plays a major role during gestation, which may be viewed as a complex process in which the mother has to support a semi-allograft. To facilitate the pregnancy, the cytokine environment in the placenta favours the regulatory Th-2-type cytokines, whose role is to counteract the pro-inflammatory Th1-type immune responses. Protective immunity to *N. caninum*, similar to many other intracellular parasites, involves Th1-type immune responses, which may become a problem for a cow trying to control the infection during pregnancy (Innes 2007). An excessive Th1 response can induce loss of the pregnancy and may therefore form one of the elements in the abortion process associated with neosporosis.

Abortion occurs in mid-gestation, usually between the fourth and sixth month, with no clinical signs of disease in the dam. The aborted foetuses are usually autolysed with no gross lesions, and placentas are not retained. The brain, heart, liver, placenta, and body fluids or serum are the best specimens for diagnosis, and diagnostic rates are higher if multiple tissues are examined. Although lesions of neosporosis are found in several organs, foetal brain is the most consistently affected organ. The most characteristic lesion of neosporosis is focal encephalitis characterized by necrosis and non-suppurative inflammation (Dubey 2003; Dubey et al., 2007).

Herds infected with neospora can exhibit both endemic and epidemic patterns of abortion. The most important feature is that the parasite persists in the female as a chronic infection, which can then be passed to the foetus during pregnancy. Two methods of within herd transmission have been postulated. The horizontal route involves a two-host life cycle of the parasite with the cow becoming infected by the ingestion of protozoan oocysts, which are shed by a definitive host – a dog. Vertical, transplacental, transmission also occurs as foetal infection frequently fails to result in abortion, the foetus surviving as a persistently infected carrier. Heifers resulting from such pregnancies can abort when they become pregnant themselves. By contrast with ovine toxoplasmosis, cows that abort a neospora-infected foetus may carry infected foetuses in subsequent pregnancies.

The major economic losses associated with neosporosis in cattle are caused by reduced reproductive performance (abortions, stillbirth, repeat breeding, increased culling rate for reproductive failure). Indirect costs include veterinary expenses associated with the diagnostic investigation, and the cost of replacement if affected cows are culled.
There is some evidence that seropositive herds achieve lower milk production than seronegative ones (Hernandez et al., 2001; Romero et al., 2005)

Diagnosis is by histopathology and immunohistochemistry of aborted foetuses and serology of the dam or the foetus (indirect fluorescent antibody test (IFAT), enzyme linked immunosorbent assay (ELISA) and direct agglutination test (DAT)).

To date there is no evidence for the venereal transmission of *N. caninum* in cattle. Studies reported by Serrano-Martinez et al. (2007) and Ferre et al. (2008) demonstrated the presence of *N. caninum* DNA in the semen and blood of experimentally infected bulls. Their observations indicated an intermittent presence of *N. caninum* in low numbers in semen, associated with a chronic stage of the infection. Nonetheless, the protozoa could not be isolated from mice inoculated with PCR-positive semen samples, and there was no seroconversion in heifers inseminated with pooled semen samples. The possible consequences in terms of disease transmission are still to be fully elucidated.

Although it has been possible to induce vertical transmission of *N. caninum* following experimental infection of rhesus macaque monkeys (Barr et al., 1994a), there is no conclusive evidence to date that *N. caninum* can infect and cause disease in humans.

Control of neospora-associated abortions may involve vaccination (Romero et al., 2004) and/or test-and-cull, aimed at eliminating infected individuals from the herd (Hall et al., 2005). Both of these approaches have limitations to their use. Test-and-cull may only be applicable in herds in which the number of infected animals is relatively small. All neospora control programs should, however, always include measures aimed at reducing the exposure of the breeding animals to the infectious forms of the parasite. This involves prompt detection and removal of the aborted foetus and afterbirth, as well as limiting the access of domestic dogs and wild canines to the cattle feed stores and pasture.

More information can be found in **www.neosporosis.com**

Influence of BVDV infection around insemination time on future fertility in cattle
In cattle, pre- and postnatal infection with BVD virus is associated with a variety of disease syndromes including immune suppression, congenital defects, abortion and mucosal disease. In several surveys, BVD was the most commonly diagnosed virus disease in bovine abortion cases. The pathology of BVD in the developing foetus is complex. Infection of the foetus before 125 days of gestation can cause foetal death and abortion, resorption, mummification, developmental abnormalities, or foetal immunotolerance and persistent infection. After 125 days of gestation, BVD may cause abortion, or the foetal immune response may clear the virus. There is increasing evidence that the influence of infection with BVD virus on reproductive performance does not limit itself to the induction of foetal death followed by abortion.
A reduction in conception rates in cattle with acute BVDV infection has been reported and is very often a major complaint in herds in which BVD is identified (Houe et al., 1993; McGovan et al., 1993). Viraemia induced experimentally during the follicular phase has resulted in a 50% reduction in pregnancy rate and a deterioration in the quantity and quality of embryos recovered after superovulation (McGowan et al., 1993; Kafi et al., 1997).

Morphological changes induced by BVD virus in the ovaries of acutely infected cattle
Ssentongo et al. (1980); Grooms et al. (1998) and McGowan et al. (2003) described inflammatory changes (lymphocytic oophoritis) within the reproductive ovarian tissue associated with acute infection with BVDV and viraemia. The inflammatory lesions already mentioned were demonstrated both in the follicles and the forming corpora lutea of infected cows and

clearly contributed to the functional disorders leading to inadequate follicular and luteal function and in consequence fertility failure.

Functional consequences of morphological changes induced by BVDV in the ovaries

1. *Impaired follicular growth*
   Grooms et al. (1998) reported that the maximum diameter and growth rate of dominant anovulatory and ovulatory follicles were significantly reduced during two oestrous cycles, subsequent to infection of seronegative cattle with a noncytopathogenic bovine pestivirus isolate. This was further confirmed by the work of Fray et al. (1999; 2000; 2002) who showed that in the cows infected with BVD virus the pattern of follicular growth was clearly disrupted with a smaller diameter being attained by the preovulatory follicle and also lesser maximum diameter of the ovulatory follicle, in comparison to non-infected cows.
   Kafi et al. (1997) described a significant decrease in the ovulation rate of superovulated heifers inoculated with non-cytopathogenic bovine pestivirus 9 days prior to AI.
2. *Inadequate oestradiol production*
   The work by Fray et al. (1999; 2000, 2002) clearly demonstrated that a cell-free viraemia around the time of breeding has a profoundly negative impact on the reproductive endocrine functions in both cows and heifers. The differences in the follicular growth in the infected cows were associated with disrupted oestradiol secretion pattern with generally lower oestradiol levels and especially delayed pre-ovulatory oestradiol peak (Fray et al., 1999; 2002).
3. *Delay in heat expression and delayed LH peak resulting from disrupted oestradiol production*
   A changed pattern of oestradiol production might, in turn, explain a delay in the onset of oestrus behaviour and the poorer expression of oestrus signs observed by Kafi et al. (1997) and McGowan et al. (2003) in heifers infected with BVDV. Furthermore, in the same experimental series, McGowan et al. (2003) observed an erratic LH pattern in the infected cows of which only a few showed a normal preovulatory surge, while in the remaining infected individuals a delayed or low amplitude preovulatory LH

peak was detected. Examination of endocrine profiles of the infected heifers in this study revealed that a majority (83%) had no normal preovulatory peaks of oestradiol and LH (McGowan et al., 2003). This could be interpreted as a direct result of inadequate follicular growth, and oestradiol secretion incapable of stimulating the proper LH secretion. A delayed and inadequate preovulatory LH surge can lead to delayed ovulation which may negatively affect the quality of oocytes and also the developmental potential of embryos.

4. *Inadequate progesterone production resulting in early embryonic losses*
   In the experiments reported by Fray et al. (1999; 2000; 2002) and McGowan et al. (2003) cows and heifers experiencing a cell-free viraemia around the time of breeding showed a delay in the post ovulatory rise in progesterone as well as generally lower progesterone concentrations between 3 and 11 days after ovulation.

It is possible that suppressed plasma progesterone concentrations observed in the BVDV infected animals compromise fertility by retarding embryo development. The delayed and inadequate preovulatory LH peak observed in BVDV viraemic cows and heifers can also cause retardation of embryonic development and affect embryo quality. This, in turn, can reduce the ability of the embryo to produce interferon-τ and prevent luteolysis. This may be supported by the results of a large scale statistical analysis of the effects of BVDV infection on fertility in dairy herds in Brittany, in which cows in herds exposed to an ongoing BVDV infection had a significantly higher risk of late return to service (later than 21 days) than cows in herds presumed to be not infected for a long time or not recently infected (Robert et al., 2003).

One of the basic approaches to reducing the reproductive losses associated with BVDV infection in cattle is the implementation of tight biosecurity measures, limiting the exposure of the animals to the virus, and vaccination with products which will prevent the cell-free viraemia and transplacental infection.

2.4.9 Unwanted pregnancy

While better avoided altogether, the accidental mating of young heifers is a common reason for terminating pregnancy. Feedlot operators also have reason to abort pregnant heifers. If pregnant at slaughter, heifers achieve lower prices and, in any case, feed efficiency is better if they are not carrying calves, and calving difficulties are avoided. Up to about day 150 of pregnancy, the corpus luteum is the only source of progesterone in the pregnant animal. Luteolysis with prostaglandins will result in abortion. If the mating is observed, prostaglandin can be injected 10-16 days later, or alternatively, it can be administered to mismated animals that do not return to oestrus after 3 weeks.
Between 100 and 150 days of pregnancy, the efficacy of prostaglandin is reduced to less than 90%, because some pregnancies become less dependent on the CL for absolute support. Thus an injection of prostaglandin is never guaranteed to terminate pregnancy. It is always wise to advise pregnancy diagnosis at least 10 days after the use of prostaglandin, and repeat the injections until all the animals have been aborted.

After day 150, the placenta produces sufficient progesterone to maintain the pregnancy on its own. The combination of 25 mg of dexamethasone and a dose of prostaglandin $F_{2\alpha}$ usually induces abortion at all stages of pregnancy. However, Thomas (1991) reported an increased mortality in feedlot heifers treated with the dexamethasone/prostaglandin combination.

2.5 Induction of parturition

The main reasons for choosing to induce parturition are:
- To advance calving to reduce the calving interval or to tighten the calving pattern.
- To reduce the incidence of dystocia by preventing foetal oversize.
- To terminate abnormal pregnancies.
- To advance the date of calving in late-conceiving cows, where breeding and production is seasonal (New Zealand).

In the cow, progesterone is necessary for the maintenance of pregnancy. As already noted, in the first 150 days of gestation and during the last few days before parturition, the corpus luteum is the main source of progesterone. In the period between, the placenta produces sufficient progesterone to maintain pregnancy. Parturition is triggered by an increase in foetal cortisol production. This initiates a rise in placental oestrogen production and of prostaglandins ($PGF_{2\alpha}$). The corpus luteum regresses and the plasma progesterone level drops sharply. Research has focused on the use of prostaglandins, corticosteroids or a combination of the two to induce parturition.

Corticosteroids

The administration of a short-acting dexamethasone (Dexadreson®; 15 ml) shortly before, or at term, mimics the rise in foetal cortisol and thus initiates the calving process. Most cows will calve within 72 hours.

When induction is attempted more than 7-10 days before the expected time of parturition, the response is more variable and induction fails more frequently. This can be overcome by priming the animal with a medium-acting corticosteroid preparation (Dexafort®; 10 ml), and about a week later giving a short-acting product (Dexadreson®; 10-15 ml). It is worth noting that 10-30% of cows will calve within a week in response to the priming injection.

Prostaglandins

Injection of a standard dose of prostaglandin $F_{2\alpha}$ during the week prior to the expected date of calving will also induce parturition, most cows calving within 48 hours. Combinations of corticosteroids and prostaglandins may be preferable because the former are required for foetal maturation.

Data both from the literature and field experience indicate that an increased occurrence of retained foetal membranes is associated with the induction of calving with prostaglandins, regardless of the type of analogue used. It is important to know the correct service date to avoid inducing a premature birth, which would significantly reduce the viability of the calf. Good breeding records are therefore important, as is close attention to the hygiene of the calving environment.

2.6 The bull

Generally, AI centres set high standards for semen quality. A fertility index or similar measure should be provided for each bull, to help the farmer select the most appropriate sire. On farms practising natural service, the fertility of the bull is of major importance to herd fertility. Sub-fertility in bulls leads to delays in conception, prolonged calving intervals, reductions in the calf crop, and maybe even to increased culling for reproductive failure. Annual evaluation of each bull's suitability for breeding is strongly recommended.

2.6.1 Evaluation of suitability for breeding

The standards for evaluating a bull's suitability for breeding are provided by the Society for Theriogenology (www.therio.org). It should be borne in mind that, at present, there is no single measurement or test available that could reliably predict the fertility of a bull, so several criteria are usually evaluated in concert in the general examination of bulls for suitability for breeding (Kastelic and Thundathil 2008). The final assessment is based on a physical evaluation and basic semen evaluation.

The examination of the fertility potential of a bull consists of four elements:
- General examination
- Examination of the genital tract
- Semen evaluation
- Assessment of libido

General examination
Having checked the bull's age and identification, special attention should be paid to the locomotory system, while the animal is standing and when moving over a hard surface. For bulls kept under extensive conditions, eyesight is also of importance.

Examination of the genital tract

A complete examination must include the penis and scrotum as well as rectal palpation. The penis must be inspected and palpated. However, some defects such as spiral deviation or erection failure are only detectable during mating.

The scrotum is inspected for abnormalities such as inguinal hernia, excess fat, gross disparity between the testes, and their size and consistency, which should be resilient. The epididymis must feel normal, with a soft tail. The scrotum must be well developed. There is a direct relationship between scrotal circumference, which reaches a maximum at 4-6 years of age, and sperm production.

Structures assessable by rectal examination include the urethra, prostate, vesicular glands, ampullae, vas deferens and internal inguinal rings. The most common abnormality is seminal vesiculitis, the aetiology and pathogenesis of which are poorly understood. *A. pyogenes, B. abortus, E. coli, Streptococcus spp.* and several others have been isolated. Response to long term treatment is variable and unreliable.

Semen evaluation

Most bulls can be made to ejaculate with an electro-ejaculator, which is a simple and safe method of enabling semen collection. Some fail to ejaculate or produce only a 'watery' urethral fluid, in which case a supervised mating utilising an artificial vagina may be more useful. The gross motility of semen is evaluated at 37°C, by placing a large drop of semen on a pre-heated microscope slide for examination under low power magnification. Gross motility is graded as 1) rapid, vigorous waves, 2) slower waves, 3) no waves but general oscillation, 4) occasional flickering only. Because gross motility also depends on sperm density, a more accurate estimate of sperm motility can be assessed using phase-contrast microscopy.

Sperm evaluation under a light microscope is able to detect gross abnormalities but unlikely to provide any information about more subtle variations in motility that could possibly affect the fertility of the examined bull. A computer-assisted semen analysis (CASA) is a far more objective method which can measure specific motion characteristics associated with the functional status of spermatozoa.

Morphology can be examined at 1000x magnification using fresh semen stained with eosin-nigrosin.
The threshold for a Satisfactory Potential Breeder is 30% of progressively motile and 70% morphologically normal sperm.

Libido
A simple test for libido is to pen a cow or heifer in oestrus and then turn the bull in for 10 -15 minutes. If he manages one or more services in this time, his libido is unlikely to be a problem. If the bull fails, he should be re-tested. Failure on both occasions gives serious grounds to question his libido.

Several new methods based on molecular biology and germ cell interaction are being studied with the intention of employing them in the future testing of fertility in bulls (Petrunkina et al., 2007; Kastelic and Thundathil 2008).

2.6.2 Infertility

Male infertility may be due to failure to mount, failure of intromission or failure of fertilization. A diagnosis can generally be made after careful examination following the above guidelines. Subfertility is much more difficult to diagnose. Testicular infections normally carry a very poor prognosis. Testicular degeneration may be caused by stress, toxins, heat and nutritional deficiencies. Diagnosis often relies on semen examination, and recovery is variable. The semen of some bulls may return to normal within 8 weeks, while for others it may take up to 6 months. Again semen testing is essential.

The hormonal treatment of infertile bulls is of limited value. PMSG acts like FSH and will stimulate spermatogenesis. hCG stimulates testosterone production because of its LH activity. GnRH will induce a short term increase of FSH and LH levels. A good history and clinical examination will assist in arriving at the correct diagnosis. Only then can a specific treatment, or a change in management (including rest), be decided upon.

Several pathogens can cause infertility in bulls or transmit infection via their semen (Givens et al., 2006; 2008). Some of them can directly affect a bull's fertility by causing disease of the reproductive tract or associating with spermatozoa to prevent fertilization. Viral pathogens that can reduce sperm quality and/or affect the bull's reproductive tract include bovine herpesvirus I (BHV-I, the agent of IBR), bovine viral diarrhoea virus (BVDV). Other viruses that can be transmitted in semen include foot-and-mouth disease virus, vesicular stomatitis virus, rinderpest virus, and lumpy skin disease virus. The risk of transmitting bovine immunodeficiency virus and bovine leukosis virus via semen appears to be very low. Bluetongue virus (BTV) can be detected sporadically in the semen of viraemic bulls and might result in venereal transmission.

Tritrichomonas foetus and *Campylobacter fetus venerealis* are sexually transmitted; they do not cause disease in the bull but can survive in frozen semen, thus it is extremely important that breeding bulls, especially those used for natural service, should be regularly tested for these two pathogens. Other micro-organisms that can be transmitted in semen and might be associated with infertility or the transmission of infection include *Brucella abortus, Leptospira spp., Histophilus somnus, Ureaplasma diversum, Mycobacterium avium subsp. Paratuberculosis, Chlamydia, Mycobacterium bovis, Coxiella burnetii, and Mycoplasma mycoides ssp. Mycoides.*

The World Organization for Animal Health (OIE) sets standards for disease control associated with semen production. Bulls placed in AI and semen collection centres should be annually tested for brucellosis, tuberculosis, BVDV, *T. foetus, C. foetus*, and BHV-1. Pre-quarantine and quarantine testing should confirm the bull to be free of brucellosis, tuberculosis, BVDV, as well as BHV-1 if the herd or AI centre is to be considered BHV-1-free. Additionally, Certified Semen Services recommend that bulls should be tested for Leptospirosis.

2.7 Embryo Transfer (ET)

Artificial insemination helps to achieve the rapid genetic improvement of a herd by making more effective use of top quality sires. The maximum reproductive capacity of the cow is one calf per year. Multiple ovulation and embryo transfer (MOET or ET) techniques increase the reproductive potential of the dam, thus enhancing the effect of the female in cattle breeding.

Some of the reasons for using ET are:
- To obtain more calves from a valuable, high quality cow.
- To increase the rate of genetic improvement of a herd.
- To facilitate international shipment of animals.
- To prevent acclimatisation problems when exporting cattle to tropical areas.
- In (International) bull breeding programmes.
- For the induction of twinning.
- To obtain purebred beef calves from the lower quality end of the dairy herd.
- To obtain offspring from cows with fertility problems.

Traditional ET technology provides relatively consistent results today, and many practitioners have 20 or more years experience in a mature industry (Scherzer et al., 2008). The exact size of the ET industry is somewhat difficult to determine. More than half a million bovine embryos were reported to have been transferred in 2003, 40% of them after freezing and thawing, and 18% having been produced in vitro (Betteridge et al., 2006). North America is still the centre of most activity (45% of transfers) with Europe and South America each accounting for 20% of the transfers in 2003. Recently, countries such as Brazil and China have become prominent in the production of bovine embryos. Bovine embryo production in vitro is now a well-established and reasonably efficient procedure. More than 100,000 embryos produced this way were transferred in 2003, almost 60% of them in South America.
In 2005, the latest year for which data are available, the number of transfers of embryos whether derived in vivo or IVP continued to rise. However, of just over 600,000 in vivo embryos transferred worldwide, approximately half were transferred fresh and half frozen. By contrast, about 260,000 IVP embryos were transferred in the same year, most of which (about 70%) were transferred fresh.

Extensive reviews of the steps involved in embryo production and transfer in cattle were provided by Mapletoft and Hasler (2005) and Sirard and Coenen (2006).

There are eseentially two sources of embryos used for transfer in cattle:

- *Embryos produced in vivo flushed from the reproductive tract of a donor cow*
  These embryos are produced in the full knowledge of the genetic potential and health history of the parental animals thus ensuring the optimal possibility for rapid genetic improvement in the herd. Nonetheless the efficacy of this system is relatively limited by factors such as: the ovulation rate after pharmacologically induced superovulation in the donor, fertilization rate and embryo recovery rate. These embryos can be transferred directly to synchronized recipients or frozen and stored in liquid nitrogen for future use.
- *Embryos derived by in vitro maturation (IVM) and in vitro fertilization (IVF) of oocytes*
  These embryos can be derived either from oocytes originating from known, selected donors and harvested by aspiration from the pre-ovulatory follicles (the so-called ovum pick-up procedure) or after the in vitro maturation of immature oocytes harvested from ovaries obtained from a slaughterhouse. The latter system, though the most efficient, poses certain problems such as the (usually) unknown genetic status of the donor cows and numerous health considerations.

It is well recognised that bovine embryos derived in vivo are of superior quality compared to those derived from in vitro maturation, fertilization and culture. Despite the high rate of nuclear maturation obtained, the developmental competence of bovine oocytes matured in vitro is variable. One likely reason for much of this variation could be the intrinsic quality of the oocytes recovered from the ovaries. Moreover, one negative consequence of both IVP and somatic cell nuclear transfer (SCNT) in cattle, and other species, is that embryos, foetuses, placentas and offspring can differ significantly in morphology and developmental competence compared with those from embryos produced in vivo (Farin et al., 2004; 2006; Lonergan and Farin

2008). Collectively, these abnormalities have been referred to as 'large offspring syndrome' or 'large calf syndrome'. As the current diagnostic possibilities for detecting possible anomalies in the in vitro derived embryos are limited, further research is needed both to evaluate the physiological background and to define future preventive strategies.

Oocyte maturation in vitro and embryo culture techniques are integral to the process required for cloning, and facilitating the breeding of transgenic cattle for the production of valuable pharmaceutical proteins in their milk. The cloning of adult cattle through nuclear transfer and the production of cloned, transgenic cattle has been achieved technically. However, it is an expensive and inefficient technology which, at this stage in its development, could only be used by the pharmaceutical industry and research community (Mapletoft and Hasler 2007; Galli and Mazzari 2008). In vitro fertilization by intra-cytoplasmic sperm injection, so prominent a feature in assisted human reproduction, is feasible in cattle, even with freeze-dried semen, but is not yet widely used. A few laboratories have reported very modest successes in producing pregnancies from embryos produced in vitro based on oocytes harvested from calves, which offers the potential for increasing the rate of genetic improvement by reducing the generation intervals.

The International Embryo Transfer Society issues a series of carefully defined procedures, especially in respect of the zoosanitary and epidemiological aspects of embryo production and transfer. Infectious factors such as BVD and IBR were identified as potentially transferable with embryos, which led to the adoption of specific procedures to ensure the safety of ET in respect of these pathogens. A comprehensive review provided by Givens et al. (2008b) summarised the current health recommendations for bovine embryo transfer, while emphasising recent research to develop and validate novel approaches to biosecurity. Most of the commercial embryo production systems use culture media supplemented with various animal-derived sources of nutrients. Although many preventive measures are applied (screening of sources, pre-treatment with high temperatures, and addition of antibiotics) such systems increase the health risks, especially for in vitro embryos (Givens et al., 2008). A system based on defined components, free from cell consituents or elements derived from blood, would be ideal from the viewpoint of health and quality control. Moreover, chemically defined conditions without serum or serum proteins, allow for more precise observation of the effects of growth or other embryotrophic factors in any given medium.

Reports are available on the use of media for which every component is semi-defined, or fully defined, chemically (Feugang et al., 2009).

2.7.1 Management of the donor cow

Under natural conditions, the cow usually has only one ovulation per cycle. Gonadotrophic stimulation of the ovaries can induce multiple ovulation (superovulation). Although embryo transfer techniques are widely used around the world, variability in response to the superstimulatory treatments remains an important limitation. Variability in ovarian response has been related to differences in superovulatory treatments, such as gonadotrophin preparation, batch, and total dose, duration and timing of treatment, and the use of additional hormones in the program, and individual variation between animals cannot be ruled out.

The recent development of protocols capable of controlling the follicular wave emergence and ovulation has not yet completely eliminated the variability in superovulatory response. Nonetheless, these treatments have had a positive impact on the application of commercial, on-farm embryo transfer, by permitting the initiation of treatments at a pre-determined time. Moreover, protocols that synchronize ovulation tightly, allow for the insemination of donor cows at a fixed time, thereby eliminating the necessity of oestrus detection during the superstimulatory protocol.

From information generated by ultrasonography, it has been established that approximately 8–12 days after oestrus (equivalent to 7–11 days after ovulation) the second follicular wave emerges in cows exhibiting two- or three-wave cycles, and a cohort of growing follicles should be available for the stimulation of multiple ovulation at that time. However, it has been shown that superovulatory response is better when gonadotrophin treatments are initiated precisely at the emergence of the follicular wave rather than later.

Three different types of gonadotrophins have been used to induce superovulation in the cow: gonadotrophins from pituitary extracts of pigs or other domestic animal (extraction FSH); equine chorionic gonadotrophin (eCG)/pregnant mares serum gonadrotrophin (PMSG); and human menopausal gonadotrophin (hMG). At present, the most notable gonadotrophins used in the ET industry in cattle to achieve multiple ovulation are pregnant mare serum gonadotrophin (PMSG) and follicle stimulating hormone (FSH). Both are administered during the mid-luteal phase, usually of a synchronized oestrous cycle, as it has been shown that the superovulatory response is higher when gonadotrophin treatment is institued precisely when the follicular wave emerges, rather than later. Therefore it is usual in normally cycling cattle to use treatments that control the timing of the follicular wave.

FSH

Natural FSH preparations are available, of porcine and ovine origin. Because FSH has a relatively short half-life, it is generally administered twice daily.

The usual regimen involves 4 or 5 days of twice daily treatments with 400 mg of purified extraction FSH (e.g. Folltropin®-V). $PGF_{2\alpha}$ is injected to induce luteolysis, 48 or 72 hours after the start of treatment. Oestrus occurs between 36 and 48 hours after the prostaglandin injection, and ovulation between 24 and 36 hours later.

PMSG/eCG

Pregnant mare serum gonadotrophin – PMSG also called equine chorionic gonadotrophin - eCG (Folligon®) has been shown to have a half-life of 40 hours and to persist for up to 10 days in bovine circulation, so a single injection is sufficient. Recommended doses of eCG/PMSG range from 1500 to 3000 IU, with 2500 IU the most commonly selected. 48 Hours after the PMSG injection, regression of the corpus luteum is induced with a dose of prostaglandin. Donaldson (1983) reported a better luteolytic effect with natural $PGF_{2\alpha}$ when two or three injections were given, but when using analogues, a single dose was sufficient. The continued stimulant effect of high doses of PMSG may have a negative effect on ovulation and cause the emergence of a second wave of follicles.

Factors affecting the success rate in embryo collection and transfer were evaluated in dairy herds by Chebel et al. (2008).

Animal-related
- Stage of the cycle. Best results are obtained when superovulation is initiated during the mid-luteal phase (day 9-13).
- Follicular status at the time of superovulation. The presence of a large dominant follicle at the time of superovulation reduces the response
- General health and nutritional status
- Lactation phase

Management and environment related
- General management of the animals (avoiding stress, adequate housing)
- External temperature and humidity

Procedure related
- Synchronization and induction system (type of system used and compliance)
- Semen/insemination. Use of high quality semen and AI at 12-24 hours after the onset of standing oestrus. Repeated inseminations do not appear to give better fertilization rates. Differences have been reported between bulls.
- Embryo harvesting and processing technique

The use of progestagens such as Crestar® provides an efficient way of ensuring a tight oestrus synchronization in embryo and oocyte donors, with the advantages of exposure to progestagen being the quality of the harvested oocytes/embryos, and the possibility of a fixed time insemination. The basic Crestar® synchronization programme can be thus combined with a single PMSG (Folligon®) injection or sequential FSH (Folltropin V®) injections, to achieve the induction of multiple ovulation.

2.7.2 Management of the recipient

Due to the high variability of embryo recovery, it is very common to find that either too many or too few recipients have been prepared. Surplus embryos may be frozen and stored in liquid nitrogen, but only good quality embryos should be selected for freezing. They can be transferred during a normal cycle or, of more practical use, during a controlled cycle. There is no difference in the pregnancy rates of recipients between transfer during a natural or a controlled cycle.
The administration of a GnRH analogue (Receptal®, Fertagyl®; 2.5 ml) at the beginning of oestrus can be used to induce and complete the ovulation in recipient cows at an oestrus synchronized using prostaglandin analogues: with a plentiful supply of suitable recipients, better results are expected, with more precise timing of ovulation and improved development of corpora lutea.

Among the factors influencing the success of embryo transfer in recipients (measured as the pregnancy/calving rate) the following are the most relevant (Peterson and Lee 2003; Looney et al., 2006; Vasconcelos et al., 2006):
- Quality of the embryo and adequate transfer technique
- Adequate timing of the transfer in relation to the recipients' oestrous cycles
- Adequate progesterone concentrations in the recipients' circulation around the time of the transfer (often correlated with milk production)
- Management of heat stress and other stress factors (management, nutrition, housing etc.)

Even if only excellent quality embryos are transferred, the resulting pregnancy rates can vary cosiderably among recipients. McMillan (1998) developed a model that allowed for the separation of the embryo's and the recipient's contribution to the survival of transferred embryos during the first 60 days of pregnancy. This model demonstrated that it is the variation in the ability of a recipient to carry the pregnancy to term (recipient quality), rather than the ability of the embryo to survive and develop, that leads to this variation in pregnancy rates after ET. Interestingly enough, the quality of the recipient does not contribute, to any great extent, to foetal losses after 60 days of pregnancy. It is important to recognise that the model proposed by McMillan suggets that there may be superior recipients within herds, and in practice, many veterinary surgeons specialising in ET strive to identify such animals, and use them repeatedly to introduce desired genetic material into the herd.

2.8 Use of sex-sorted semen in cattle breeding

The application of sexed semen allows dairy producers to select from their herd's potential dams and produce replacement heifers from only the genetically superior animals.

The current technology to sort X and Y chromosome-bearing sperm populations requires individual identification and selection of spermatozoa in a modified high-speed flow cytometer (reviewed by Seidel 2007; Garner and Seidel 2008). The demand for female calves has grown rapidly, which encourages the demand for sex-sorted semen from bulls of high genetic value. The success of the technology will depend mainly on the fertilizing capacity of the sorted spermatozoa, as this is the factor which has the most effect, and is therefore the most economically relevant.

To date, fertility is still variable and is quite dependent on processing after sorting. New processing techniques are under investigation and will likely be able to improve the fertility rates for sex-sorted semen. Selection of the most appropriate bulls and testing the sorted samples on a routine basis are very important to success.

The possibilities of DNA damage to the spermatozoa during the sorting procedure, with resulting abnormalities in embryos/foetuses, has placed a major question mark over the wider use of sexed semen in cattle. The procedure of sperm sorting has proved to be safe for the sperm's genetic material so far, however. Furthermore, large-scale studies have found no increase in the abortion rate, or differences in gestation length, neonatal death, calving difficulty, birth weight, weaning weight, or live births when sexed sperm is used for AI, compared to the use of unsexed control sperm. Therefore, it appears that genetic damage to sperm during sex-sorting is probably minimal or even non-existent.

Commercially available sex-sorted semen is often used primarily in heifers because of their inherently higher fertility and the limited amount of sexed sperm available. Conception rates obtained in dairy herds have been reported ranging from 30% to 70%, with the average level of fertility in a given herd, and managerial factors, greatly influencing the outcome of AI (Garner and Seidel 2008).

2.9 Twinning

In the dairy cow, twins are associated with higher calf mortality, retained placenta, longer calving to conception intervals and reduced milk yield. If these problems can be controlled by careful management, the induction of a twin pregnancy may have economic advantages. In beef cattle, in which milk yield is not the primary source of income, twinning has been shown to have interesting advantages.

The use of gonadotrophins to induce a 'mild superovulation' increases not only the frequency of twins but can also lead to a few instances of triplets and quadruplets.

The transfer of two embryos, or the transfer of a single embryo into inseminated animals, increases the total number of calves born and the proportion (40 to 60%) of twin pregnancies. In this case the economic outcome of the technique depends largely on the cost of the embryo in relation to the price of the calf.

2.10 References

Al-Katanani YM., Paula-Lopes FF., Hansesn PJ. Effects of season and exposure to heat stress on oocyte competence in Holstein cows. J Dairy Sci 2002;85:390-396

Almier M., De Rosa G., Grasso F., Napolitana F., Bordi A. Effect of climate on the response of three oestrus synchronisation techniques in lactating dairy cows. Anim Reprod Sci 2002;71:157-168

Ambrose JD., Schmitt EJP., Lopes FL., Mattos RC., and Thatcher WW. Ovarian and endocrine responses associated with the treatment of cystic ovarian follicles in dairy cows with gonadotropin releasing hormone and prostaglandin $F_{2\alpha}$, with or without exogenous progesterone. Can Vet J. 2004 ; 45: 931–937.

Ambrose JD., Kastelic JP., Rajamahendran R., Aali M., Dinn N. Progesterone (CIDR)-based timed AI protocols using GnRH, porcine LH or estradiol cypionate for dairy heifers: Ovarian and endocrine responses and pregnancy rates. Theriogenology 2005;64:1457–1474.

Ambrose DJ., Radke B., Pitney PA., Goonewardene LA. Evaluation of early conception factor lateral flow test to determine nonpregnancy in dairy cattle. Can Vet J 2007;48:831-835

Anderson ML., Blanchard PC., Barr BC., Dubey JP., Hoffman RL., Conrad PA. Neospora-like protozoan infection as a major cause of abortion in california dairy cattle. J. Am Vet Med Assoc 1991; 198: 241-244

Anderson ML., Andrianarivo AG., Conrad PA. Neosporosis in cattle. Anim Reprod Sci 2000; 60-61: 417-431

Anderson ML. Infectious causes of bovine abortion during mid- to late-gestation. Theriogenology 2007;68: 474–486

Arbel R., Bigun Y., Ezra E., Sturman H., Hojman D. The Effect of Extended Calving Intervals in High Lactating Cows on Milk Production and Profitability. J Dairy Sci 2001; 84:600–608

Arechiga CF., Staples CR., McDowell LR and Hansen PJ. Effects of timed insemination and supplemental β-carotene on reproduction and milk yield of dairy cows under heat stress. J Dairy Sci 1998;81:390-402

Armstrong DV. Heat stress interaction with shade and cooling. J Dairy Sci 1994;77:2044-2050

Aroyo A., Yavin S., Arav A., Roth Z. Hindering of cleavage timing in bovine parthenotes duirng the hot season. Reprod Fertil Dev 2007;19:203, Abstract 173

Ayad A., Sousa NM., Sulon J., Hornick JL., Iguer-Ouada M., Beckers JF. Correlation of five radioimmunoassay systems for measurement of bovine plasma pregnancy-associated glycoprotein concentrations at early pregnancy period. Res Vet Sci 2009 (in press)

Barber JS., Gasser RB., Ellis J., Reichel MP., MacMillan D., Trees AJ. Prevalence of antibodies to Neospora caninum in different canid populations. J Parasitol 1997;83:1056-1058

Barlund CS., Carruthers TD., Waldner CL., Palmer CW. A comparison of diagnostic techniques for postpartum endometritis in dairy cattle. Theriogenology 2008;69::714–723

Barr BC., Conrad PA., Sverlow KW., Tarantal AF., Hendrickx AG. Experimental fetal and transplacental Neospora infection in the nonhuman primate. Lab. Invest. 1994; 71:236–242.

Bartolome JA., Archbald LF., Morresey P., et al. Comparison of synchronization of ovulation and induction of estrus as therapeutic strategies for bovine ovarian cysts in the dairy cow. Theriogenology. 2000;53:815–825

Bartolome J A., Silvestre FT., Arteche ACM., Kamimura S., Archbald LF., and Thatcher WW. The use of Ovsynch and Heatsynch forre-synchronization of cows open at pregnancy diagnosis by ultrasonography. J. Dairy Sci.2002;85 (Suppl. 1):99. (Abstr.)

Bartolome JA., Santos JEP., Pancarci SM., Melendez P., Arteche et al. Induction of ovulation in non lactating dairy cows and heifers using different doses of a desloreline implant. Theriogenology 2004;61:407-19

Bartolome JA., Silvestre FT., Kamimura S., Arteche ACM et al. Resynchronisation of ovulation and timed insemination in lactating dairy cows I: use of Ovsynch and Heatsynch protocols after non-pregnancy diagnosis by ultrasonography. Theriogenology 2005a;63:1617-1627

Bartolome JA., Sozzi A., McHale J., Melendez P., Arteche ACM., Silvestre FT., Kelbert D., Swift K., Archbald LF., Thatcher WW. Resynchronization of ovulation and timed insemination in lactating dairy cows, II: assigning protocols according to stages of the estrous cycle, or presence of ovarian cysts or anestrus. Theriogenology 2005b;63:1628–1642

Bartolome JA., Sozzi A., McHale J., Swift K., Kelbert D., Archbald LF., Thatcher WW. Resynchronization of ovulation and timed insemination in lactating dairy cows III. Administration of GnRH 23 days post AI and ultrasonography for nonpregnancy diagnosis on day 30. Theriogenology 2005c;63: 1643–1658

Bartolome JA,. Thatcher WW., Melendez P., Risco CA., Archbald LF. Strategies for the diagnosis and treatment of ovarian cysts in dairy cattle. JAVMA 2005d;227:1409-1414

Bech-Sabat G., Lopez-Gatius F., Garcia-Ispierto I., Santolaria JP., Serrano B., Nogareda C., Sousa, de NM., Beckers JF., Yaniz J. Pregnancy patterns during the early fetal period in high producing dairy cows treated with GnRH or progesterone. Theriogenology 2009; 71:920–929

Berisha B., Schams D. Ovarian function in ruminants. Domest Anim Endocrinol 2005;29:305-317

Betteridge KJ. Farm animal embryo technologies: Achievements and perspectives. Theriogenology 2006; 65: 905–913

Binelli M., Thatcher WW., Mattos R., Baruselli PS. Antiluteolytic strategies to improve fertility in cattle. Theriogenology 2001;56:1451-1463

Bloch A., Folman Y., Kaim M., Roth Z., Braw-Tal R., Wolfenson D. Endocrine Alterations Associated with Extended Time Interval Between Estrus and Ovulation in High-Yield Dairy Cows. J Dairy Sci 2006; 89:4694–4702

Bonnet BN., Martin SW., Meek AH. Associations of clinical findings, bacteriological and histological results of endometrial biopsy with reproductive performance of post partum dairy cows. Prev Vet Med 1993;15:205-20

Breuel KF., Spitzer JC., Henricks DM. Systemic progesterone concentration following human chorionic gonadotroin administration at various times during the estrous cycle in beef heifers. J Anim Sci 1989;67:1564-1572

Bridges PJ., Brusie MA., Fortune JE. Eleveated temperature (heat stress) in vitro reduces androstenedione and estradiol and increases progesterone secretion by follicular cells from bovine dominant follicles. Dom Anim Endocrinol 2005;29:508-522

Brito LF., Silva AE., Barbosa RT. Testicular thermoregulation in Bos indicus, crossbred and Bos taurus bulls: relationshiop with scrotal, testicular vascular cone and testicular morphology and effects on semen quality and sperm production. Theriogenology 2004;61:511-528

Britt JH., Harrison DS., and Morrow DA. Frequency of ovarian follicular cysts, reasons for culling and fertility in Holstein-Friesian cows following postpartum treatment with gonadotrophin releasing hormone at two weeks after parturition. Am J Vet Res 1977;50:749-51.

Bucklin RA., Turner LW., Beede DK., Bray DR., Hemken RW. Methods to relieved heat stress for dairy cows in hot, humid climates. Appl Eng Agric 1991;7:241-247

Burton NR., Lean IJ. Investigation by meta-analysis of the effect of prostaglandin F_{2a} administered post partum on the reproductive performance of dairy cattle. Vet Rec 1995;136:90-4

Butler J E., Hamilton WC., Sasser RG., Ruder CA., Hass GM, and R. J. Williams. Detection and partial characterization of two bovine pregnancy-specific proteins. Biol Reprod 1982; 26:925–933.

Buttler WR., Calaman JJ., Beam SW. Plasma and milk urea nitrogen in relation to pregnancy rate in lactating dairy cattle. J Anim Sci 1996;74:858-865

Butler WR. Nutritional interactions with reproductive performance in dairy cattle. Anim Reprod Sci 2000; 60-61:449-457

Buxton D., Maley SW., Pastoret PP., Brochier B., Innes EA. Examination of red foxes (Vulpes vulpes) from Belgium for antibody to Neospora caninum and Toxoplasma gondii. Vet Rec 1997;141:308-309

Cabaj W., Moskwa B., Pastusiak K., Gill J. Antibodies to Neospora caninum in the blood of European bison (Bison bonasus bonasus L) living in Poland. Vet Parasitol 2005;128:163-168

Calder MD., Salfen BE., Bao B., Youngquist RS., Garverick HA. Administration of progesterone to cows with ovarian follicular cysts results in a reduction in mean LH and LH pulse frequency and initiates ovulatory follicular growth. J Anim Sci. 1999;77:3037–3042

Cambell MH., Miller JK. Effect of supplemental dietary Vitamin E and zinc on reproductive performance of dairy cows and heifers fed excess iron. J Dairy Sci 1998;81:2693-9

Cartmil JA., Hensley BA., El-Zarkouny SZ., Rezell TG., Smith JF., Stevenson JS. An alternative AI-breeding protocol during summer heat stress. J Dairy Sci 1999;82:48 (abstr).

Cartmill JA., El-Zarkouny SZ., Hensley BA., Lamb GC., and Stevenson JS. Stage of cycle, incidence and timing of ovulation and pregnancy rates in dairy cattle after three timed breeding protocols. J. Dairy Sci. 2001;84:1051–1059

Cavalieri J., Hepworth G., Fitzpatrick LA., Shaphard RW., Macmillan KL. Manipulation and control of the oestrous cycle in pasture-based dairy cows. Theriogenology 2006;65:45-64

Cavalieri J., Smart VM., Hepworth G., Ryan M., Macmillan KL. Ovarian follicular development and hormone concentrations in inseminated dairy cows with resynchronized estrous cycles Theriogenology 2008;70: 946–955

Cerri RLA., Rutigliano HM., Bruno RGS., Santos JEP. Progesterone concentration, follicular development and induction of cyclicity in dairy cows receiving intravaginal progesterone inserts. Anim Reprod Sci 2009;110:56–70

Chagas e Silva J., Diniz P., Lopes da Costa L. Accessory corpora lutea indiced by hCG treatment enhance survival of half embryos in high yielding lactating dairy cows. Proceedings of the 16th ICAR, Budapest 2008;

Chebel RC., Demetrio DGB., Metzger J. Factors affecting success of embryo collection and transfer in large dairy herds. Theriogenology 2008;69:98–106

Colazo MG., Ree TO., Emmanuel DGV., Abrose DJ. Plasnam luteinizing hormone concentrations in cows given repeated treatments or three different doses of gonadotropin releasing hormone. Theriogenology 2009;71:984-992

Coleman DA., Bartol FF., Spencer TE., Floyd JG., Wolfe DF., and Brendemuehl JP. Effects of a potent GnRH agonist and hormonal profiles, synchronization of estrus and fertility in beef cattle. J Anim Sci 1991; 69(Suppl. 1): 396

Chebel RC., Santos JEP., Cerri RLA., Galvao KN., Juchem SO., Thatcher WW. Effect of resynchronisation with GnRH on day 21 after artificial insemination on pregnancy rate and pregnancy loss in lactating dairy cows. Theriogenology 2003;60:1389-99

Chenault JR., Kratzer DD., Rzepkowski RA., Goodwin MC. LH and FSH response of Holstein heifers to fertirelin acetate, gonadorelin and buserelin. Theriogenology 1990;34:81-98

Cordoba MC., and Fricke PM. Initiation of the breeding season in a grazingbased dairy by synchronisation of ovulation. J Dairy Sci 2002;85:1752-1763

Cordoba MC., Sartori R., Fricke PM. Assessment of a commercially available early conception factor (ECF) test for determining pregnancy status of dairy cattle. J Dairy Sci 2001; 84:1884–1889

Curran, S., Kastelic JP., and Ginther OJ. Determining sex of the bovine fetus by ultrasonic assessment of the relative location of the genital tubercle. Anim. Reprod. Sci. 1989;19:217–227.

Davies CJ., Hill JR., Edwards JL., Schrick FN., Fisher PJ., Eldridge JA., Schlafer DH. Major histocompatibility antigen expression on the bovine placenta: its relationship to abnormal pregnancies and retained placenta. Anim Reprod Sci 2004;82–83: 267–280

DeJarnette JM., Day ML., House RB., Wallace RA., Marshall CE. Effect of GnRH pretreatment on reproductive performance of post partum suckled beef cows following synchronisation of oestrus using GnRH and $PGF_{2\alpha}$. J Anim Sci 2001a;79:1675-1682

DeJarnette JM., Salverson RR., Marshall CE. Incidence of premature estrus in lactating dairy cows and conception rates to standing estrus or fixed-time inseminations after synchronisation using GnRH and $PGF_{2\alpha}$. Anim Reprod Sci 2001b;67:27-35

DeJarnette JM., Marshall CE. Effects of presynchronisation using combinations of $PGF_{2\alpha}$ and (or) GnRH on pregnancy rates of Ovsynch and Cosynch treated lactating Holstein cows. Anim Reprod Sci 2003;77:51-60

De Rensis F., Marconi P., Capelli T., Gatti F., Facciolongo F., Frazini S., Scaramuzzi RJ. Fertility in postpartum dairy cows in winter or summer following oestrus synchronisation and fixed time AI after induction of an LH surge with GnRH or hCG. Theriogenology 2002;58:1675-1687

Dijkhuizen AA., Huirne RBM., Renkema JA. Modelling animal health economics. Department of Farm Management, Wageningen Agricultural University. 1991.

Dijkstra, T., Eysker, M., Schares, G., Conraths, F.J., Wouda, W., Barkema, H.W. Dogs shed Neospora caninum oocysts after ingestion of naturally infected bovine placenta but not after ingestion of colostrums spiked with Neospora caninum tachyzoites. Int. J. Parasitol. 2001;31:747–752

Diskin MG., Austin EJ., Roche JF. Exogenous hormonal manipulation of ovarian activity in cattle. Dom Anim Endocrinol 2002;23:211-228

Donofrio G., Herath S., Sartori C., Cavirani S., Flammini CF., Sheldon IM. Bovine herpesvirus 4 (BoHV-4) is tropic for bovine endometrial cells and modulates endocrine function. Reproduction 2007;134:183–197.

Dosogne H., Hoeben D., Burvenich V., Lohouis JACM. Effect of cephapirin and mecillinam on the phagocitic and respiratory burst activity of neutrophil leukocytes isolated from bovine blood. J Vet Pharmacol Therap 1998; 21:421-427

Drilrich M., Beetz O., Pfuzner A., Sabin M., Sabin HJ et al. Evaluation of a systemic antibiotic treatment of toxic puerperal metritis in dairy cows.J Dairy Sci. 2001;84:2010-7.

Drilrich M., Mahlstedt M., Reichert U., Tenhagen BA., Heuwieser W. Strategies to improve the therapy of retained fetal membranes in dairy cows.J Dairy Sci. 2006;89:627-35

Drillich M., Voigt D., Forderung D., Heuwieser,W. Treatment of acute puerperal metritis with flunixin meglumine in addition to antibiotic treatment. J Dairy Sci 2007;90: 3758–3763.

Drost M., Ambrose JD., Thatcher MJ., Cantrell CK., Wolsdorf KE., Hasler JF., Thatcher WW. Conception rates after artificial insemination or embryo transfer in lactating dairy cows during summer in Florida. Theriogenology 1999;52:1161-1167

Dubey JP., Lindsay DS. Neospora caninum induced abortion in sheep. J Vet Diagnost Invest 1990;2:230-233

Dubey JP., Acland HM., Hamir AN. Neospora caninum (Apicomplexa) in stillborn goat. J Parasitol 1992;78:532-534

Dubey JP. Review of Neospora caninum and neosporosis in animals. Korean J. Parasitol. 2003; 41: 1-16

Dunne LD., Diskin MG., Sreenan JM. Embryo and foetal loss in beef heifers between day 14 gestation and full term. Anim Reprod Sci 2000; 58: 39-44

Ealy AD., Drost M., Hansen PJ. Developmental changes in embryonic resistance to adverse effects of maternal heat stress in cows. J Dairy Sci 1993;76: 2899-2905

Ealy AD., Arechiga CF., Bray DR., Risco CA., Hansen PJ. Effectiveness of shortterm cooling and vitamin E for alleviation of infertility induced by heat stress in dairy cows. J Dairy Sci 1994;77:3601-3607

Eiler H. Retained placenta. In: Youngquist, R.S. (Ed.), Current Therapy in Large Animal Theriogenology. W.B. Saunders Co., 1997 Philadelphia, PA, pp. 340–348.

Ellington JE., Foote RH., Farrell PB., Hasler JF., Webb J., Henderson WB., Mc- Grath AB. Pregnancy rates after the use of a gonadotrophin releasing hormone agonist in bovine embryo transfer recipients. Theriogenology 1991;36:1035-1042

Etherington WG., Kelton DF., and Adams JE. Reproductive performance of dairy cows following treatment with fenprostalene, dinoprost, or cloprostenol between 24 and 31 Days post partum: A field trial. Theriogenology 1994; 42: 739-752

El-Zarkouny SZ., Cartmill JA., Hensley BA.,. Stevenson JS. Pregnancy in dairy cows after synchronized ovulation regimens with or without presynchronization and progesterone. J Dairy Sci 2004;87:1024–1037.

Esslemont D., Kossaibati M. The cost of Poor Fertility and Disease in UK Dairy Herds. Daisy Research Report, 2002

Farin PW., Ball L., Olson JD., Mortimer RG., Jones RL., Adney WS., McChesney AE. Effect of Actinomyces pyogenes and gram-negative anaerobic bacteria on the development of bovine pyometra. Theriogenology 1989;31:979-89.

FarinCE.,FarinPW.,PiedrahitaJA. Developmentoffetusesfrominvitro–produced and cloned bovine embryos. J Anim Sci 2004. 82(E. Suppl.):E53–E62

Farin PW., Piedrahita JA., Farin CE. Errors in development of fetuses and placentas from in vitro-produced bovine embryos. Theriogenology 2006;65:178-91

Fernandes C., Alves B., Oliveira E., Viana J., Figueiredo A., Gioso M., Oba E. Efficiancy of different cloprostenol doses in the postpartum period of Zebu (Bos indicus) beef cows. Proceedings of the XXV WBC, Budapest 2008a; Book of Abstracts, Abst. 855; p. 190

Fernandes C., Figueiredo A., Alves B., Oliveira E., Viana J., Gioso M. Use of florfenicol associated or not to Cloprostenol in puerperal disturbances in dairy cows. Proceedings of the XXV WBC, Budapest 2008a; Book of Abstracts, Abst. 857; p. 191

Ferre I., Serrano-Martinez E., Martinez A., Osoro K., Mateos-Sanz A., del-Pozo I., Aduriz G., Tamargo C., Hidalgo CO., Ortega-Mora LM. Effects of re-infection with Neospora caninum in bulls on parasite detection in semen and blood and immunological responses. Technical note. Theriogenology 2008;69: 905–911

Feugang JM., Camargo-Rodriguez O., Memili E. Culture systems for bovine embryos. Livestock Sci 2009;121: 141–149

Fortune JE., Rivera GM., Evans ACO., Turzillo AM. Differentiation of Dominant Versus Subordinate Follicles in Cattle. Biol Reprod 2001; 65: 648–654

Franco M., Block J., Jousan FD., Castro e Paula, de LA., Brad AM., Franco JM., Grisel F., Monson RL., Rutledge JJ., Hansen PJ. Effect of transfer of one or two in vitro-produced embryos and post-transfer administration of gonadotropin releasing hormone on pregnancy rates of heat-stressed dairy cattle. Theriogenology 2006a; 66: 224–233

Franco M., Thompson PM., Brad AM., Hansen PJ. Effectiveness of administration of gonadotropin-releasing hormone at Days 11, 14 or 15 after anticipated ovulation for increasing fertility of lactating dairy cows and non-lactating heifers. Theriogenology 2006b;66: 945–954

Frazer GS. A rational basis for therapy in the sick postpartum cow. Veterinary Clinics of North America: Food Animal Practice 2005;21, 523–568.

Fricke PM., Scanning the Future—Ultrasonography as a Reproductive Management Tool for Dairy Cattle. J Dairy Sci 2002; 85: 1918–1926 Fray MD., Mann GE., Clarke MC., Charleston B. Bovine viral diarrhoea virus: its effects on oestradiol, progesterone and prostaglandin secretion in the cow. Theriogenology 1999;51:1533-1546

Fray MD., Mann GE., Clarke MC., Charleston B. Bovine viral diarrhoea virus: its effects on ovarian function in the cow. Vet Microbiol 2000;77:185-194

Fray MD., Mann GE., Bleach ECL., Knight PG., Clarke MC., Charleston B. Modulation of sex hormone secretion in cows by acute infection with bovine viral diarrhoea virus. Reproduction 2002;123:281-289

Fricke PM. Guenther JN., and Wiltbank MC. Efficacy of decreasing the dose of GnRH used in a protocol for synchronization of ovulation and timed AI in lactating dairy cows. Theriogenology 1998;50:1275–1284

Friedrich M., Holtz W. Establishment of an ELISA for Measuring Bovine Pregnancy-Associated Glycoprotein in Serum or Milk and Its Application for Early Pregnancy Detection. Reprod Domest Anim 2009 (in press)

Fuji TU., Kasai N., Nisi SA., Dubey JP., Gennari SM. Seroprevalence of Neospora caninum in female water buffaloes (Bubalus bubalis) from the south eastern region of Brazil. Vet Parasitol 2001;99:331-334

Galli C., Lazzari G. The manipulation of gametes and embryos in farm animals. Repro Domest Anim 2008;43(Suppl.2):1-7

Garcia FEO., Cordero MJL., Hizarza EA., Peralta OJG., Ortega CME., Cárde nas M., Gutierrez CG., Sánchez TEMT. Induction of a new follicular wave in Holstein heifers synchronized with norgestomet. Animal Reprod Sci 2004;80: 47–57

Galvao KN., Santos JEP., Cerri RL., Chebel RC., Rutigliano HM., Bruno RG., Bicalho RC. Evaluation of Methods of Resynchronization for Insemination in Cows of Unknown Pregnancy Status. J. Dairy Sci 2007; 90:4240–4252

Garcia-Ispierto I., Lopez-Gatius F., Santolaria P., Yaniz JL., Nogareda C., Lopez-Bejar M., De Rensis F. Relationship between heat stress during the peri-implantation period and early fetal loss in dairy cattle. Theriogenology 2006;65: 799–807

Garner DL., Seidel GE., Jr. History of commercializing sexed semen for cattle Theriogenology 2008;69:886-895

Garverick HA. Ovarian follicular cysts in dairy cows. J Dairy Sci 1997;80:995- 1004

Geary TW., Wittier JC., Downing ER., LeFever DG., Silcox RW., Holland MD., Nett TM., and Niswender GD. Pregnancy rates of postpartum beef cows that were synchronized using Syncro-Mate B or the Ovsynch protocol. J. Anim. Sci.1998;76:1523–1527

Geary TW., Downing ER., Bruemmer JE., Whittier JC. Ovarian and estrous response of suckled beef cows to the select synch estrous synchronisation protocol. Prof Anim Sci 2000;16:1-5

Gilbert RO., Shin ST., Guard CL., Erb HN. Incidence of endometritis and effects on reproductive performance of dairy cows. Theriogenology 1998

Gilbert RO., Shin ST., Guard CL., Erb HN., Frajblat M. Prevalence of endometritis and its effects on reproductive performance of dairy cows. Theriogenology 2005; 64:1879-1888

Ginther OJ., Bergfelt DR., Kulick LJ., Kot K. Selection of the dominant follicle in cattle: role of estradiol. Biol Reprod 2000; 63:383–389.

Ginther OJ., Bergfelt DR., Kulick LJ., Kot K. Selection of the dominant follicle in cattle: role of two-way functional coupling between follicle stimulating hormone and the follicles. Biol Reprod 2000; 62:920–927.

Givens MD. A clinical, evidence-based approach to infectious causes of infertility in beef cattle. Theriogenology 2006;66: 648–654

Givens MD., Marley MSD. Pathogens that cause infertility of bulls or transmission via semen. Theriogenology 2008;70:504–507

Givens MD., Marley SD. Approaches to biosecurity in bovine embryo transfer programs. Theriogenology 2008b;69: 129–136

Gondim LFP., McAllister MM., Pitt WC., Zemlicka DE. Coyotes (Canis latrans) are definite hosts of Neospora caninum. Int J Parasitol 2004;34:159-161

Green JA., Parks TE., Avalle MP., Telugu BP., McLain AL., Peterson AJ, et al. The establishment of an ELISA for the detection of pregnancy-associated glycoproteins (PAGs) in the serum of pregnant cows and heifers. Theriogenology 2005;63:1481–503.

Green MP., Hunter MG., Mann GE. Relationship between maternal progesterone secretion and embryo development on day 5 of pregnancy in dairy cows. Anim Reprod Sci 2005;88:179-189

Greve T., Lehn-Jensen H. The effect of hCG administration on pregnancy rate following non-surgical transfer of viable bovine embryos. Theriogenology 1982;17:91 (abstract)

Groenendaal H., Galligan DT, and H. A. Mulder. 2004. An economic spreadsheet model to determine optimal breeding and replacement decisions for dairy cattle. J Dairy Sci 2004; 87:2146–2157.

Grooms DL., Brock KV., Pate JL., day ML. Changes in ovarian follicles following acute infection with bovine viral diarrhoea virus. Theriogenology 1998;49:595-605

Gröhn YT., Hertl JA., Harman JL. Effect of early lactation milk yield on reproductive disorders in dairy cows. A. J Vet Res 1994; 55:1521-1528

Gupta S., Gupta HK., Soni J. Effect of Vitamin E and selenium supplementation on concentrations of plasma cortisol and erythrocyte lipid peroxides and the incidence of retained fetal membranes in crossbred dairy cattle. Theriogenology 2005;64:1273-1286

Guzeloglu A., Erdem H., Saribay MK., Thatcher WW., Tekeli T. Effect of the administration of flunixin meglumine on pregnancy rates in Holstein heifers. Vet Rec 2007;160: 404-406

Guzeloglu A., Erdem H., Cinar M., Kilic K., Talmac M., Gorgundur A., Gumen A. Effect of ketoprofen administration 15 and 16 days after AI on conception rates in lactating dairy cows. Proceedings of the 16th ICAR, Budapest 2008; Abst. p. 43

Hall CA., Reichel MP., Ellis JT. Neospora abortions in dairy cattle: diagnosis, mode of transmission and control. Veterinary Parasitology 2005;128: 231–241

Hansen PJ. Effects of environment on bovine reproduction. In: Youngquist RS (ED), Current Therapy in Large Animal Theriogenology, WB Saunders, Philadelphia, PA, 1997, pp. 403-415

Hansen PJ., Drost M., Rivera RM., Paula-Lopes FF., Al-Katanani YM., Krininger CE., Chase CC Jr. Adverse impact of heat stress on embryo production: causes and strategies for mitigation. Theriogenology 2001;55:91-103

Hansen PJ. Physiological and cellular adaptations of zebu cattle to thermal stress. Anim Reprod Sci 2004;82-83:349-360.

Hatler TB., Hayes SH., Laranja da Fonseca LF., Silvia WJ. Relationship between endogenous progesterone and follicular dynamics in lactating dairy cows with ovarian follicular cysts. Biol Reprod. 2003;69:218–223

Hendricks KEM., Bartolome JA., Melendez P., Risco C., Archbald LF. Effect of repeated administration of $PGF_{2\alpha}$ in the early post partum period on the prevalence of clinical endometritis and probability of pregnancy at first insemination in lactating dairy cows. Theriogenology 2005 in press

Hernandez J., Risco C., Donovan A. A between exposure to Neospora caninum and milk production in dairy cows. JAVMA 2001;219:632-635

Hernandez-Ceron J., Chase Jr CC., Hansen PJ. Differences in heat tolerance between preimplantation embryos from Brahman, Romosinuano and Angus Breeds. J Dairy Sci 2004;87:53-58

Haugejorden G., Waage S., Dahl E., Karlberg K., Beckers JF., Ropstad E. Pregnancy associated glycoproteins (PAG) in postpartum cows, ewes, goats and their offspring. Theriogenology 2006;66: 1976–1984

Heuwieser W., Ferguson JD., Guard CL., Foote RH., Warnick LD., Breickner LC. Relationship between administration of GnRH, body condition score and fertility in Holstein dairy cattle. Theriogenology 1994;42:703-714

Heuwiesser W., Tenhagen BA., Tischer M., Luhr J., Blum H. Effect of three programmes for the treatment of endometritis on the reproductive performance of a dairy herd. Vet Rec 2000;146:338-41

Hill J., Gilbert R. Reduced quality of bovine embryos cultured in media conditioned by exposure to an inflamed endometrium. Aust Vet J 2008; 86:312-6.

Houe H., Myrup Pedersen K., Meyling A. The effect of bovine viral diarrhoea virus infection on conception rate. Prev Vet Med 1993;15:117-123

Humblot P. Use of pregnancy specific proteins and progesterone assays to monitor pregnancy and determine the timing, frequencies and sources of embryonic mortality in ruminants. Theriogenology 2001;56:1417-1433

Innes EA., Wright S., Bartley P., Maley S., Macaldowie C., Esteban-Redondo I., Buxton D. The host–parasite relationship in bovine neosporosis. Vet Immunol Immunopathol 2005; 108: 29–36

Innes EA. The host-parasite relationship in pregnant cattle infected with Neospora caninum. Parasitology 2007;134:1903-10

Jonsson NN., McGowan MR., McGuigan K., Davison TM., Hussain AM., Kafi M. Relationship among calving season, heat load, energy balance and post partum ovulation of dairy cows in subtropical environment. Anim Reprod Sci 1997;47:315-326

Jolly PD., McDougall S., Fitzpatrick LA., Macmillan KL., Entwistle K. Physiological effects of undernutrition on post partum anestrous in cows. J Reprod Fertil 1995; Suppl 49: 477-492

Kafi M., McGowan MR., Kirkland PD., Jillela D. The effect of bovine pestivirus infection on the superovulatory response of Fresian heifers. Theriogenology 1997;48:985-996

Kaim M., Bloch A., Wolfenson D., Braw-Tal R., Rosenberger M., Voet H., Folman Y. Effect of GnRH administered to cows at the onset of oestrus on timing of ovulation, endocrine responses and conception. J Dairy Sci 2003;86:2012-2021

Kaneda Y., Domeki I., Kamomae H., Otake M., Watanabe F., Nishikata K. Effects of additional injection of hCG on the formation of the corpus luteum and fertility of oestrus synchronised dairy heifers by stimulus injection of prostaglandin F_{2a} and estradiol benzoate. Jpn J Anim Reprod 1981;27:89-91

Kasimanickam R., Duffield TF., Foster RA., Gartley CJ., Leslie KE., Walton JS et al. Endometrial cytology and ultrasonography for the detection of subclinical endometritis in postpartum dairy cows. Theriogenology 2004;62:9-23

Kasimanickam R., Duffield TF., Foster RA., Gartley CJ., Leslie KE., Walton JS., and. Johnson WH. The effect of a single administration of cephapirin or cloprostenol on the reproductive performance of dairy cows with subclinical endometritis. Theriogenology, 2005; 63: 818-830

Kastelic JP and Thundathil JC. Breeding soundness Evaluation and Semen Analysis for Predicting Bull Fertility. Reprod Domest Anim 2008;43 (Suppl.2):368-373

Kharche SD., Srivastava SK. Dose dependent effect of GnRH analogue on pregnancy rate of repeat breeder crossbred cows. Animal Reproduction Science 2007; 99: 196–201

Keister ZO., DeNise SK., Armstrong DV., Ax RL., and Brown MD. Pregnancy outcomes in two commercial dairy herds following hormonal scheduling programs. Theriogenology 1999;51:1587–1596.

Kindahl H., Ondensvik K., Aiumlamai S., and Fredriksson G. Utero-ovarian relationship during the bovine postpartum period. Anim Reprod Sci 1992; 28:

Kornmatitsuk B., Chantaraprateep P., Kornmatitsuk S., Kindahl H. Different types of postpartum luteal activity affected by the exposure of heat stress and subsequent reproductive performance in Holstein lactating cows. Reprod Domest Anim 2008;43:515-519

Lamming GE., Darwash AO., Back HL Corpus luteum function in dairy cows and embryo mortality. J Reprod Fertil 1989; Suppl 37:245-252

Lane EA., Austin EJ., Crowe MA. Oestrous synchronisation in cattle-Current options following the EU regulations restricting use of oestrogenic compounds in food-producing animals: A review. Anim Reprod Sci 2008;109: 1–16

LeBlanc SJ., Diffield TF., Leslie KE., Bateman KG., Keefe GP., Walton JS., Johnson WH. Defining and diagnosing post partum clinical endometritis and its impact on reproductive performance in dairy cows. J Dairy Sci 2002;85:2223-2236

LeBlanc SJ., Duffield TF., Leslie KE., Bateman KG, Keefe GP., Walton JS., Johnson WH. The Effect of Treatment of Clinical Endometritis on Reproductive Performance in Dairy Cows. J Dairy Sci 2002b;85:2237–2249

LeBlanc SJ., Herdt T., Seymour W., Duffield T., Leslie K. Factors associated with peripartum serum concentrations of vitamin E, retinol, and (-carotene in Holstein dairy cattle, and their associations with periparturient disease. J Dairy Sci 2004;87, 609–619.

LeBlanc SJ. Postpartum uterine disease and dairy herd reproductive performance: A review. Vet J 2008;176: 102–114

Lee C., Maurice R., Pennington JA., Hoffman WF., Brown MD. Efficacy of gonadotrophin-releasing hormone administration at the time of artificial in semination of heifers and post partum repeat breeder dairy cows. AM J Vet Res 1983;44:2160

Lewis GS., Caldwell DW., Rexroad CE., Dowlen HH., Owen JR. Effect of gonadotrophin-releasing hormone and human chorionic gonadotrophin on pregnancy rate in dairy cattle. J Dairy Sci 1990;73:66-72

Lewis GS. Uterine health and disorders. J Dairy Sci 1997;80:984-94

Lewis GS. Steroidal regulation of uterine immune defenses. Anim Reprod Sci 2004; 82–83: 281–294

Lincke A., Drillich M., Heuwieser W. Subclinical endometritis in dairy cattle and ist effect on reproductive performance - a review on recent publications. Berl Munch Tierarztl Wochenschr 2007;120:245-250

Lindsay DS., Kelly EJ., McKown R et al. Prevalence of Neospora caninum and Toxoplasma gondii antibodies in coyotes (Canis latrans) and experimental infections of coyotes with Neospora caninum. J Parasitol 1996;82:657-659

Lindsay DS., Spencer J., Rupprecht CE., Blagburn BL. Prevalence of agglutinating antibodies to Neospora caninum in racoons. J Parasitol 2001;87:1197-1198

Lonergan P., Fair T. In vitro-produced bovine embryos—Dealing with the warts. Theriogenology 2008; 69: 17–22

Looney CR., Nelson JS., Schneider HJ., Forrest DW. Improving fertility in beef cow recipients. Theriogenology 2006;65:201–209

Lopez H., Satter LD., Wiltbank MC. Relationship between level of milk production and oestrus behaviour of lactating dairy cows. Anim Reprod Sci 2004,81:209-23

Lopez H, Caraviello DZ, Satter LD, Fricke PM, Wiltbank MC. Relationship between level of milk production and multiple ovulations in lactating dairy cows. J Dairy Sci 2005;88:2783–93.

Lopez-Gatius F., Lopez-Bejar M. Reproductive performance of dairy cows with ovarian cysts after different GnRH and cloprostenol treatments. Theriogenology 2002;58:1337-1348

Lopez-Gatius F., Santolaria P., Martino A., Delatang F., De Rensis. The effects of GnRH treatment at the time of AI and 12 days later on reproductive performance of high producing dairy cows during the warm season in northestern Spain. Theriogenology 2006;65:820-830

Lopez-Gatius F., Hunter RHF., Garbayo JM., Santolaria P., Yaniz J., Serrano B., Ayad A., de Sousa NM., Beckers JF. Plasma concentrations of pregnancy-associated glycoprotein-1 (PAG-1) in high producing dairy cows suffering early fetal loss during the warm season. Theriogenology 2007;67: 1324–1330

Lucaci E. Effects of flunixin meglumine (FM) on reproductive events in fixed timed artificial inseminated cows. Proceedings of the 16th ICAR, Budapest 2008, Abstr. P. 50

Lynch R A., Alexander BM., and R. G. Sasser. The cloning and expression of the pregnancy-specific protein B. Biol Reprod 1992; 46 (Suppl. 1):72. (Abstr.)

Macmillan KL., Taufa VK., Day AM. Effects of an agonist of gonadotrophin releasing hormone (buserelin) in cattle III. Pregnancy rates after a post-insemination injection during metoestrus or dioestrus. Anim Reprod Sci 1986;11:1-10.

Macmillan KL., Laen IJ., Westwood CT. The effects of lactation on the fertility of dairy cows. Aust Vet J 1996; 73: 141-147

Macmillan KL.,Segwagwe BE., Pino CS. Associations between the manipulation of patterns of follicular development and fertility in cattle. Animal Reprod Sci 2003;78:327–344

Malayer JR., Hansen PJ. Differences between Brahman and Holstein cows in heat-shock induced alteration of protein secretion by oviducts and uterine endometrium. J Anim Sci 1990;68:266-280

Mann GE., Lamming GE., Fray MD. Plasma oestradiol and progesterone during early pregnancy in the cow and the effects of treatment with buserelin. Anim Reprod Sci 1995; 37: 121-131

Mann GE., Mann SJ., Lamming GE. The interrelationship between the maternal hormone environment and the embryo during the early stages of pregnancy. J Reprod Fertil 1996; Abstr Series 17:55

Mann GE., Lamming GE., Fisher PA. Progesterone control of embryonic interfeton-Tproduction during early pregnancy in the cow. J Reprod Fertil 1998;Abst Series 21:37

Mann GE., Payne JH., Lamming GE. Hormonal regulation of oxytocin-induced prostaglandin $F_{2\alpha}$ secretion by the bovine and ovine uterus in vivo. Dom Anim Endocrinol 2001;21:127-141

Mapletoft RJ., Hasler JF. Assisted reproductive technologies in cattle: a review. Rev Sci Tech 2005;24:393-403
Matsui M., Shimada A., Yagi K., Kida K., Miyamoto A., Miyake YI. The characteristics of ovarian function and endocrine status in pregnant cows duirng early period after insemination. Proceedings of the 16th ICAR, Budapest 2008; Abst. p. 52
McDougall S., Cullum AA., Anniss FM., and Rhodes FM. Treatment of anovulatory anoestrus postpartum dairy cows with a gonadotrophin-releasing hormone (GnRH), prostaglandin $F_{2\alpha}$ GnRH regimen or with progesterone and oestradiol benzoate. N.Z. Vet. J. 2001 ;49:168–172.
McDougal S., Compton CWR., Annis FM. Effect of exogenous progesterone and oestrdaiol on plasma progesterone concentrations and follicle wave dinamics in anovulatory anoestrus post partum cattle. Anim Reprod Sci 2004;84:303-14
McGowan MR., Kirkland PD., Richards SD., Littlejohns IR. Increased reproductive losses in cattle infected with bovine pestivirus around the time of insemination. Vet Rec 1993;133:39-43
McGowan MR., Kafi M., Kirkland PD., Kelly H., Occhio MD., Jillella D. Studies of the pathogenesis of bovine pestivirus-induced ovarian dysfunction in superovulated cattle. Theriogenology 2003;59:1051-1066
McMillan WH. Statistical models predicting embryo survival to term in cattle after embryo transfer. Theriogenology 1998;50:1053-1070
Mee MO, Stevenson JS, Scoby RK, Folman Y. Influence of gonadotrophin-releasing hormone and timing of insemination relative to estrus on pregnancy rate of dairy cattle at first service. J Dairy Sci 1990; 73: 1500-1507
Mee MO., Stevenson JS., Alexander BM., Sasser RG. Administration of GnRH at estrus influences pregnancy rates, serum concentrations of LH, FSH, estradiol 17B, Pregnancy-specific protein B and progesterone, proportion of luteal cell types and in vitro production of progesterone in dairy cows. J Anim Sci 1993;71:185-198
Mee JF., Ryan PD., and Condon T. Ultrasound diagnosis of pregnancy in cattle. Vet. Rec. 1994;134:532.
Mejia ME and Lacau-Mengido IM. Endometritis treatment with a $PGF_{2\alpha}$ analog does not improve reproductive performance in a large dairy herd in Argentina. Theriogenology 2005;63:1266-1276
Melendez P., Gonzalez G., Aguilar E., Loera O., Risco C., Archbald LF. Comparison of Two Estrus-Synchronization Protocols and Timed Artificial Insemination in Dairy Cattle. J Dairy Sci 2006;89:4567–4572
Merrill ML., Ansotegui RP., Burns PD., MacNeil MD., Geary TW. Effects of flunixin meglumine and transportation on establishment of pregnancy in beef cows. J. Anim. Sci. 2007. 85:1547–1554
Mihm M., Deletang F., Roche JF. The gonadotrophin and ovarian response to an intermediate or low dose of gonadorelin in beef heifers: influence of dose, follicle status and progesterone environment. J Reprod Fertil Abstr Ser 1998;21:74
Mihm M., Bleach ECL. Endocrine regulation of ovarian antral follicle development in cattle. Anim Reprod Sci 2003; 78: 217–237
Mihm M., Evans ACO. Mechanisms for dominant follicle selection in monovulatory species: a comparison of morphological, endocrine and intraovarian events in cows, mares and women. Reprod Domest Anim 2008;43 (Suppl. 2):48-46
Moreira F., Orlandi C., Risco CA., Mattos R., Lopes F., Thatcher WW. Effects of presynchronisation and bovine somatotropin on pregnancy rates to a timed artificial insemination protocol in lactating dairy cows. J Dairy Sci 2001;84:1646-59

Morgan WF., and Lean IJ. Gonadotrophin-releasing hormone treatment in cattle: a meta-analysis of the effects on conception at the time of insemination. Austral Vet J 1993;70:205209
Morton JM., Tranter WP., Mayer DG., Jonsson NN. Effects of Environmental Heat on Conception Rates in Lactating Dairy Cows: Critical Periods of Exposure. J Dairy Sci 2007;90:2271–2278
Murray RD., Allison JD., Gard RO. Bovine endometritis: comparative efficacy of alfaprostol and intra-uterine therapies, and other factors influencing clinical success. Vet Rec 1990;127:86-90
Nakao T., Gamal A., Osawa T., Nakada K., Moriyoshi M., Kawata K. Postpartum plasma PGF metabolite profile in cows with dystocia and/or retained placenta, and effect of fenprostalene on uterine involution and reproductive performance. J Vet Med Sci 1997;59:791-4
Nebel RL and Jobst SM. Symposium: gonadotropin-releasing hormone and prostaglandin for estrus detection. Evaluation of Systematic Breeding Programs for Lactating Dairy Cows: A Review. J Dairy Sci 1998; 81:1169-1174
Nishigai M., Kamomae H., Tanaka T., Kaneda Y. The effect of administration of human chorionic gonadotropin in enhancing bovine corpus lutea luteinization and luteal function. J Reprod Dev 2001;47:283-94
Nishigai M., Kamomae H., Tanaka T.,Kaneda Y. Improvement of pregnancy rate in Japanese Black cows by administration of hCG to recipients of transferred frozen-thawed embryos. Theriogenology 2002;58:1597-1606
Nobel RL., Jobst SM., Dransfield MBG., Pandolfi SM., Balley TL. The use of radio frequency data communication system, Heat Watch, to describe behavioural estrus in dairy cattle. J Dairy Sci 1997;179 (abstract) Olynk NJ., Wolf CA. Economic Analysis of Reproductive Management Strategies on US Commercial Dairy Farms. J Dairy Sci 2008; 91:4082–4091
Olynk NJ., Wolf CA. Stochastic economic analysis of dairy cattle artificial insemination reproductive management programs. J Dairy Sci 2009; 92:1290–1299
Opsomer G., Mijten P., Coryn M., and de Kruif A. Post-partum anoestrus in dairy cows: a review. Vet Quart 1996;18: 68-75
Opsomer G., Grohn YT., Hertl J., Coryn M., Deluyker H., de Kruif A. Risk factors for post partum ovarian disfunction in high producing dairy cows in Belgium: a field study. Theriogenology 2000;53:841-857
Padula AM., Borman JM., Wright PJ., Macmillan KL. Restoration of LH out-put and 17B oestradiol responsiveness in acutely ovariectomised Holstein dairy cows pre-treated with a GnRH agonist (deslorelin) for 10 days. Anim Reprod Sci 2002;70:49-63
Padula AM., Macmillan KL. Oestradiol 17B responsiveness, plasma LH profiles, pituitary LH and FSH concentrations in long terms ovariectomised Holstein cows at 24h, 48h and 21 days following treatment with an absorbable GnRH agonist implant. Anim Reprod Sci 2005;85:27-39
Pancarci SM., Jordan ER., Risco CA., Schouten MJ., Lopes FL., Moreira F., and Thatcher WW. Use of estradiol cypionate in a presynchronized timed artificial insemination program for lactating dairy cattle. J. Dairy Sci. 2002;85:122–131
Paula-Lopes FF., Chase Jr, CC., Al-Katanani YM., Krininger III CE., et al. Genetic divergence in cellular resistance to heat shock in cattle: differences between breeds developed in temperate versus hot climates in responses of preimplantation embryos, reproductive taract tissues and lymphocytes to increased culture temperatures. Reproduction 2003;125:285-294s
Peter AT., Vos PLAM., Ambrose DJ. Postpartum anestrus in dairy cattle. Review. Theriogenology 2009; in press
Peters AR., Drew SB., Mann GE., Lamming GE., Beck NF. Experimental and practical approaches to the establishment and maintenance of pregnancy. J Physiol Pharmacol 1992; 43 (4 Suppl 1): 143-152

Peters AR., Ward SJ., Warren MJ., Gordon PJ.., Mann GE, Webb R. Ovarian and hormonal responses of cows to treatment with an analogue of gonadotrophin releasing hormone and prostaglandin $F_{2\alpha}$. Vet Rec 1999; 27: 343-346

Peters AR., Martinez TA., Cook AJC. A meta-analysis of studies of the effect of GnRH 11-14 days after insemination on pregnancy rates un cattle. Theriogenology 2000;54:1317-1326

Peterson AJ., Lee RSF. Improving successful pregnancies after embryo transfer. Theriogenology 2003;59: 687-697

Petrunkina AM., Waberski D., Gunzel-Apel AR., Topfer-Petersen E. Determinants of sperm quality and fertility in domestic species. Reproduction 2007;134: 3–17

Phatac AP., Whitmore HL., Brown MD. Effect of gonadotrophin-releasing hormone on conception rate in repeat-breeder dairy cows. Theriogenology 1986;26:605

Pieterse MC., Szenci O., Willemse AH., Bajcsy CSA., Dieleman SJK., Taverne MAM. Early pregnancy diagnosis in cattle by means of linear-array real-time ultrasound scanning of the uterus and a qualitative and quantitative milk progesterone test. Theriogenology 1990; 30(3):697-707.

Pösö J., Mäntysaari EA. Genetic relationships between reproductive disorders, operational days open and milk yield. Livest Prod Sci 1996; 46: 41-48

Pursley JR., Mee MO., and Wiltbank MC. Synchronization of ovulation in dairy cows using $PGF_{2\alpha}$ and GnRH. Theriogenology 1995;44:915–923.

Pursley JR., Kosorok MR., Wiltbank M.C. Reproductive management of lactating dairy cows using synchronization of ovulation. J. Dairy Sci. 1997;80: 301–306.

Rabiee AR., Lean IJ., Stevenson MA. Efficacy of Ovsynch program on reproductive performance in dairy cattle: a meta analysis. J Dairy Sci 2005;88:2754-2770

Rajamehendran R and Sianangama PC. Effect of human chorionic gonadotrophin on dominant follicles in cows: formation of accessory corpora lutea, progesterone production and pregnancy rates. J Reprod Fertil 1992;95:577-584

Rensis de F., Marconi P., Capelli T., Gatti F., Facciolongo F., Franzini S., Scaramuzzi RJ. Fertility in post partum dairy cows in winter or summer following oestrus synchronisation and fixed time AI after the induction of an LH surge with GnRH or hCG. Theriogenology 2002;58:1675-1687.

Rensis de F., Scaramuzzi RJ. Heat stress and seasonal effects on reproduction in the dairy cow-a review. Theriogenology 2003;60:1139-1151

Rensis de F., Valentini R., Gorrieri F., Bottarelli E., Lopez-Gatius F. Inducing ovulation with hCG improves the fertility of dairy cows during the warm season. Theriogenology 2008;69: 1077–1082

Rhoads ML., Rhoads RP., Gilbert RO., Toole R., Butler WR. Detrimental effects of high plasma urea nitrogen levels on viability of embryos from lactating dairy cows. Animal Reprod Sci 2006;91:1-10

Rhodes FM., Burke CR., Clark BA., Day ML., Macmillan KL. Effect of treatment with progesterone and oestradiol benzoate on ovarian follicle turnover in postpartum anoestrus cows and cows which have resumed oestrous cycles. Anim Reprod Sci 2002;69:139-150

Robert A., Beaudeau F., Seegers H., Joly A., Philipot JM. Large scale assessment of the effect associated with bovine viral diarrhoea virus infection on fertility of dairy cows in 6149 dairy herds in Brittany (Western France). Theriogenology 2003;61:17-127

Robinson RS., Hammond AJ., Wathes DC., Hunter MG., Mann GE. Corpus luteum-endometrium-embryo interactions in the dairy cow: underlying mechanisms and clinical relevance. Reprod Domest Anim 2008;43 (Suppl. 2):104-112

Roche JF., Boland MP., McGeady TA. Reproductive wastage following artificial insemination in cattle. Vet Rec 1981; 109: 95-97

Roelofs JB., Graat EAM., Mullaart E., Soede NM., Voskamp-Harkema W., KempB. Effects of insemination–ovulation interval on fertilization rates and embryo characteristics in dairy cattle. Theriogenology 2006;6: 2173–2181

Romano JE., Thompson JA., Kraemer DC., Westhusin ME., Forrest DW., Tomaszewski MA. Early pregnancy diagnosis by palpation per rectum: Influence on embryo/fetal viability in dairy cattle. Theriogenology 2007; 67:486–493

Romero JJ., Perez E., Frankena P. Effect of a killed whole Neospora caninum techyzoite vaccine on the crude abortion rate of Costa Rican dairy cows under field conditions. Vet Parasitol 2004;123:149-159

Romero JJ., Van Breda S., Vargas B., Dolz G., Frankena P. Effect of neosporosis on productive and reproductive performance of dairy cattle in Costa Rica. Theriogenology 2005;64:1928-1939

Ronchi B., Stradaioli G., Verini Supplizi A., Bernabuci U., Lacetera N., Accorsi PA. Influence of heat stress or feed restriction on plasma progesterone, oestradiol 17-Beta, LH, FSH, prolactin and cortisol in Holstein Heifers. Livestock Prod Sci 2001;68:231-241

Rosenberger M., Chun SY., Kaim M., Herz Z., Folman Y. The effect of GnRH administered to dairy cows during oestrus on plasma LH and conception in relation to the time of treatment and insemination. Anim Reprod Sci 1991;24:13-24

Roth Z., Meidan R., Braw-Tal R., Wolfenson D. Immediate and delayed effects of heat stress on follicular development and its association with plasma FSH and inhibin concentration in cows. J Reprod Fert 2000;120:83-90

Roth Z., Meidan R., Shaham-Albalancy A., Braw-Tal R., Wolfenson D. Delayed effect of heat stress on steroid production in medium sized and preovulatory bovine follicles. Reproduction 2001a;121:745-751

Roth Z., Arav A., Bor A., Zeron Y., Braw-Tal R., Wolfenson D. Improvement of quality of oocytes collected in the autumn be enhanced removal of impaired follicles from previously heat-stressed cows. Reproduction 2001b;122:737-744

Rukkwamsuk T., Wensing T., Kruip TAM. Relationship between triacyloglycerol concentration in the liver and first ovulation in post partum dairy cows. Theriogenology 1998; 51: 1133-1142

Rutledge JJ. Use of embryo transfer and IVF to bypass effects of heat stress. Theriogenology 2001;55:105-111

Ryan DP., Prichard JF., Kopel E., Godke RA. Comparing early embryo mortality in dairy cows during hot and cool seasons of the year. Theriogenology 1993;39:719-737

Saacke RG. Insemination factors related to timed AI in cattle. Theriogenology 2008;70:479–484

Sangsritavong S., Combs DK., Sartori R., Wiltbank MC. High feed intake increases blood flow and metabolism of progesterone and oestradiol-17B in dairy cattle. J Dairy Sci 2002;85:2831-42

Santos JE., Thatcher WW., Pool L., Overton MW. Effect of human chorionic gonadotropin on luteal function and reproductive performance of high producing lactating Holstein dairy cows. J Anim Sci 2001;79:2881-2894

Santos JEP., Bartolome JA., Cerri RLA., Juchem SO., Hernandez O., Trigg T et al. Effect of a deslorelin implant in atimed artificial insemination protocol on follicle development, luteal function and reproductive performance of lactating dairy cows. Theriogenology 2004;61:421-35

Sartori R., Sartor-Bergfelt R., Mertens SA., Guenther JN., Parrish JJ., Wiltbank MC. Early embryonic development during summer in lactating dairy cows and nulliparous heifers. Biol Reprod 2000; 62:155

Sartori R., Rosa GJM., Wiltbank MC. Ovarian structures and circulating steroids in heifers and lactating cows in summer and lactating and dry cows in winter. J Dairy Sci 2002;85:2813-2822

Scherzer J., Fayrer-Hosken RA., Ray L., Hurley DJ., Heusner GL. Advancement in large animal embryo transfer and related biotechnologies. Reprod Domest Anim 2008;43:371-6.

Schmitt EJP, Diaz T, Barros CM, de la Sota RL, Drost M, Fredriksson EW, et al. Differential response of the luteal phase and fertility in cattle following ovulation of the first-wave follicle with human chorionic gonadotropin or an agonist of gonadotropin-releasing hormone. J Anim Sci 1996a;74:1074–83.

Schmitt EJ-P., Barros CM., Fields PA., Fields MJ., Diaz T., Kluge JM. A cellular and endocrine characterisation of the original and induced CL after administration of gonadotropin'releasing hormone agonist or human chorionic gonadotropin on day 5 of the estrus cycle. J Anim Sci 1996;74:1915-29

Schmitz W., Driancourt MA., Hoppe S., Friedrich M., Erhardt G., Gauly M., Holtz W., Schmitz W. A modified Co-Synch protocol for timed artificial insemination in beef cattle. Abst. Proc. 16th ICAR, 2008, Budapest.

Sedlak K., Bartova E. Seroprevalences of antibodies to Neospora caninum and Toxoplasma gondii in zoo animals. Veterinary Parasitology 2006; 136:223–231

Seidel GE.,Jr. Overview of sexing sperm. Theriogenology 2007;68:443-446

Serrano-Martnez E., Ferre I., Martinez A., Osoro K., Mateos-Sanz A., del-Pozo I., Aduriz G., Tamargo C., Hidalgo CO., Ortega-Mora LM. Experimental neosporosis in bulls: Parasite detection in semen and blood and specific antibody and interferon-gamma responses. Theriogenology 2007;67:1175–1184

Sheldon IM., Noakes DE. Comparison of three treatments for bovine endome tritis Vet Rec 1998; 142:575-9

Sheldon IM., Noakes DE., Rycroft AN., Pfeiffer DU., Dobson H. Influence of uterine bacterial contamination after parturition on ovarian dominant follicle selection and follicle growth and function in cattle.
Reproduction 2002;123:837-845

Sheldon, I.M., Rycroft, A.N., Zhou, C. Association between postpartum pyrexia and uterine bacterial infection in dairy cattle. Vet Rec 2004a;154, 289–293.

Sheldon IM., Dobson H. Postpartum uterine health in cattle. Animal Reprod Sci 2004b;82-83:295-306

Sheldon IM., Noakes DE., Rycroft AN., Dobson H. Effect of intrauterine administration of oestradiol on postpartum uterine bacterial infection in cattle. Anim Reprod Sci 2004c;81:13–23

Sheldon IM., Bushnell M., Montgomery J., Rycroft AN. Minimum inhibitory concentrations of some antimicrobial drugs against bacteria causing uterine infections in cattle. Vet Rec 2004d;155: 383-387

Sheldon IM., Lewis GS., LeBlanc S., Gilbert R. Defining post partum uterine disease in cattle. Theriogenology in 2006;65:1516-1530.

Sheldon IM., Williams EJ., Miller ANA., Nash DM., Herath S. Uterine diseases in cattle after parturition. Vet J 2008;176:115–121

Shephard R. Investigation of a whole herd controlled breeding program using GnRH and prostaglandin in commercial seasonally-calving dairy herds. Aust Cattle Vet 2002;23:24-28

Shrestha HK., Nakao T., Suzuki T., Higaki T., Akita M. Effects of abnormal ovarian cycles duirng pre-service period postpartum on subsequent reproductive performance of high producing Holstein cows.
Theriogenology 2004;61:1559-1571

Sianangama PC., Rajamahendran R. Effect of human chorionic gonadotropin administered at specific times following breeding on milk progesterone and pregnancy in cows. Theriogenology 1992;38:85

Singh J., Murray RD., Mshelia G., Woldehiwet Z. The immune status of the bovine uterus during the peripartum period. Review. Vet J 2008;175:301–309
Silcox RW., Powell KL., and Kiser TE. Ability of dominant follicles (DF) to respond to exogenous GnRH administration is dependent on their stage of development. J Anim Sci 1993; 71(Suppl. 1): 219
Silva E., Sterry RA., Kolb D., Mathialagan N., McGrath MF., Ballam JM., and P. M. Fricke. Accuracy of a Pregnancy-Associated Glycoprotein ELISA to Determine Pregnancy Status of Lactating Dairy Cows Twenty-Seven Days After Timed Artificial Insemination. J Dairy Sci 2007;90:4612–4622
Silvia WJ., Lewis GS., McCracken JA., Thatcher WW., Wilson L. Hormonal regulation of uterine secretion of prostaglandin F2alpha during luteolysis in ruminants. Biol Reprod 1991;45:655-63
Silvia WJ., Halter TB., Nugent AM., Laranja da Fonseca LF. Ovarian follicular cysts in dairy cows: an abnosrmality in folliculogenesis.Dom Anim Endocrinol 2002;23:167-177
Silva JRV., Figueiredo JR., van den Hurk R. Involvement of growth hormone (GH) and insuline-like growth factor (IGF) system in ovarian folliculogenesis. Theriogenology 2009;71:1193-1208
Skarzynski DJ., Ferreira-Dias G., Okuda K. Regulation of luteal function and coprus luteum regression in cows: hormonal control, immune mechanisms and intercellular communication. Reprod Domest Anim 2008;43 (Suppl. 2):57-65
Sirard MA., Coenen K. In vitro maturation and embryo production in cattle. Methods Mol Biol 2006;348:35-42
Small JA., Ambrose JD., McCaughey WP., Ward DR., Sutherland WD., Glover ND., Rajamahendran R. The effects of gonadotrophin releasing hormone in prostaglandin $F_{2\alpha}$-based timed insemination programs for beef cattle. Can J Anim Sci 2001;81:335-343
Sota de la, R. L., Burke JM.,, Risco CA., Moreira F., DeLorenzo MA., and Thatcher WW. Evaluation of timed insemination during summer heat stress in lactating dairy cattle. Theriogenology 1998;49:761–770
Sousa NM., , Ayad a., Beckers JF., Gajewski Z. Pregnancy-associated glycoproteins (pag) as pregnancy markers in the ruminants. J Physiol Pharmacol 2006;57 (Suppl.8):153-171
Ssentongo YK., Johnson RH., Smith JR. Association of bovine viral diarrhoea-mucosal disease virus with ovaritis in cattle. Aust Vet J 1980;56:272-273
Sterry RA., Welle ML., Fricke PM. Treatment with Gonadotropin-Releasing Hormone After First Timed Artificial Insemination Improves Fertility in Noncycling Lactating Dairy Cows. J Dairy Sci 2006;89:4237–4245
Stevens RD., Dinsmore RP., Cattle MB. Evaluation of the use of intra-uterine infusions of oxytetracycline, subcutaneous injections of fenprostalene, or a combination of both, for the treatment of retained fetal membranes in dairy cows. J Am Vet Med Assoc. 1995; 207:1612-5
Stevenson JS., Call EP., Scoby RK., Phatak AP. Double insemination and gonadotrophin-releasing hormone treatment of repeat breeding cattle. J Dairy Sci 1990; 73: 1766-1772
Stevenson JS., Frantz KD., Call EP. Conception rates in repeat breeders and dairy cattle with unobserved estrus after prostaglandin $F_{2\alpha}$ and gonadotrophinreleasing hormone. Theriogenology 1988;29:451
Stevenson JS., Phatak AP., Call EP., Scoby RK. Double insemination and GnRH treatment of repeat breeding Holsteins. J Dairy Sci 1989; Suppl 72:352
Stevenson JS., Kobayashi Y., and Thompson KE. Reproductive performance of dairy cows in various programmed breeding systems including Ovsynch and combination of gonadotropin-releasing hormone and prostaglandin $F_{2\alpha}$. J. Dairy Sci. 1999; 82:506–515

Stevenson JS., Smith JF., and Hawkins DE. Reproductive outcomes for dairy heifers treated with combinations of prostaglandin $F_{2\alpha}$, norgestomet and gonadotropin-releasing hormone. J. Dairy Sci. 2000;83:2008–2015

Stevenson JS., Thompson KE., Forbes WL., Lamb GC., Grieger DM., Corah LR. Synchronizing estrus and (or) ovulation in beef cows after combinations of GnRH, norgestomet, and prostaglandin $F_{2\alpha}$ with or without timed insemination. J. Anim. Sci. 2000. 78:1747–1758

Stevenson JS., Tiffany SM., Lucy MC. Use of estrdaiol cypionate as a substitute for GnRH in protocols for synchronising ovulation in dairy cattle. J Dairy Sci 2004;87:3298-305

Stevenson JS.,. Pursley JR., Garverick HA., Fricke PM., Kesler DJ.,. Ottobre JS, Wiltbank MC. Treatment of cycling and noncycling lactating dairy cows with progesterone during Ovsynch. J Dairy Sci 2006;89:2567–2578.

Stevenson JL., Dalton JC., Santos JEP., Sartori R., Ahmadzadeh A., Chebel RC. Effect of Synchronization Protocols on Follicular Development and Estradiol and Progesterone Concentrations of Dairy Heifers. J Dairy Sci 2008;91:3045–3056

Thatcher WW., Meyer MD., Danet-Desnoyers G. Maternal recognition of pregnancy. J Reprod Fertil 1995; Suppl 49:15-28

Thatcher WW., Moreira F., Pancarci SM., Bartolome JA., Santos JEP. Strategies to optimize reproductive efficiency by regulation of ovarian function. Dom Animal Endocrinol 2002;23: 243–254

Thomas JC. Induced abortion - a therapeutic disaster. Proceedings of the AACV Pan Pacific Conference; Sydney 1991:35-6.

Thompson KE., Stevenson JS., Lamb GC., Grieger DM., Loest DE. Follicular, Hormonal, and Pregnancy Responses of Early Postpartum Suckled Beef Cows to GnRH, Norgestomet, and Prostaglandin $F_{2\alpha}$. J. Anim. Sci. 1999. 77:1823–1832

Tieman JCH., Rodrogues AAR., de Souza SLP., Barbanti Duarte JM., Gennari SM. Occurrence of anti-Neospora caninum antibodies in Brazilian cervids kept in captivity. Vet Parasitol 2005;129:341-343

Todoroki J, Yamakuchi H, Mizoshita K, et al. Restoring ovulation in beef donor cows with ovarian cysts by progesterone-releasing intravaginal silastic devices. Theriogenology. 2001;55:1919–1932

Torres-Junior de JRS., Pires de MFA., Sa de EF., Ferreira de AM., et al. Effect of maternal heat-stress on follicular growth and oocyte competence in Bos indicus cattle. Theriogenology 2008; 69: 155–166

Twagiramungu HL., Guilbault A.., Proulx J, Villeneuve P., and Dufour JJ. Influence of an agonist of gonadotropin-releasing hormone (buserelin) on oestrus synchronisation and fertility in beef cows. J Anim Sci 1992; 70:1904

Ullah G., Fuquay JW., Keawkhong T., Clark BL., Pogue DE., Murphey EJ. Effect of gonadotrophin-releasing hormone at estrus on subsequent luteal function and fertility in lactating Holsteins during heat stress. J Dairy Sci 1996;79:1950-1953

White CR., Keister ZO., McCauley TC., AX RL. Hormonal therapy in dairy cows: Five ways to improve reproductive efficiency. Vet Med 1996;6: 571-575

Willard S., Gandy S., Bowers S., Graves K., Elias A., Whisnant C. The effects of GnRH administration postinsemination on serum concentrations of progesterone and pregnancy rates in dairy cattle exposed to mild summer heat stress. Theriogenology 2003;59:1799-1810

Williams SW., Stanko RL., Amstalden M., and Williams GL. Comparison of three approaches for synchronization of ovulation for timed artificial insemination in Bos indicus-influenced cattle managed on the Texas gulf coast. J. Anim. Sci. 2002;80:1173–1178

Wiltbank MC., Gtimen A., and Sartori R. Physiological classification of anovulatory conditions in cattle. Theriogenology 2002;57:21-52

Wiltbank M., Lopez H., Sartori R., Sangsritavong S., Gumen A. Changes in reproductive physiology of lactating dairy cows due to eleveted steroid metabolism. Theriogenology 2006;65:17-29

Wolf D., Schares G., Cardenas O., Huanca W., Cordero A., Barwald A., Conraths FJ., Gauly M., Zahner H., Bauer C. Detection of specific antibodies to Neospora caninum and Toxoplasma gondii in naturally infected alpacas (Lama pacos), llamas (Lama lama) and vicuñas (Lama vicugna) from Peru and Germany. Vet Parasitol 2005;130:81-87

Wolfenson D., Lew BJ., Thatcher WW., Graber Y., Meidan R. Seasonal and acute heat stress effects on steroid production by dominant follicles in cows. Anim Reprod Sci 1997;47:9-19

Wolfenson D., Roth Z., Meidan R. Impaired reproduction in heat-stressed cattle: basic and applied aspects. Anim Reprod Sci 2000;60-61:535-547.

Wolfenson D., Sonego H., Bloch A., Shaham-Albalancy A., Kaim M., Folman Y., Meidan R. Seasonal differences in progesterone production by luteinised bovine thecal and granulosa cells. Domest Anim Endocrinol 2002;22:81-90

Vanholder T., Opsomer G., Kruif de A. Aetiology and pathogenesis of cystic ovarian follicles in dairy cattle: a review. Reprod Nutr Dev 2006a;46:105–119

Vanholder T., Leroy JLMR., Coryn M., Fiers T., de Kruif A., Opsomer G. Effects of -OHbutyrate on bovine granulosa and theca cell function in vitro. Reprod Domest Anim 2006b;41:39-40.

Vasconcelos JLM., Silcox RW., Lacerda JA., Pursley JR., and WiltbankMC. Pregnancy rate, pregnancy loss, and response to heat stress after AI at two different times from ovulation in dairy cows. Biol. Reprod. 1997;56 (Suppl 1):140. (Abstr.)

Vasconcelos JLM., Silcox RW., Rosa GJ., Pursley JR., Wiltbank MC. Synchronisation rate, size of the ovulatory follicle and pregnancy rate after synchronisation of ovulation beginning on different days of the oestrous cycle in lactating dairy cows. Theriogenology 1999;52:1067-1078

Vasconcelos JLM., Demetrio DGB., Santos RM., Chiari JR., Rodrigues CA., Sa Filho OG. Factors potentially affecting fertility of lactating dairy cow recipients. Theriogenology 2006;65:192–200

Vasconcelos JL., Sa Filho OG., Campos Perez G., Takiguchi Nogueira Silva A. Intravaginal progesterone device and/or temporary weaning on reproductive performance of anestrous crossbred Angus×Nelore cows. Anim Reprod Sci 2009;111:302–311

Vries de A. Economic Value of Pregnancy in Dairy Cattle. J Dairy Sci. 2006a;89:3876–3885

Vries, de A., Crane MB., Bartolome JA., Melendez P., Risco CA., Archbald LF. Economic Comparison of Timed Artificial Insemination and Exogenous Progesterone as Treatments for Ovarian Cysts. J Dairy Sci 2006b; 89:3028–3037

De Vries A., Overton M., Fetrow J., Leslie K., Eicker S., G. Rogers G. Exploring the Impact of Sexed Semen on the Structure of the Dairy Industry. J Dairy Sci 2008;91:847–856

Xie S., Low BG., Nagel RJ., Kramer KK., Anthony RV., Zoli AP., Beckers JF., and R. M. Roberts. Identification of the major pregnancy-specific antigens of cattle and sheep as inactive members of the aspartic proteinase family. Proc Natl Acad Sci 1991; USA 88:10247–10251.

Xu ZZ., Verkerk GA., Mee JF., Morgan SR., Clark BA., Burke CR., and Burton LJ. Progesterone and follicular changes in postpartum noncyclic dairy cows after treatment with progesterone and estradiol or with progesterone, GnRH, $PGF_{2\alpha}$ and estradiol. Theriogenology 54:273–282and estradiol. Theriogenology 2000;54:273–282

Yavas Y., Walton JS. Induction of ovulation in post partum suckled beef cow: a review. Theriogenology 2000a;54:1-23

Yavas Y., and Walton JS. Postpartum acyclity in suckled beef cows: a review. Theriogenology 2000b;54:25-55

Younas M., Fuquay JW., Smith AE., Moore AB. Estrous and endocrine responses of lactating Holsteins to forced ventilation during summer. J Dairy Sci 1993;76:430-436s

Zerbe H., Schneider N., Leibold W., Wensing T., Kruip TA., Schuberth HJ. Altered functional and immunophenotypical properties of neutrophylic granulocytes in post partum cows associated with fatty liver. Theriogenology 2000; 54: 771-786

Zerbe H., Ossadnik C., Leibold W., Schuberth HJ. Influence of E. coli and Arcanobacterium pyogenes isolated from bovine puerperal uteri on phenotypic and functional properties of neutrophils. Vet Microbiol 2001;79:351-365

Zerbe H., Ossadnik C., Leibold W., Schuberth HJ. Localsecretions of Escherichia coli- or Arcanobacterium pyogenesinfected bovine uteri modulate the phenotype and the functional capacity of PMN granulocytes. Theriogenology 2002;57: 1161–1177.

3 Equine Reproduction

3.1 Physiology

3.1.1 Physiology of the oestrous cycle

Reproductive activity in the horse is seasonal; the natural breeding season for mares extends from early spring to late summer, which in the Northern Hemisphere means April to September, and in the Southern Hemisphere, October to March. Horses are called 'long-day' breeders because their normal cyclic activity is primarily activated by the increase in daylight length (i.e. longer photoperiod) in early spring, while in the late summer and early autumn, shortening of the daylight length (i.e. shorter photoperiod) triggers the termination of the breeding season.
Secondary factors in the spring, such as increasing temperature and improving dietary intake, hasten the onset of the breeding season. There is a strong relationship between photoperiod and the occurrence of ovulation. Figure 1 clearly shows the association between changes in photoperiod and the seasonality of reproduction.
Ovulation in the mare is minimal or absent during the winter and occurs at its maximum frequency in the summer. Spring and autumn are considered to be transitional periods and are characterized by frequent irregular oestrous cycles, varying in both the duration of the cycle and the timing of ovulation.

Figure 1 Association between photoperiod and reproductive seasonality.

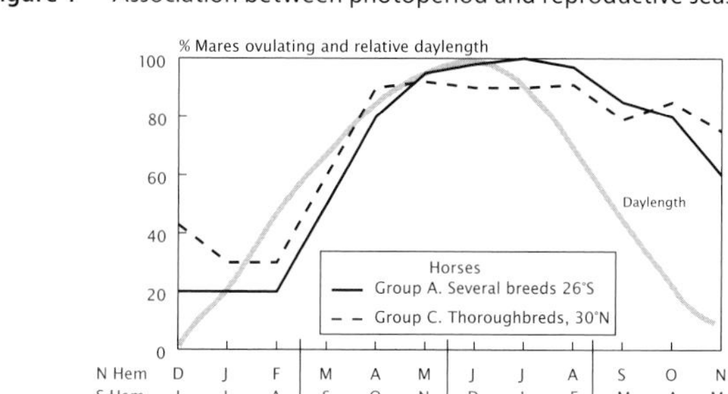

During the reproductive season, mares will come into heat on average every 21 (18-24) days; though ponies have a longer cycle on average (25 days). In mares, both follicle stimulating hormone (FSH) and luteinizing hormone (LH) secretion is driven specifically by bursts of gonadotrophin-releasing hormone. During the oestrous cycle of the mare, the concentrations of FSH rise twice. The first rise takes place from day 8 to 14 of the cycle and the second from day 15 until day 2 of the next cycle. Follicular waves in mares are of two types, major waves (with dominant and subordinate follicles) and minor waves (in which the largest follicle never attains the diameter of a dominant follicle).
Growth rates of the future ovulatory and non-ovulatory follicles of the ovulatory follicular wave begin to deviate when the diameter of the future ovulatory follicle reaches an average of 22.5mm (Ginther et al., 2008a). The ovulatory follicle grows at a rate of 3mm/day, reaching 35mm at day 4 (ovulation being day 0) or at the beginning of the pre-ovulatory period.
There are profound differences in wave patterns observed during the oestrous cycle in various breeds. In some breeds (e.g. quarter horses, ponies), only one major wave can usually be detected in late dioestrus which leads on to oestrus and ovulation. In other breeds (e.g. thoroughbreds), a secondary wave frequently develops in early dioestrus. The dominant follicle of this wave will either ovulate or be anovulatory.

LH is secreted in pulses from day 16 of the cycle until day 3 of the next cycle. Both the oestradiol and LH peri-ovulatory surges begin approximately 10 days before the peri-ovulatory period or near the end of luteolysis, and a day or two before follicle deviation. The prolonged ascending arm of the LH surge (10 days) with a peak occurring after ovulation, contrasts with the short ascending arm in cattle (about 4 hours) with the peak prior to ovulation (Ginther et al., 2008a).
Oestradiol is believed to be a key factor in generating a full LH surge in mares. It increases LH synthesis (Sharp et al., 1991; Robinson et al., 1995), induces the formation of pituitary GnRH receptors, and may augment GnRH secretion. Oestradiol from the dominant follicle creates a surge in the plasma that peaks on day 2 and then wanes. There is much evidence to indicate that the LH surge cannot begin until the dominant follicle secretes sufficient oestradiol, and cannot occur while oestrogen

positive feedback is inadequate (Irvine et al., 2000). A slight but significant increase in circulating progesterone can be detected consistently in mares on the day ovulation is detected.

Incidence of double ovulation
The incidence of double ovulation is thought to be strongly affected by breed, reproductive status, age, and repeatability in individual mares. The estimated double-ovulation rates among breeds and types are Thoroughbreds: 25%, Standardbreds: 15%, lactating and non-lactating Quarter Horses: 7 and 14% respectively, and ponies: 2% (Ginther et al., 2008a). It is also well documented that mares which have double ovulations, and therefore two corpora lutea, have higher circulating progesterone concentrations.

It is important for the equine veterinary practitioner to realize that there is a high level of repeatability in respect of many aspects of the oestrous cycle, follicle population, and gonadotrophin concentrations in individual mares (Jacob et al., 2009). These include the repeatability of double ovulations and a tendency for the pre-ovulatory follicle to reach a diameter characteristic for any particular individual.

Passage of fluid into the abdominal cavity at ovulation
Recent studies indicate that considerable hormone-laden follicular fluid passes through the fimbriae of the oviduct into the peritoneal cavity at ovulation (Ginther et al., 2008b). These hormones are absorbed from the peritoneal cavity and alter the circulating concentrations of oestradiol and inhibin, which in turn alter the concentrations of LH and FSH. King et al., (2008) postulated that prolactin in this fluid could be a contributor to the peri-ovulatory prolactin surge.

Oestrus lasts for about 5 (3-9) days and ovulation takes place 24-48 hours before the end of oestrus. Horses display a longer period of oestrus during the spring and autumn (7-10 days), than during the midsummer (4-5 days). Unlike the developing follicle, the corpus luteum is insensitive to day length, and dioestrus behaviour last 14-15 days consistently throughout the ovulatory season. Some studies have demonstrated slightly longer dioestrus during midsummer (16 days) than spring or late autumn (13 days) whereas others have detected no difference at all.

Season also has a pronounced effect on the sperm output and sexual behaviour of the stallion. Seasonal influence has been demonstrated on the reaction time (time between first visual contact and copulation) and the duration of copulation. Sperm production is at its maximum between late May and July. It is possible to bring sperm production forward by manipulating the photoperiod, but the effect does not usually last throughout the breeding season. The greatest sexual activity in stallions (in the Northern Hemisphere) is observed from March to the end of October.

3.1.2 Fertilization and pregnancy maintenance

Fertilization in mares takes place in the oviduct and is possible up to 30 hours after ovulation. Transport of the ovum through the oviduct into the uterus takes about 6 days. When it finally reaches the uterus, the equine embryo remains spherical in shape and migrates freely throughout the uterine lumen until day 17 after ovulation. This is the time when the primary maternal recognition of pregnancy takes place.

Thanks to extensive research, it is now quite clear that the constant movement of the equine embryo throughout the uterus between days 7 and 17 is necessary to ensure that maternal recognition of pregnancy is achieved in every part of the uterus (Allen 2001a). Therefore, for maintenance of early pregnancy, the endometrium needs to be in good condition (see 3.4.2) with no physical barriers to prevent the conceptus from moving freely through the lumen. Pathological changes within the endometrium, as well as large endometrial cysts or septa, can contribute to insufficient maternal recognition of the embryo and subsequent loss of the pregnancy.

By some mechanism, not yet clearly understood, mares suppress the normal cyclical upregulation of oxytocin receptors in the endometrium, and thereby prevent the release of the luteolytic prostaglandin $PGF_{2\alpha}$ in response to oxytocin release from the endometrium (Stout et al., 2000). Having escaped luteolysis

between days 14-16 after insemination, the function of the mare's corpus luteum is retained, but its progesterone production decreases steadily over the next 20 days. The progesterone supply is then supplemented by additional corpora lutea induced by chorionic gonadotrophin.
Between days 25 and 35 after ovulation, trophoblast cells begin to multiply, and around 36 to 38 days, they migrate deep into the maternal endometrium to form structures, unique to the equidae, known as endometrial cups. These are actively secretory and play a crucial part in the maintenance of pregnancy until the placenta can supply sufficient progesterone on its own at about day 100. Large amounts of equine chorionic gonadotrophin (eCG, also called pregnant mare serum gonadotrophin/PMSG) are produced and secreted by the endometrial cups between days 40 and 70 of pregnancy (Allen 2001a). In conjunction with pituitary FSH, eCG stimulates the development of accessory corporalutea, providing an additional source of progesterone. After day 70 of pregnancy, the endometrial cups begin to degenerate and the levels of eCG steadily decrease. Finally, at around 100 to 120 days, the necrotic cups detach from the surface of the endometrium, remaining free within the uterine lumen, where they sometimes lodge in the allantochorion to form the so-called allantochorionic pouch.
It is not until as late as day 40 after ovulation that the non-invasive trophoblast of the allantochorion begins to establish a stable, microvillous attachment to the luminal epithelial cells of the endometrium. The primary haemotrophic exchange unit of the non-invasive allantochorionic placenta, the microcotyledon, is formed by day 120 of pregnancy. Pregnancy in the mare lasts for 11 months (310-365 days).

The first oestrus after parturition, also called the 'foal heat', occurs at 5 to 15 days post partum. Although the fertility of this first heat is generally believed to be low, some horse owners attempt to breed the mare at this time. One of the reasons for this is the unpredictable duration of sexual inactivity in lactating mares.
When the mare is not pregnant, or when the pregnancy is not recognised, the uterine endometrium starts to secrete prostaglandin $PGF_{2\alpha}$ from day 14 to 16. The release of $PGF_{2\alpha}$ causes luteolysis of the corpus luteum, allowing the release of gonadotrophin, and the mare returns to oestrus.

3.1.3 Seasonal regulation of reproductive activity in the mare

Normal seasonal changes in reproductive activity of the mare are triggered by changes in the photoperiod, as well as by temperature and nutritional factors. The crucial transmission of the light signals to the hypothalamic-pituitary axis occurs via melatonin, a neurotransmitter secreted by the pineal gland; synthesis and release of melatonin is directly modulated by the photoperiod. Although the effect of photoperiod is well documented, the site of action of melatonin has not been studied extensively in horses. From studies in other species however, it is known that melatonin does not directly influence the secretion of GnRH, but acts through a complex neuro-endocrine network (Malpaux et al., 1999). Elevated concentrations of melatonin are only present in blood during the hours of darkness. At the end of the breeding season, the daylight length shortens, and temperature and natural food availability are reduced. Long periods of short days stimulate the production of melatonin, which in turn affects the release of GnRH from the hypothalamus. In contrast, at the beginning of breeding season, there is an inhibition of melatonin secretion because of the increasing daily photoperiod.

The neuro-endocrine mechanisms governing seasonality are assumed to involve modulation of the GnRH pulse frequency and, through this, the direct gonadotrophin signal to the ovaries. In the mare, the frequency of FSH and LH pulses increases gradually during the weeks preceding the first ovulation in the spring.

In mid-summer, two releases of FSH occur during each oestrous cycle: one in late oestrus or early dioestrus, and the second in mid-dioestrus. Similar to the observations in ponies, a change also appears to take place in the FSH profile in thoroughbred mares during the autumn transition period (from two surges to one surge per cycle) (Irvine et al., 2000). It has been proposed that, in mares, exposure to two periods of increased FSH concentrations is required for dominant follicles to mature. Thus, it may be that the absence of the early dioestrus surge in the autumn oestrous cycles is the reason for the reduced follicular development at the end of the season.

Although the final failure to ovulate is supposedly associated with the lack of a proper LH surge, corpus luteum function and

follicular oestrogen production are compromised several cycles earlier. It is possible that the FSH priming of the developing follicle becomes inadequate as the season progresses (Irvine et al., 2000).
Many studies have reported that the first failure to ovulate in autumn is associated with the absence of an LH surge and that the last surge is smaller in most of the mares studied (Nequin et al., 1998; Ginther et al., 2003). Reduction of the LH surge in cycles during the autumn may also affect corpus luteum function. A similar situation, but in reverse order, takes place during the transition from anoestrus to the breeding season. In approximately 50% of mares, sequential anovulatory follicular waves then develop, with the dominant follicle reaching a diameter similar to that of a pre-ovulatory follicle. These follicles fail to ovulate because of the suppression of GnRH secretion by neuronal mechanisms that inhibit LH stimulation. Furthermore, these large transitional follicles are thought to be unable to produce steroid hormones in sufficient quantity, though the reason for this is not clear.

Prolactin may also play a part in seasonal breeding in mares. Prolactin concentrations are high in the summer and low in the winter months (Evans et al., 1991). Treating mares with prolactin or drugs that stimulate prolactin secretion (e.g. sulpride) can hasten the first ovulation of spring (Besognet et al., 1997). In cycles in summer, sudden spikes of plasma prolactin concentration are observed shortly after luteolysis, closely followed by an increase in oestrone concentration (Shand et al., 1998). This could indicate the possible role of prolactin in follicular growth and maturation.

During seasonal anoestrus in the mare, the ovaries are deprived of gonadotrophin stimulation and remain small, compact and hard at rectal palpation, with indiscernible inner structures, and there is little tone in either the cervix or the body of the uterus. However, with the start of the breeding season, the ovaries become softer and several small follicles can usually be palpated easily.

At the beginning of the breeding period, mares often experience a transitory period of decreased ovarian activity, with small follicles which undergo atresia and are replaced by new developing ones. In March and April, approximately 70% of mares will show oestrus, although only 50% will ovulate at this time. In May and June, most mares clearly demonstrate oestrus, of shorter duration (5-6 days) which almost always leads to ovulation.

3.2 Reproductive management

3.2.1 Oestrus detection

The most common method of detecting oestrus in mares is called 'teasing', when exposing the mare to a stallion causes her to exhibit the external signs of oestrus. A mare in oestrus tolerates and even encourages the advances of a stallion. She squats, raises her tail, urinates, everts the clitoris ('clitoral wink') and stands still, as the stallion calls, nibbles, licks, even bites or threatens her. As the stallion nibbles her stifles and hocks, the mare may tilt her pelvis further. The posture of the oestrus mare, with the rounded back (kyphosis) is unlike the oestrus posture of other animals (e.g. cats, dogs, cattle, and rodents) which arch their backs (lordosis).
These signs can be vague at the beginning of the breeding season and early in oestrus, but will gradually become more evident as the season progresses, and towards the time of ovulation. Other external stimuli can reduce the demonstration of oestrus signs, such as the presence of a foal or an unfamiliar environment. In these circumstances, the judicious use of a 'twitch' can lead to the signs being more obvious.

If not in heat, mares approached from behind by an interested stallion, will pull back their ears, keep their tails down and try to kick him.

Nowadays, rectal ultrasound scanning to monitor the reproductive activity of mares is becoming commonplace in large breeding facilities, well-run stud farms and even with owners with a single mare. This technique allows for the timing of ovulation to be estimated with some precision, and for the early detection of many abnormalities within the reproductive tract. The number of natural services or artificial inseminations (AI) can thus be reduced, reducing the likelihood of venereally transmitted infections.

3.2.2 Mating

Ovulation takes place 24-48 hours before the end of oestrus and, since the length of oestrus can vary according to the season and the individual, prediction of the precise timing of ovulation (without the use of repeated ultrasound scanning) is practically impossible.

Mares can be inseminated from 30 hours before, to 12 hours after ovulation. Later insemination may result in pregnancy but early embryonic mortality becomes more likely.

3.2.3 Artificial insemination

Artificial insemination (AI) is becoming more common, as it offers certain advantages both in terms of management and health:

- a larger number of mares can be bred to a single stallion
- the mare can be bred at home, thus reducing the risks associated with transport and gathering horses from different locations
- the cost of transport and insurance are eliminated
- no need to risk injury transporting the new-born foal
- the risk of injury to mare, stallion and handlers, inevitable with natural mating, is much reduced
- reduced opportunities for the spread of venereal disease
- reduces the risk of mating causing contamination in 'problem' mares

Artificial insemination can be carried out with fresh, cooled or frozen-thawed semen. The first is used when the stallion and mare are housed close to each other so that the time from sperm collection to AI can be less than an hour. The second is suitable for AI with a 24-48 hour gap between collection and AI, and usually results in a conception rate similar to that obtained with fresh semen. The use of cooled semen is now a well-established technique, and many stallion owners have made cooled semen available in response to breeder demand. Some limitations still exist in that not all stallions produce ejaculates suitable for cooling, and the logistics of insemination must be very well managed, because of the relatively brief viability of cooled semen (24-48 hours).

The quality of the semen, the breeding status of the mare and her management during the oestrus period are the three factors with the greatest impact on pregnancy rates achieved in a frozen semen breeding programme.
Mares to be bred with frozen semen should be monitored beforehand for regular and normal cyclicity. All mares (except maidens <6 years old) should have their uterus sampled for culture and cytology at least once. Maiden mares with any evidence of fluid accumulation must undergo the same procedure. When breeding mares with frozen semen, ovulation should be induced with hCG, for example (Chorulon®), to optimize the use of semen by minimizing the number of inseminations per oestrus.
Due to the wide range in the timing of ovulation, when mares are treated with hCG, they should be examined by rectal palpation and ultrasonography every 6–8 hours after the injection, so that they can be inseminated when ovulation is imminent or as soon as it has been detected.

One of the most important reasons that frozen equine semen is not more widely used is the variation in the capacity of sperm from different stallions to tolerate freezing and thawing. It is thought that only 25% of stallions will support pregnancy rates comparable with those of fresh semen AI, or natural mating, even with healthy mares inseminated at the best time (Vidament et al., 1997). When properly used, the average pregnancy rate per cycle with frozen semen is around 30–40% with 1.8–2 cycles per pregnancy.
However, pregnancy rates per cycle commonly vary between 0 and 100% (Loomis 2001; Samper 2001).

There is still some controversy about whether mares should be bred just prior to or just after ovulation. It is becoming evident that more than one insemination with frozen semen in the same cycle results in a slightly, but consistently, higher pregnancy rate compared to a single insemination (Vidament et al., 1997). Although there is no actual consensus for the recommended timing of insemination with frozen semen, 19/21 laboratories suggest breeding between 6 hours before and 6 hours after ovulation (Samper and Morris 1998). A retrospective study by Barbacini et al. (1999) suggested that there is no significant difference in pregnancy rates when mares are bred 6 hours prior to or 6 hours after ovulation.

For many years, the standard procedure when inseminating mares with frozen semen has been to deposit the semen in the uterine body. However, several groups have recently reported differences in pregnancy rates when mares were bred with reduced sperm numbers at the utero-tubal junction ipsilateral to the ovary which contained the pre-ovulatory follicle. It appears that breeding deep in the uterine horn or close to the uterotubal junction maximizes sperm usage, increases the number of sperm in the oviduct which could result in higher pregnancy rates of mares bred with frozen semen.

The number of spermatozoa per inseminate for fresh, cooled and frozen semen have been established. Mares are typically inseminated with 500 million progressively motile spermatozoa (PMS) immediately after collection, or one billion PMS that have been cooled and stored for 24 hours at 5°C. The typical dose for mares inseminated with frozen semen varies from 400 to 800 million spermatozoa. There are occasions when semen is limited and insemination with fewer sperm is advantageous. Low-dose deposition of equine sperm can be carried out either with a guiding hand inserted in the rectum or by using an endoscope. Hysteroscopic insemination with small numbers of fresh or frozen spermatozoa is now being used to obtain pregnancies by stallions whose semen is in short supply.

3.2.4 Embryo transfer

Embryo transfer (ET) in horses is a technique developed relatively recently, which allows more than one foal per year to be obtained from valuable mares. The major candidates for embryo transfer include older mares unable to carry a foal themselves, and those competing in racing, polo or other sports. Their genetic potential can be used to produce foals carried by surrogate mares.
The majority of equine embryos currently collected originate from spontaneous single ovulations. They are usually collected by flushing the donor's uterine lumen between 7 and 8 days after ovulation (Squires et al., 2003). The procedure is performed with an appropriate culture media including protein and antibiotics to ensure a high rate of embryo survival and eliminate possible bacterial contamination. The embryos are evaluated to check their morphology and suitability before they are transferred.
As in other species, the success of embryo transfer is heavily dependent on the management of the recipient. The highest pregnancy rates are obtained when the recipient ovulates either the day before the donor, or up to 3 days after the donor mare.
At present it is possible to cool and store embryos at 5°C, which allows them to be transported over longer distances. But the conservation of equine embryos at low temperatures has not been pursued as dynamically as in cattle. Most of the equine breed registers do not approve of foals which have developed from frozen embryos.
Moreover, as superovulation is not yet well established, and yields poor results, there are only very few frozen embryos from which to benefit. There are technical difficulties also, since equine embryos are enclosed in an acellular protein capsule which allows only limited penetration of the cryoprotectant, which restricts the ability to freeze them.

Numerous attempts have already been tried to induce multiple ovulations in mares, including the administration of eCG/PMSG, GnRH, porcine FSH and equine pituitary extract, as well as immunization against inhibin (Squires et al., 2003; 2007). So far, however, no procedure or product has produced good enough, or repeatable enough, results in mares.

A recent publication by Logan et al. (2007) reported on the use of equine FSH (eFSH) in superovulation protocols in mares. The study evaluated the effect of pre-treatment with progesterone and oestradiol on the follicular response to eFSH, and compared doses of eFSH and ovulatory agents on follicular development and ovulation. The number of pre-ovulatory follicles was greater for mares given 12.5 mg of eFSH compared to those given 6.25 mg. The number of ovulations was greatest in mares given 12.5 mg of eFSH twice daily followed by hCG administration. However, there was no advantage in treating them with progesterone and oestradiol prior to eFSH administration.

3.3 Control of oestrus

The natural breeding season in horses in the Northern Hemisphere is from April to October, but there are several reasons to try to influence the normal patter of reproduction. In racehorses and trotters the performance of 'two-year-olds' and 'three-yearolds' is important. The age of the horse is always measured from 1st January onwards and, therefore, in the racing industry, it is important that foals are born as early as possible after the 1st of January so that they can reach as much of their mature body weight (and strength) as possible by the time they compete as two and three year olds. On stud farms, it can be advantageous to synchronize oestrus to enable the better planning of the process. Oestrus synchronization maximizes the number of cycles per year in which a mare can be bred. In the case of ET, it is necessary to synchronize recipients with donors, of course.

3.3.1 Transition period

Several methods have been investigated to hasten the onset of the breeding season in the mare. Breeders are under economic pressure to breed mares as early as possible in the year to have a 'real-time' age advantage over foals born later in the year (as explained in 3.3). Recently foaled mares generally have few problems coming into oestrus early in the season, because of the hormonal activity at the end of pregnancy. Induction of cyclicity in maiden or barren mares is a far more difficult task, however.

Photoperiodic stimulation
Most of the work in recent decades has focused on the role of the photoperiod in reproduction. It has been demonstrated that artificially simulating long days can be used to advance the time of the first oestrus and ovulation (Nagy et al., 2000). Even though increasing daylight length is the natural means of inducing cyclic ovarian activity in early spring, the artificial stimulation of the same process needs to begin as early as December. Even then there is considerable individual variation in the interval from the start of the treatment to the first ovulation.

The success of the management of the photoperiod depends not so much on the total number of hours of light per day but much more on the pattern of light over the 24-hour period. Many observations have indicated that, as in other seasonally breeding species, mares have a photosensitive phase during the normal period of darkness. The presence or absence of light 9.5 hours after the onset of darkness, rather than the total hours of light and dark, are important for the response. Cyclic ovarian activity can be induced in seasonal anoestrus mares by applying a 1- to 2-hour period of artificial light approximately 9.5 - 10 hours after the abrupt beginning of the dark phase.

The combination of manipulation of the photoperiod and GnRH treatment (see later in this section) has been reported to produce better results than are achieved with the former technique alone (Lowis et al., 1991). Traditionally, the recommended intensity of light to use is about 100 lux and the treatment needs to be continued beyond the first ovulation.

Progestagens
The basis of the use of progestagens to induce oestrus and ovulation is the inhibitory effect of exogenous progestagens on the hypothalamic-pituitary axis. They have been widely used in an attempt to hasten the onset of cyclic ovarian activity and to minimize the occurrence of irregular or prolonged oestrus periods in mares during the transition period (Squires 1993; Nagy et al., 1998a,b). Administration of altrenogest (Regumate Equine®) for 2-3 days is required to eliminate the signs of oestrus, but they will return 2 days after the withdrawal of the

progestagen. As mares may ovulate during treatment, it is recommended that $PGF_{2\alpha}$ (e.g., Estrumate®) be given at the end of the treatment if the mare is intended for immediate breeding.
Regardless of the type of progestagen, it has been shown on numerous occasions that only mares in the middle-to-late transition period (generally defined as those with follicles of 25 mm in diameter or larger) respond favourably to progestin treatment.

Recent publications have also reported attempts to use progesterone-releasing intravaginal devices in mares which were developed for use in cattle (Ataman et al., 2000; Klug et al., 2001; Handler et al., 2006). Although a degree of oestrus induction and synchronization has been obtained, the use of these products in the field is reported to be associated with a variable degree of vaginal discharge, and low retention rate. Moreover, these products are not authorized for use in horses.

Gonadotrophin-releasing hormone
The use of GnRH seems to be the most successful method for inducing oestrus early in the transition period, especially when combined with photoperiodic stimulation (Lowis 1991). Ever since the earliest studies, GnRH has received a great deal of interest because of the applications in the modern equine breeding industry due to its capacity to stimulate follicular growth and ovulation.
Alexander and Irvine (1991) showed that LH pulses occurred 2-3 times daily during dioestrus and 30 times a day during oestrus. Portable, programmable, battery-operated minipumps are available to simulate this pattern artificially. Experiments have demonstrated that low doses of GnRH given hourly, or every 8 hours, can induce the development of pre-ovulatory follicles, though more frequent injections are required to induce ovulation.
In one of the trials, injections of GnRH given three times daily between January to March, followed by hCG administration, induced oestrus within 12 days in all the 49 mares studied. Pregnancy rate was about 50%. Ginther and Berfelt (1990) injected anoestrus mares twice daily with GnRH analogue and advanced the time of ovulation in responsive mares by an

average of 40 days, compared to the controls. Studies by Harrison et al. (1990) noted encouraging results when a synthetic GnRH analogue, buserelin (Receptal®), was administered to anoestrus mares twice daily over a prolonged period.

3.3.2 Breeding season

Oestrus is often induced during the breeding season in order to treat fertility disorders (see 3.4). Other than for therapeutic purposes, induction during the breeding season (reviewed by Squires et al., 2008) can be used for the following indications:

- *Shortening of the first post partum luteal phase in order to hasten the onset of the oestrus after the 'foal heat'.*
  There has been much discussion about breeding mares at the foal heat. Because of puerperal infections, and inadequate uterine involution, the second oestrus after foaling is usually more fertile. By inducing the second oestrus at 20 days post partum, the usual 21 days lost waiting for it to occur naturally after the foal oestrus can be reduced.
  A single dose of $PGF_{2\alpha}$ or its analogue (e.g. Estrumate®) can be administered 4 to 6 days after the ovulation of the foal heat.

- *Induction of oestrus when the previous ovulation dates are known*
  Specific indications for this procedure might include a missed breeding, diagnostic or therapeutic considerations, and synchronization of oestrus with the availability of the stallion or ET. A single dose of $PGF_{2\alpha}$ analogue is usually administered 4 to 6 days after the previous ovulation.

- *Induction of oestrus when the previous ovulation dates are unknown*
  This technique has a practical application in the synchronization of a group of mares for breeding or for ET, for example. In this regimen, two doses of $PGF_{2\alpha}$ are administered 14 to 18 days apart.

- *Induction of oestrus following synchronization based on progestagen programmes.*
  A single dose of $PGF_{2\alpha}$ analogue is administered on the last day of progestagen treatment to ensure the complete elimination of luteal tissue. This can be followed 4-5 days later by hCG (e.g. Chorulon®, 1500-3000 IU) administration to ensure the proper timing of ovulation.

In the majority of mares, the corpus luteum is sensitive to exogenous $PGF_{2\alpha}$ by the 4th day after ovulation (Meyers 1991). The follicular status of the ovary also has an effect on the possible interval between treatment with $PGF_{2\alpha}$ and the onset of oestrus and ovulation. Spontaneous dioestrus ovulation takes place in approximately 5% of equine oestrous cycles. In some cases, they may account for the failure of luteolysis following the use of $PGF_{2\alpha}$. Nonetheless, it can be concluded that in the majority of mares, the administration of $PGF_{2\alpha}$ or its analogues on day 5 after ovulation will lead to the onset of oestrus and subsequent ovulation within 3-4 days, and the effect of administration on day 9 after ovulation, will be within 9-10 days.
A recent study reported by Newcombe et al. (2008) evaluated the effect of a cloprostenol (Estrumate®) dose on the interval before ovulation in mares treated in dioestrus. The results demonstrated a significant effect of both dose and follicular diameter at the time of cloprostenol administration on the interval between treatment and ovulation. The shortest mean interval (2.4 days) was observed after the administration of higher doses in mares with follicles 36 mm or larger, whereas the longest (4.9 days) occurred after the treatment with smaller doses when follicles were 28 to 31 mm in diameter. Moreover, these authors stressed that mares with large follicles at the time of the administration of PGF should be monitored closely to ensure that the ovulation is not missed.

3.3.3 Induction of ovulation

Oestrus normally lasts for 5 to 7 days in the breeding season, and ovulation takes place 24 to 48 hours before the end of the oestrus period. Mares are most fertile just before, or around the time of ovulation. Since the time of ovulation cannot be reliably predicted, mares are usually bred every second day until ovulation has occurred.

Being able to time an ovulation has many advantages for the equine practitioner, including (1) reduction in the number of matings needed by highly popular stallions; (2) increased accuracy in the timing of breeding when using imported frozen semen or stallions whose fresh semen is viable for a short time only; (3) reduction in the number of matings or inseminations with problem or difficult mares; and (4) optimization of the use of desirable but sub-fertile stallions.

Currently there are two types of hormone used to induce ovulation in mares, human chorionic gonadotropin (hCG) and gonadotrophin releasing hormone (GnRH), both of which have been used for many years (reviewed by Samper 2008; Squires 2008). For hCG the typical dose is 2500 IU given intravenously when the mare is in behavioural oestrus and has a follicle greater than 35 mm. Ovulation occurs in the next 48 hours with a 83-89% response rate (Duchamp et al., 1987, Barbacini et al., 2000; Grimmert and Perkings 2001).

Human chorionic gonadotrophin has been demonstrated to induce antibodies with high doses and frequent dosing. However, repeated administration of normal doses (1500-3000 IU), even in 5-6 consecutive cycles, did not interfere with fertility (Roser et al., 1979; Wilson et al., 1990). Although there is no evidence that hCG has a direct positive effect on pregnancy rate, several studies report a better pregnancy rate in hCG-treated mares: when treated before ovulation, pregnancy rates were 66% versus 50% in the controls (Woods et al., 1990). The higher rates were probably the result of the tighter synchronization of ovulation and mating/AI.

The efficacy of hCG treatment and ovulatory response are heavily dependent on the ovulatory follicle diameter at the time of the treatment. It is advisable to treat mares only when the ovulatory follicle has reached the diameter of 3.5mm or more.

Gonadotrophin-releasing hormone has also been recommended for the induction of ovulation in cyclic mares. Various regimes of GnRH administration have been studied involving intermittent injection (Bott et al., 1996; McKinnon et al., 1997; Barrier-Battut et al., 2001), pulsatile administration (Johnston, 1986; Becker and Johnston, 1992), slow-release implants (Meyers et al., 1997) and a single injection (Duchamp et al., 1987). Barier-Battut et

al. (2001) observed that most mares treated twice daily with an intravenous dose of 20 or 40 mcg of buserelin ovulated within 48 hours. Similar results were obtained by Camillo et al. (2004), but these authors claimed a more closely compact ovulation when hCG was used. A recently reported study by Levy and Duchamp (2007) concluded that a single administration of buserelin induces ovulation in the mare during the breeding season, a treatment suitable for the usual conditions of veterinary practice.
Recently, the use of the GnRH analogue deslorelin (Ovuplant®) as an implant has been approved for the induction of ovulation in mares. It is indicated for use in mares displaying behavioural oestrus and with a follicle of at least 30mm in diameter (McKinnon et al., 1993, 1997).The results of the study reported by Vandervall et al. (2001) confirmed previous reports that although the ovulatory response and fertility were no different for hCG- and Ovuplant®-treated mares, any of the latter group which failed to become pregnant, had a significantly delayed return to oestrus and prolonged inter-ovulatory interval. In the study reported by Blanchard (2002) treatment of mares with either hCG or deslorelin resulted in similar ovulatory responses and pregnancy rates. Deslorelin-treated mares, however, had fewer ovarian follicles ≥ 20mm in diameter 16 days after treatment, than did hCG treated mares.

A recent study by Berezowski et al. (2004) compared efficacy and tightness of the ovulations induced by hCG (Chorulon®), deslorelin implant (Ovuplant®) and deslorelin injection. All three products produced an acceptable response for use in clinical practice, with no differences between them in the proportion of mares ovulating within 2 days of treatment.

Suppression of oestrus in performance mares
Oestrus behaviour can sometimes be a problem in show mares. Progestagen therapy with altrenogest (Regumate Equine®) is effective in suppressing oestrus behaviour. If the mare is in oestrus when treatment is begun, oestrus behaviour is usually suppressed in 2-3 days. When therapy with progestagens is considered for performing animals, any local regulations for the use of pharmaceutical products in competing horses should be taken into consideration.

3.4 Reproductive disorders

3.4.1 Retained placenta

Blanchard et al. (1990) gave an overview on the management of dystocia in the mare, in which the problem of retained placenta was also discussed. In mares, the placenta is normally expelled 30 minutes to 3 hours after parturition. When it takes longer than this, there are risks of toxic metritis, septicaemia, toxaemia, laminitis and even death, which increase with time. The risk of these complications depends to a large extent on the management of the mare. Observations involving 3500 well managed Standard bred mares revealed that 10.6% suffered from retained placenta, but none of them developed toxic metritis or laminitis.

Retained placenta may result in the delayed involution of the uterus and impaired fertility at the foal heat.

Treatment of retained placenta is usually by the administration of oxytocin, alone or in combination with other medications. Oxytocin can be administered subcutaneously or intramuscularly at a dose of 20 IU, and can be repeated every few hours. The placenta is normally expelled within 1-2 hours after administration (Blanchard and Varner 1993). Larger doses of oxytocin will lead to intense spasmodic uterine contractions and may cause considerable distress to the mare. The administration of 60 IU in an intravenous infusion of 1-2 litres saline solution leads to expulsion in 75% of cases.

In addition, gentle traction on the placenta can be applied, but any more forceful traction which might damage the uterus, tear the placenta or lead to uterine prolapse, should be strictly avoided. Uterine lavage results in a more complete separation of the chorionic villi and removes small pieces of the placenta and debris which may be present in the uterus. Uterine lavage can be combined with oxytocin treatment. Intra-uterine and/or systemic antibiotic treatment can prevent the development of septicaemia. Should signs of toxaemia occur, non-steroidal anti-inflammatory drugs (NSAID) are indicated (Blanchard and Varner 1993).

3.4.2 Endometritis/Endometriosis

The majority of mares that do not become pregnant after mating suffer, or have already suffered, from various disorders of the endometrium. Degenerative changes in the uterus are associated with advancing age, and bacterial and other infections can lead to inflammatory changes. Contagious Equine Metritis (CEM) plays an important role. However, it is not appropriate to discuss CEM here; it is a specialised topic, and many countries have their own statutory regulations to control the disease.

Endometritis after mating

A transient endometritis always occurs in mares after mating, due to the inevitable contamination and the irritant effect of semen (Watson 2000; LeBlanc and Causey 2008). Whether bred by natural mating or artificial insemination, breaching the cervix at breeding results in a similarly intense inflammatory response in genitally normal mares.

However, some mares go on to develop persistent endometrial inflammation. Sperm induced persistent endometrial inflammation has been suggested as contributory to fertility problems in mares because of the altered uterine environment and consequently reduced embryonic survival.

The most critical factor in the uterine defences against infection is the rapid, physical clearance of inflammatory debris from the uterus after mating or foaling. Typically, mares with persistent inflammation have been subject to a number of predisposing factors such as poor perineal conformation, a dependent uterus, and delayed expulsion of uterine debris due to suboptimal myometrial contractility. Several studies link susceptibility to infection with the impaired clearance of debris. Mares experimentally unable to fight off an intra-uterine bacterial challenge with *Streptococcus equi zooepidemicus* within 96 hours are described as susceptible to endometritis (Card 2005). Mares able to clear the bacterial contamination are considered to be resistant to endometritis. Uterine myo-electrical activity is markedly delayed and activity is less intense in susceptible mares, compared with those in resistant mares after intrauterine inoculation with *S. equi ssp. zooepidemicus*.

Peak endometrial inflammation is reached usually 12-24h after breeding (Katila 2001). Susceptible mares accumulate uterine fluid and retain endometrial oedema for 3-5 days post-insemination. If inflammation persists, there can be a long-standing influx of lymphocytes and plasma cells into the endometrium, possibly contributing to chronic degenerative changes and impairment of endometrial function.

Changes in the conformation of the vulva predispose the mare to uterine infection. Vulvoplasty for the closure of the upper vulvar lips improves fertility and is a well established procedure (Hemberg et al., 2005). Repeated foaling and breeding can cause anatomical defects, such as poor perineal conformation, an incompetent vagino-vestibular sphincter, vaginal stretching, an incompetent cervix or a pendulous uterus, as well as degenerative changes, such as an abnormal myometrium, periglandular fibrosis, vascular degeneration, lymphangiectasia, scarring and atrophy of endometrial folds or damage to the mucociliary apparatus. Any of these defects can interfere with uterine drainage and thus play an important part in the pathogenesis of endometritis (Hurtgen 2006).

To improve pregnancy rates in susceptible mares requires the early detection of inflammatory changes by means of rectal palpation, ultrasound examination and/or endometrial cytology, and timely intervention to manage the persistent endometrial inflammation. A typical sign of inflammation is the accumulation of fluid in the uterus, seen during ultrasound examination. The diagnosis of endometritis should be confirmed by cytology. The histological characteristics of endometritis involve infiltration by polymorphonuclear leukocytes (PMN), lymphocytes and macrophages (Card 2005; LeBlanc and Causey 2008). Although there are several schemes for interpreting cytological findings, in general the presence of >5% neutrophils is considered indicative of endometrial inflammation (Card 2005).
Endometrial biopsy is a valuable tool for identifying the cause of subclinical endometritis and especially for determining treatment success (LeBlanc and Causey 2008). Histopathological changes can be classified as inflammatory (acute, subacute or chronic) and non-inflammatory, including endometrial hypoplasia, hyperplasia and chronic degenerative conditions of the uterus.

Severe degenerative processes, such as elastosis, lymphangiectasia, excessive exudate, loss of epithelium and epithelial hyperplasia, will interfere with a mare's ability to become pregnant (LeBlanc and Causey 2008).

The decision to treat a mare for persistent post-mating inflammation should be based on history and clinical signs such as poor uterine tone, intra-uterine accumulation of fluid, exfoliative endometrial cytological evaluation and bacterial culture/sensitivity. Mares presented for breeding which are considered to be susceptible to endometritis (predisposing factors, history of endometritis after previous matings) should be examined by ultrasound every day or every other day during oestrus and especially for 1–2 days after breeding, to identify any patterns of uterine oedema, the presence and location of intrauterine fluid accumulations, to monitor response to therapy and to record ovulations.

Treatment of endometritis

The treatment of endometritis in mares is generally aimed at physically assisting the uterus to clear inflammatory debris and other contaminants. Other therapeutic objectives are the correction of defects in the uterine defences, neutralizing virulent bacteria and controlling post-breeding inflammation (LeBlanc and Causey 2008).

- *Uterine lavage (flushing)*

  Uterine lavage assists in removing the contaminated uterine contents. There is no risk of development of resistance, and uterine contractions are stimulated. It can be performed pre- or post-mating. Uterine irrigation conducted as early as 4 h post-mating has no harmful effect on pregnancy rates. It is most commonly performed in repeat breeder mares and in mares with more than 2 cm of intrauterine fluid post-mating.

  One litre three times a day for three days is advisable, and it should be continued until the fluid returning from the uterus is seen to be clear. Following the final flush, 20 IU oxytocin (e.g. Intertocine -S®) can be given to assist the evacuation of the uterine contents. Saline can be used for flushing, or a stock solution of povidone iodine, diluted (1:1000) in distilled water, as an alternative as it is effective against some bacterial and yeast infections.

- *Hormone therapy.*

  The most common approach involves single or multiple oxytocin injections, 3-12 hours after mating (Pycock 1996; Watson 2000). Oxytocin injection is often accompanied by the local administration of antibiotics or uterine lavage.

  Oxytocin does not appear to be effective in all mares that accumulate intrauterine fluid. Factors that may affect the response include an inadequate number of endometrial receptors, a pendulous uterus, a closed cervix and an excessive dose resulting in inappropriate contractions, the abnormal propagation of uterine contractions or prolonged inflammation. If a clinician suspects that oxytocin does not stimulate appropriate drainage, it may be beneficial to administer cloprostenol instead.

  During oestrus the uterus is better able to resolve uterine infections. If a corpus luteum is present, $PGF_{2\alpha}$ treatment will bring mares into oestrus, providing an extra physiological stimulus to address the infection, without the risk of introducing micro-organisms by intra-uterine treatment. The use of prostaglandin after AI proved to be efficient in eliminating accumulated uterine fluid, but seemed to go on to affect the developing corpus luteum as well (Troedsson et al., 2001; Brendemuehl et al., 2002). Administration of cloprostenol more than 12 hours after ovulation is associated with a decrease in plasma progesterone concentrations decreased pregnancy rates have also been reported when cloprostenol was given 2 days after ovulation. Therefore, it is advisable to limit the treatment time to within 12 hours of ovulation.

  Oestrogens have been used with success in a daily dose of 6-10 mg intramuscularly, starting during oestrus and continuing for 3 days after ovulation. The treatment can be combined with antibiotics or uterine lavage.

- *Antibiotics.*

  Antibiotics of known suitability for intra-uterine use should be chosen on the basis of sensitivity testing. Endometritis is commonly treated by the intrauterine infusion of an appropriate antibiotic for 3–5 days during oestrus. Antibiotic infusions should be preceded by uterine irrigation because exudate in the uterine lumen may inactivate or dilute the

infused antibiotic to a sub-therapeutic concentration. Intrauterine antibiotic treatment should be avoided during dioestrus, as treatment during the progesterone phase has resulted in the development of resistant bacterial and fungal infections (McDonnell and Watson 1992).
Disinfectants and antibiotics can induce severe local reactions, resulting in persistent fibrosis and intra-uterine adhesions. In case of suspected hypersensitivity, the uterus should be flushed with large volumes of distilled water solution. Systemic antibiotics have also been used to treat endometritis because uterine irritation and the potential for the introduction of bacterial contamination to the endometrium are avoided, and the duration of treatment is not dictated by the oestrous cycle. Moreover, systemic therapy eliminates the need to invade the vestibule, vaginal canal and cervix. Pycock and Newcombe (1996) demonstrated positive results with combined antibiotic and oxytocin therapy achieving subsequent pregnancy rates higher than those achieved with the use of intravenous oxytocin or intra-uterine antibiotics on their own.

Embryo transfer could represent a management technique invaluable as a method of obtaining foals from mares with persistent chronic endometritis, a history of repeated early embryonic death or abortion, and non-responsive, persistent mating-induced endometritis.

Endometriosis
The term endometriosis was introduced by Kenney (1992) who summarized the specific alterations of the equine endometrium, and was modified by Schoon et al. (1992). Currently the condition is defined as an active or inactive periglandular and/or stromal endometrial fibrosis including glandular alterations within fibrotic foci.
Until now, little has been known about the aetiology and pathogenesis of this major cause of equine infertility. The degree of endometriosis in mares increases with age, but there is no association with the number of foalings. A recent study reported by Hoffmann et al. (2009) suggested that all fibrotic foci were independent of the hormonal control mechanism of the uterus. These authors concluded that cyclic and seasonal endocrine changes seemed to have no effect on the progression of the disease, and that various types of endometriosis therefore

represent different stages in the fibrotic process, possibly leading to the destruction of the glands and the subsequent development of a stromal fibrosis.

The diagnosis of endometriosis is made by histopathological examination of a uterine biopsy, when the features are likely to be periglandular fibrosis, cystic dilation of endometrial glands and glandular necrosis. The first sign of endometriosis is atypical morphological and functional differentiation of periglandular endometrial stromal cells.
There can often be 2-3 layers of fibrotic tissue around glands, but as many as 10 in severe cases. The initial stage of fibrosis is characterized by the presence of large polygonal periglandular stromal cells (type I) that produce collagen fibres. In advanced fibrosis, the histological picture is dominated by metabolically active or inactive stromal cells (type II), without signs of collagen synthesis, as well as myofibroblasts. The contractibility of the latter may lead to a constriction of uterine glands resulting in glandular dilatation. Additionally, myofibroblasts may be able to affect the composition and extent of the extracellular matrix by secreting different mediators.
With an internationally accepted scoring system (Kenney and Doing 1986), a reliable prognosis can be made about the possibility of the mare conceiving and carrying to term (Table 1).

Table 1 Expected foaling rates in mares according to the histological classification of the endometrium.

Mare category	Degree of endometrial pathology	Expected foaling rate (%)
I	absent	80-90
IIA	mild	50-60
IIB	moderate	10-50
III	severe	< 10

Treatment of endometriosis
Endometriosis is more or less irreversible, though treatment has been attempted by physical and chemical curettage. Although the anatomy of the equine uterus does not allow for complete

curettage, it has been possible to demonstrate an improvement in conception rate. Chemical curettage has been carried out with a variety of different products: DMSO (50 ml of a 30 or 50% solution), collagenase (100 mg in 50 ml physiological saline), povidone iodine solutions or filtered *Streptococcus* cultures. In each case, the treatment induces a transient inflammation and activation of the endometrial glands.

Placentitis

Equine placentitis and the resulting loss of pregnancy are becoming an increasingly recognised problem in the breeding industry. The majority of placental infections are caused by ascending infections from the environment. The most commonly isolated microorganisms include: *Streptococcus equi zooepidemicus, Escherichia coli, Pseudomonas aeruginosa, Klebsiella pneumoniae* and *nocardioform species* (Giles et al., 1993). The placenta can also become infected by viruses and fungi, but these organisms usually cause abortion earlier in gestation.

Although bacterial infection initiates disease, it has been postulated, based on recent work from an experimental model of ascending placentitis in pony mares, that premature delivery may occur secondary to inflammation of the chorion rather than as a consequence of foetal infection (Macpherson et al., 2008).

The most common clinical presentation for the mare with placentitis is premature udder development, with or without vulval discharge (Macpherson et al., 2008). However, vulval discharge is a particularly inconsistent clinical finding in mares with bacterial placentitis.

Transrectal ultrasonographic examination of the caudal reproductive tract has become a commonplace tool in the diagnosis of placentitis. Mares with placental infection or inflammation exhibit an increased CTUP (combined thickness of the uterus and placenta). Separation of the membranes from the endometrium can also be observed. In some individuals, purulent hyperechoic material may accumulate in pockets between the chorioallantois and the endometrium. Thickening of the amnion may also indicate inflammation.

Treatment options include broad spectrum antibiotics in an attempt to eliminate the bacterial infection, anti-inflammatory drugs such as flunixin meglumine (believed to prevent the release of prostaglandins) as well as progestagens, such as altrenogest, which is often used to sustain pregnancy in mares (Macpherson 2005). A recent review by Macpherson and Bailey (2008) provided an overview of the various therapeutic substances used in the treatment of placentitis in mares (Tab 2).

Table 2 Products commonly used to treat placentitis in the mare (adapted from Macpherson and Bailey 2008)

Action	Active substance	Dose, route, and frequency
Antimicrobial	Potassium penicillin Procaine penicillin Ceftiofur Cefazolin Trimethoprim sulfa	22,000 units/kg, i.v., qid 22,000 units/kg, i.m., bid 2.2 mg/kg, i.v. or i.m., bid 20 mg/kg, i.v., qid 15–30 mg/kg, p.o., bid
Anti-inflammatory	Flunixin meglumine Phenylbutazone Pentoxifylline	1 mg/kg, i.v., bid 2.2–4.4 mg/kg, p.o., bid 8.5 mg/kg, p.o., bid
Tocolytic/uterine quiescence	Altrenogest Isoxuprine	0.088 mg/kg, p.o., sid 1 mg/kg, sid

3.4.3 Persistent corpus luteum

A persistent corpus luteum is an important cause of infertility in the mare, which should be differentiated from true anoestrus by blood progesterone assay and ultrasound examination. Treatment with $PGF_{2\alpha}$ is simple and usually successful.

3.4.4 Post partum anoestrus

Fewer than 10% of mares fail to ovulate within 20 days of foaling, so there is no condition of lactational anoestrus, as such, in the mare (Deischel and Aurich 2005). However, there is some evidence that fertility is affected to a certain degree by lactation.

Post partum anoestrus is therefore mostly used to describe a lack of cyclicity after the foal heat, due to a persistent corpus luteum. These mares can be successfully treated with prostaglandins and bred at the next oestrus. Sometimes hCG or GnRH are used as an extra stimulus to ovulation.
Treatment of mares with inactive ovaries needs to be started early by giving, for example, between 2 and 4 doses per day of Receptal® (to a maximum of 10 ml) for 5-7 days, or until oestrus is observed.

3.4.5 Prolonged oestrus

Prolonged oestrus usually occurs at the end of the transition period and is often due to the presence of a large, persistent follicle, actively producing oestrogen. Progestagen therapy is usually successful (Allen et al., 1990) but hCG has not proved to be useful.
A progesterone-releasing intra-vaginal device (PRID®) has been successful in suppressing oestrus; a normal oestrus ensues after removal of the device, in most mares (Rutten et al., 1986). Oral progestagen (e.g. Regumate®) can also be used, and the next oestrus will usually begin 2-3 days after the withdrawal of treatment.
Synthetic analogues of GnRH can also be used, as they will shorten the duration of oestrus by inducing the ovulation of the persistent follicle.

3.4.6 Embryonic mortality and abortion

Early embryonic death is generally defined as loss of pregnancy during the first 40 days of gestation, whereas abortion is accepted as describing the loss of pregnancy between days 40 and 300.
In most field studies, the embryonic mortality rate is assessed by measuring losses occurring between the first diagnosis of pregnancy and a repeat examination at around day 40. In the literature, estimations of embryonic mortality rate range from 5 to 15%.
A study in France involving 3,740 mares, revealed an overall 8.9% embryonic mortality rate (deduced from examinations between

days 22 and 44) (Chevalier-Clément 1989). In some specific categories of mare, the incidence was much higher, for example, 24.4% for mares with endometrial cysts, and 34.8% when the conceptus appeared to be abnormal.
As described in chapter 3.2.2, the timing of mating or AI in relation to ovulation is important for the prevention of early embryonic mortality. Mares should be bred in the period from 30 hours before ovulation to 12 hours after.

Luteal insufficiency in mares as a cause of pregnancy loss
As already mentioned, adequate progesterone levels are essential for the development and maintenance of pregnancy to term. Although there is evidence in other species of luteal insufficiency being a cause of loss of pregnancy, the contribution of this condition to the embryonic/foetal mortality in the horse is still under discussion. Nonetheless more progestagens are used in an attempt to maintain pregnancy in mares than in any other species (Allen 2001).

Early luteal insufficiency
As in other species the corpus luteum verum becomes susceptible to the luteolytic action of endogenous prostaglandins from day 18 after fertilization because of the reappearance of previously suppressed endometrial oxytocin receptors (Stout and Allen 2001). It has no luteotrophic support from then until the beginning of eCG secretion at day 38-40, and it appears to be highly susceptible to luteolysis during this period.
It is well recognised that many equine pregnancies fail during this early period which was confirmed in a study by Morris and Allen (2001), surveying 1,393 closely monitored Throughbred mares. These authors determined that as many as 63% of all the pregnancy losses recorded throughout gestation in this group of mares occurred between days 15 and 45 after ovulation.

It seems probable that some form of luteal inadequacy, caused either by the failure of the proper development of the corpus luteum itself, or triggered by endotoxins released in colic, for example, or in any other disease condition, could be a common reason of early pregnancy failure in mares. It has been demonstrated, in the mare, that prostaglandin release associated with endotoxaemia of gastrointestinal or exogenous origin will cause luteolysis and pregnancy loss during the first 40 days of pregnancy (Daels et al., 1987). Furthermore, endotoxin-induced abortion can be prevented by the administration of exogenous progestagen, altrenogest (Regumate Equine®) and/or prostaglandin inhibitors such as flunixin meglumine (Daels et al., 1989).

Pharmacological support of early luteal function

Although there is little evidence in the literature of early luteal insufficiency in mares, field experience and the results of some reported studies, indicate a beneficial effect of the pharmacological support for the function of the early corpus luteum. Essentially, luteotrophic treatment can take one of two directions: induction of additional corpora lutea by the administration of GnRH at 11-12 days post insemination, or progestagen supplementation by the oral administration of altrenogest (Regumate Equine®).

In their preliminary study, Pycock et al. (1995) reported that a single use of buserelin (Receptal®), a synthetic GnRH analogue, during the late luteal phase/dioestrus period (8-11 days after mating), had improved the pregnancy rates in mares at day 28-30. Receptal® was injected intramuscularly on days 10 or 11, or subcutaneously on day 8. Both methods had the same effect in terms of the improvement of pregnancy rate. In the study by Newcombe et al. (2000), treatment of mares with 20 to 40 mcg of buserelin between days 8 and 12 after mating significantly increased pregnancy rates by approximately 10%.

There is no clear evidence that primary luteal insufficiency causes early embryonic death prior to day 25 in the mare. Treatment with GnRH in late dioestrus, before the luteolytic signal is triggered, may perhaps prevent luteal regression in mares in which the embryo alone is incapable of eliciting the proper signal for the maternal recognition of pregnancy.

Mare Reproductive Loss Syndrome

This condition was first described, and called Mare Reproductive Loss Syndrome (MRLS), during the spring of 2001, when horse farms in and around central Kentucky experienced an outbreak of early foetal loss, late-term abortions, stillbirths, and neonatal deaths (Sebastian et al., 2008). Both early and late foetal losses were characterized by the absence of specific clinical signs in aborting mares.

Overall, approximately 3,500 Thoroughbred foals and numerous foals of other breeds (approximately 1,000 Paint horses and Quarter horses) were lost due to MRLS in 2001.
In 2004, a similar equine abortion storm was reported from Australia and exposure to caterpillars was identified as a risk factor. In 2006, the syndrome was observed in Florida and New Jersey.
While it is still referred to as MRLS, it is now generally accepted that whatever causes the syndrome, also results in significant numbers of cases of ophthalmic and cardiac disease in horses of varying sex and age.
Although the precise pathogenesis of MRLS is still largely unknown, there is strong evidence to link the exposure of pregnant mares to large numbers of Eastern tent caterpillars with the loss of their pregnancies.
Research into the possible pathogenesis of MRLS is continuing. A recent report by Volkmann et al., (2008) analysed the hormonal profile of mares affected by the disease. They concluded that the results of this field study (particularly the decreased concentrations of conjugated oestrogens) suggested that the primary target of the causative agent of MRLS-induced foetal death was the chorionic portion of the placenta. Moreover, these authors postulated that the agent required very intimate contact between the maternal endometrium and the foetal chorion in order to reach its target tissue, because pregnancies of less than 35 days (prior to the development of the placenta) were largely unaffected during the MRLS outbreak.

Abortion
The overall abortion rate (between days 44 and 310) was found to be 9.1%.
Loss of pregnancy can be from infectious causes (e.g. EHV-1), or non-infectious (e.g. twinning) or of unknown origin, and prevention can only be directed against the first two, of course. Table 3 lists the most common infectious causes of abortion and infertility in mares.

Table 3 Infectious causes of infertility and abortion in horses (not luteal dependent during middle and late foetal development) (Adapted from Givens et al., 2008)

Bacterial	Fungal	Protozoan	Viral
• *Streptococcus zooepidemicus* • *Taylorella equigenitalis*	• Mycotic abortion	• *Trypanosoma equiperidum*	• *Equine herpesvirus 1* • *Equine viral arteritis virus*

Streptococcus zooepidemicus

Streptococcus zooepidemicus represents one of the bacteria most commonly isolated from mares with uterine disease. It can cause abortion as a result of ascending infection of the foetus and placenta (see placentitis). Bacterial abortions usually occur at 5–10 months of gestation. Diagnosis is based on bacterial culture as well as evidence of autolysis and inflammation of the foetus and placenta.

Taylorella equigenitalis

Taylorella equigenitalis, the causative factor of contagious equine metritis (CEM), is a gram-negative coccobacillus. The infection is highly contagious and transmitted venereally. Diagnosis is based on culture of the organism from the clitoral fossa, clitoral sinuses, and endometrium or cervix. The PCR technique can be used to identify the organism in these samples. Antibodies against *Taylorella equigenitalis* may also be detected serologically.

Equine Rhinopneumonitis (Equine Herpesvirus 1)

Equine herpesvirus 1 can cause abortion, neonatal death, respiratory disease, and neurological disease. It is transmitted by the inhalation of infectious aerosol droplets, or by direct contact with infectious secretions. As with other herspesviruses, equine herpesvirus 1 persists in a latent state that can be reactivated.

It is considered to be the most important viral cause of abortion in horses. Abortions usually take place after 7 months of gestation and are not preceded by any clinical signs in the mare. The placenta may be oedematous or normal while the aborted foetus may exhibit the following pathological changes:

subcutaneous oedema, jaundice, increased volume of thoracic fluid, and an enlarged liver with yellow-white lesions approximately 1 mm in diameter. Histologically, these lesions represent areas of necrosis containing intranuclear inclusions. Characteristic inclusion bodies are found in histological preparations of the liver lesions and necrotic lymphoid tissues. Necrotizing bronchiolitis is also a common finding. Diagnosis is performed using a fluorescent antibody test or by virus isolation from foetal tissues. Prevention is based on vaccination, as well as preventing the exposure of pregnant mares to horses attending shows or other equine events.

Equine viral arteritis (EVA)

Equine viral arteritis (EVA) is an acute, contagious, viral disease of equids caused by equine arteritis virus. The virus can cause sporadic abortions between 5 and 10 months of gestation. The infection is spread by inhalation of infectious aerosol droplets or venereally. If clinical signs of disease are apparent, they include fever, hind limb oedema, nasal and ocular discharge, urticaria and anorexia as well as respiratory signs such as coughing and dyspnoea. Diagnosis is by a history of EVA signs shortly before abortion, virus isolation from the foetal tissues, or by seroconversion of the dam. Vaccines against equine viral arteritis are available in some countries.

Trypanosoma equiperidum

Trypanosoma equiperidum is a venereally transmitted protozoa that causes Dourine.

The disease is still found in Africa, South and Central America, and the Middle East. Clinical signs of the infection include a mucopurulent vulval discharge, fever, and raised cutaneous plaques followed by ataxia, depression, severe anaemia, and death. Mortality among infected horses can reach 50–70%. The control of the disease is mainly by means of strict quarantine, and the testing and eradication of infected animals.

3.4.7 Twin pregnancy and unwanted pregnancy

Twin pregnancy is almost always an unwelcome event for the horse breeder. Twin pregnancy very often results in early embryonic death or abortion. In 9.7% of mares carrying twins, both were resorbed, while one was resorbed in 61.5% of them. Abortion took place in 52.8% of the remaining mares in which no foetal resorption had taken place. When both foals are carried to term, one or both of them are usually much smaller than single foals.

It is possible to diagnose twinning by ultrasonography, when one of the embryos can be 'crushed' and eliminated manually, through the rectal wall, or the pregnancy terminated with $PGF_{2\alpha}$. However, care should be taken if assuring the owner or breeder of the absence of twin pregnancies because, for various reasons, the technique cannot be 100% accurate, even when more than one scan is performed. Even the most experienced operators have been known to miss the presence of twins on rare occasions.

The manual reduction of twins can be performed if their vesicles are not contiguous and only if it is accomplished before day 28 of pregnancy. If it is done later, it will almost inevitably lead to the death and expulsion of both embryos.
If it needs to be attempted later, intervention is preferably performed around day 70 with an intra-cardiac injection of potassium chloride or penicillin-streptomycin aqueous suspension, with the aid of trans-abdominal ultrasound.
If signs of impending abortion are seen after the procedure, progestagen supplementation may be used until 12 days before the expected foaling date.
It may also be necessary to consider inducing abortion where a mare is bred unintentionally by the wrong stallion. Prostaglandin $F_{2\alpha}$ can be used to induce abortion in the mare before day 150 of pregnancy, after that, placental production of progesterone takes over from the corpus luteum, and the mare is unlikely to abort in response to $PGF_{2\alpha}$.

3.5 Pregnancy diagnosis

Early pregnancy diagnosis is essential in order to try again with those mares found to be not pregnant, as well as to detect the presence of twins as soon as possible.

The following methods can be used for pregnancy diagnosis in mares:

1. *Absence of subsequent oestrus behaviour*
   This method is simple but very unreliable as mares may vary in the intensity of their oestrus signs, especially when no teaser stallion is used, or there may be prolonged luteal activity (persistent corpus luteum).
2. *Measurement of hormone levels*
   Progesterone
   Plasma progesterone can be measured by radio-immunoassay or enzyme-linked immunosorbent assay (ELISA), the latter being available for use in a practice laboratory allowing a more rapid result. At 17 to 22 days post-ovulation, pregnant mares should have progesterone levels above 2 ng/ml. A prolonged luteal phase of the cycle in a non-pregnant mare will lead to a false positive result, so the test should be carried out twice, at least.
   Equine Chorionic Gonadotrophin (eCG)/Pregnant Mare Serum Gonadotrophin (PMSG)
   There are detectable concentrations of eCG/PMSG in blood from approximately 40 days after ovulation, which usually persist until 80 - 120 days after ovulation. The amount of eCG/PMSG produced varies enormously from mare to mare.
   Placental oestrogens
   From day 65 of pregnancy onwards, oestrone sulphate is detectable in serum, increasing to a peak level at around day 200, and remaining there beyond 300 days. In general, this is a reliable test and can even be performed on faeces. It is also a good indicator of foetal viability. However, its usefulness is limited by the fact that it only becomes truly reliable relatively late in pregnancy.
3. *Rectal examination of the reproductive tract and ultrasound examination*
   Rectal palpation by a veterinary surgeon, nowadays usually accompanied by ultrasound scanning, is the most accurate

and useful method of pregnancy diagnosis. Experienced practitioners can detect pregnancy in the mare using a rectal probe as early as 13-16 days after ovulation. It is possible to measure the size of the embryo and check its growth rate (Bucca et al., 2005). The extra advantages of this early method of pregnancy diagnosis are that twin pregnancies may be detected in time to take action (see 3.4.6), and barren mares can be identified early enough to optimize the opportunities to mate them again.

4. *Measurement of pregnancy specific proteins*
   Early pregnancy factor (EPF)/Early conception factor (ECF)
   Early pregnancy factor (EPF) was first identified in pregnant mice and later in sheep and cattle by using the rosette inhibition test. The EPF glycoprotein has been identified in most pregnant mammalian species investigated to date. Early pregnancy factor is a secretion with growth regulatory and immunomodulatory properties that is required for the successful establishment of pregnancy.
   Although developed originally for early pregnancy diagnosis in cattle, several EPF/ECF tests have been tried in horses with variable success. Moreover a quick mare-side test has been recently developed for a detection of equine ECF. Horteloup et al. (2005) reported the use of this test in mares on days 0, 5, 8, 11 and 18 after ovulation. The results of this study indicated that non-pregnancy status could not be determined in the early pregnant mare with any high degree of accuracy by the ECF test. A recent attempt reported by Marino et al. (2009) using a commercially available ECF™ test (EDP Biotech Company, Knoxville, TN, USA) concluded that, regardless of whether the test strips were evaluated by a human or an electronic reader, this assay was not accurate for the identification of the non-pregnant mare.

3.6 Induction of parturition

The induction of parturition can be beneficial to enable the close observation of mares during parturition, particularly in those which have had foaling problems in the past, or which have undergone surgery previously. Mares with serious problems around the time of the expected parturition (e.g. colic, endotoxaemia, etc.) may need to be induced in order to prevent the further escalation of the disease problem. Induction of parturition does, therefore, offer practical advantages, but it should only be performed when parturition is imminent and when close observation is absolutely assured.

Several methods are mentioned in the literature with varying success rates, both with regard to the induction itself as well as to later complications for the mare and foal. Meyers and Le Blanc (1991) summarized the use of hormones to induce parturition in the mare.

Induction is only recommended when the following criteria are fulfilled:

- The mammary glands should be developed and already contain colostrum. This is the most important criterion. Also, the calcium content of the udder secretion is a useful predictor of the foal's readiness to be born. At 12 hours before foaling, in spontaneously foaling mares, 95% of all mares tested were within 180 - 280 ppm (using a test strip for assessing the hardness of water).
- Gestation should have been of sufficient length. The previous gestation(s) is a good indicator. In general, gestation should be at least 320-330 days.
- The cervix and the sacro-ischiatic ligaments should be softened.

Methods for induction of parturition

- Glucocorticoids are not as effective as they are in other species. In addition, complications have been reported, such as weak foals, prolonged parturition, dystocia and poor milk production.
- Oxytocin is effective, quite reliable and fast-acting. Parturition is usually completed within 90 minutes. Although a single dose of 60-100 IU intramuscularly is very effective, it is too high because it causes considerable distress to the mare and could be dangerous. A slow intravenous drip of oxytocin in saline solution (1 IU oxytocin/min) is a more gradual and safer method, but has the disadvantage that the human involvement necessary may hinder the parturition process. Another method is to inject 10-20 IU oxytocin subcutaneously at intervals of 15-20 min, up to a maximum of 60-80 IU. Low doses of oxytocin (e.g. Intertocine-S®; 2.5-10 IU) given intravenously were successful in triggering parturition in 300- to 350-kg pony mares.

- Prostaglandin $F_{2\alpha}$ has been used. Natural $PGF_{2\alpha}$ seems to have been of limited success in horses and may be accompanied by side-effects, such as abdominal discomfort, sweating and nervousness.
- Asyntheticanalogue, cloprostenol (e.g. Estrumate®), at a dose of 250 mcg (1 ml) intramuscularly, is very effective and well tolerated in mares.
- Combinations of cloprostenol (e.g. Estrumate®) and oxytocin (e.g. Intertocine-S®; 10-20 IU) can also be used and was found efficient in practical conditions.

3.7 The stallion

Fertility in stallions is assessed by clinical examination, semen evaluation, and observation of sexual behaviour. It is critical to balance the number of mares to the particular stallion's sex drive and sperm production.

3.7.1 Reproductive performance evaluation

A stallion's reproductive evaluation begins with a clinical examination, focusing on the external genitalia, and the hind legs and back (to confirm its ability to mount a mare). The testicles should be palpated for consistency and position within the scrotum, and their circumference measured. Libido is then evaluated and, in particular, the reaction time from presentation of the mare to the time of covering. Deficiencies in libido, excessive aggressiveness toward mare or handler, and other abnormalities of behaviour are all recorded.

Semen collection

If the examination takes place before the breeding season, three consecutive collections are carried out 24 hours apart, to eliminate existing semen reserves. During the season, the stallion is rested (from sexual activity) for three days prior to testing. Semen is collected on two occasions, an hour apart, and evaluated for gel-free volume, total number of spermatozoa, percentage of progressive motile sperm (PMS), morphology and pH.

Assessment of the number of PMS of a particular stallion allows for its better management:
- in natural mating, a fertile male will usually mount twice a day, six times a week;
- with AI, sperm quality and quantity will determine how many mares can be inseminated with each ejaculate and the semen will usually be collected three times a week

Semen transportation

One of the major changes in the horse breeding industry is certainly the widespread acceptance of the transport of cooled semen. Each year the number of mares bred using cooled semen gradually increases. The major advantage of this technology is that the mare does need to be transported for breeding so there is less possibility of injury or disease to the mare or foal. Furthermore, the people involved in breeding horses have access to a greater number of desirable stallions.

Transport of cooled semen requires the semen temperature to be reduced from 37°C to 5°C. Since spermatozoa are sensitive to the damage caused by cold, several additives are used to protect them such as EDTA, egg yolk, and BHT.

To maintain the fertilising capacity, semen is diluted 1:3 with semen extenders providing energy and protection from cold shock; it is then cooled at a rate less than 0.05°C/min between 18°C and 8°C, and maintained at a low temperature (3 to 6°C) for up to 36 hours. The semen is placed in an air-tight polystyrene container with a separate cooling system, and shipped to the mare by express courier. Sperm cells should not come into contact with either the rubber plunger of a syringe or with the cooling device.

Semen conservation at low temperatures

As already mentioned, there are certain limitations to the conservation of equine semen in low temperatures mainly associated with variability in the ability of sperm from different stallions to tolerate freezing and thawing. It is thought that frozen semen from only 25% of stallions will sustain pregnancy rates comparable with that of fresh semen or natural mating, when inseminated into healthy mares at the proper time (Vidament et al., 1997).

The majority of equine semen is frozen in 0.5 ml straws at a concentration of 200–400 million sperm per ml. Typically, cooling rates in the range of 10–50°C/min are employed, with relatively low concentrations of cryoprotectants (Squires 2005).

Use of sexed semen

Although the technique of flow cytometry has proved to be an accurate method for separating X- and Y-chromosome-bearing spermatozoa, it has enjoyed minimal use in the equine industry. Factors limiting the use of sexed semen in the industry include the greater cost of the equipment, as well as the licence needed to use it. Furthermore, the fertility of sex-sorted spermatozoa is highly stallion-dependent and the logistics of having the mare, stallion and equipment in the same place are problematic.

3.7.2 Cryptorchidism

Cryptorchidism describes the condition in which one or both testes fail to descend normally into the scrotal sac and is a dual problem in horses. The condition was reviewed recently by Edwards (2008). Cryptorchidism is common (2-8% of male horses), and it is generally accepted, although not proven, to be a hereditary condition. Cryptorchidism is often a unilateral condition occurring with equal frequency on either side, but in 10-15% of cases surveyed, it occurs bilaterally. In slightly more than half of cases the testis (or testes) have been reported to be abdominal.

Some owners may want the condition to be treated but most, those that have no need for a stallion for breeding purposes, prefer the more quiet behaviour of a gelding (castrated male).
When a cryptorchid stallion is hemi-castrated leaving one testicle in the inguinal canal or abdominal cavity, the so-called 'gelding' continues to exhibit male characteristics, very often including aggressive and dangerous behaviour. Sometimes the retained testicle will even degenerate into a tumour.
If the remaining testicle can be palpated in the inguinal canal, diagnosis is easy. When the testicle is hidden within the abdominal cavity, it is more difficult.

GnRH and hCG have been used to treat cryptorchidism in man and animals. The success rate is difficult to estimate, since controlled studies have never been published. In stallions, there are also anecdotal reports of the use of hCG or GnRH treatment to induce the descent of an inguinally retained testicle into the scrotum. If this is to be attempted, it should not be delayed very long after puberty because the spermatogenic capacity of the retained testicle will be permanently damaged by the higher temperature experienced in the inguinal region. The testicle may remain small, soft and spermatogenically inactive even after it has descended.
GnRH is used to treat cryptorchidism in stallions up to 2 years of age (500 mcg twice daily for 3 weeks). Reproduction Lab., Lexington, KY (USA) advocates this treatment, reporting a 60% success rate if the testis is palpable in the inguinal canal. If the testis descends into the scrotum, therapy is continued until it reaches normal dimensions. Others suggest 2500 IU of HCG, twice a week for 4-6 weeks. But, it is not known how often testicular descent has been successfully achieved, and whether the testicle subsequently exhibits normal spermatogenic function. The treatment seems, at least, to be relatively safe, as Pawlak and Tischner (2001) reported that administering 2000 IU hCG three times a week for 16 weeks to 5–7-month old normal pony stallions failed to induce any pathological changes or damage sperm production. They only noted a transient rise in testosterone production and an earlier onset of sexual behaviour than in control animals.
Human chorionic gonadotrophin can be used to diagnose cryptorchidism in so-called 'geldings' (Lu 2005). Silberzahn et al. (1989) measured the effect of 10000 IU hCG given intravenously to geldings, stallions and cryptorchids. In the stallions and cryptorchids, maximum blood testosterone concentrations were observed 2 days after hCG injection. In real geldings, hCG injection had no effect on testosterone levels.

3.7.3 Sexual behaviour

Sexual behaviour in the stallion is influenced by many factors, including season, hormone levels, psychology and the skills of the handler. Common problems include unsympathetic handling, overuse, illness or pain (often musculoskeletal) or, in

the case of a stallion used for artificial insemination, an inadequately prepared artificial vagina (e.g. not warm enough, too little pressure).
Suboptimal libido or poor mating ability appear to be among the more common reproductive complaints in the breeding stallion. However, very few centres in the world specialize in the diagnosis and treatment of sexual disorders in stallions, and more research is needed to fully understand the complexities of the process.

Deficient libido
It is generally accepted that pharmacological treatment to stimulate libido or mating ability is a last resort, to be attempted only when clinical examination, careful management and handling, and patient attempts to train and encourage the stallion, have failed. When it is considered necessary to reduce the anxiety of a novice stallion (0.05 mg/kg diazepam slow IV, 5 min prior to breeding) or to temporarily boost its libido (50 mcg GnRH subcutaneously, at 2 hours and 1 hour before breeding), these techniques are usually only required on a limited number of occasions (mostly only once), because ejaculation is a powerful reinforcing stimulus (McDonnell 2003). Although the GnRH treatment regime aims to increase the circulating testosterone concentrations temporarily, the use of exogenous testosterone to boost libido is not recommended, because too a high a dose risks suppressing spermatogenesis and stimulating aggressive behaviour (Stout et al., 2005).

3.7.4 Testicular degeneration

Numerous factors can influence the degeneration of the testes of a stallion, including age, trauma, and infectious and parasitic disease. Diagnosis of degeneration is difficult if the results of previous examinations are unavailable and if the size and consistency of the testicles cannot be compared with previous measurements. Biopsy and histological examination of testicular tissue is possible, but can cause severe haemorrhage and the rupture of the blood/testicular barrier, causing the formation of antibodies to spermatozoa which can hamper reproductive performance.
Ultrasound imaging is a non-invasive and risk-free procedure

that allows the investigation of testicular texture. Inflammation or oedema of the scrotum can interfere with heat dissipation, resulting in an increase in scrotal and testicular temperature, severely affecting fertility. An increase of the temperature by as little as 2°C for 24 hours, if not promptly addressed, sterilizes the stallion until new spermatozoa are formed (57 days).

3.7.5 Haemospermia and urospermia

The presence of blood or urine in the ejaculate reduces fertility. Blood may be found following infection, trauma, neoplasia, habronemiasis, or the use of a rubber ring to prevent masturbation. It seems that the presence of red blood cells, as low as 20% of whole blood, is the key factor in reducing fertility, but the immediate dilution with semen extenders lessens the negative effects of blood contamination. Rest from sexual activity for up to 3 months, and treatment appropriate to the cause of disease, can lead to resolution of the problem.

Urospermia is more difficult to diagnose because clinical signs are subtle, and the reason for the dysfunction is unknown. Affected stallions may urinate during ejaculation only 30% of the time, and it takes very little urine to affect fertility. Because the condition is so sporadic, it is difficult to evaluate treatment models and results are often inconclusive.

3.8 References

Alexander SL., Irvine CHG. Control of the onset of the breeding season in the mare and its artificial regulation by progesterone treatment. J Reprod Fertil 1991;Suppl 44:307-318

Allen WR. Exogenous hormonal control of the mare's oestrus cycle. Symp. Reprod. Horse. Ghent, Belgium. 1990.

Allen WR. Fetomaternal interactions and influences during equine pregnancy. Reprod 2001a;121:513-527.

Allen WR. Luteal insufficiency and Embryo mortality in the mare. Reprod Dom Anim 2001;36:121-131

Ataman MB., Gunay A., Gunay U., Baran A., Suman M. Oestrus synchronization with progesterona impregnated device and prostaglandin $F_{2\alpha}$ combined with human chorionic gonadotrophin in transitional mares. Revue Med Vet 2000;151:1031-1034

Barbacini S., Gulden P.,Marchi V., Zavaglia G. Incidence of embryonic loss in mares inseminated before or after ovulation. Equine Vet. Ed. 1999;1:108–112.

Barbacini S., Zavaglia G., Gulden P., Marchi V., Necchi D. Retrospective study on the efficacy of hCG in an equine artificial insemination programme using frozen semen. Equine Vet. Ed. 2000;2:404–408.

Barrier-Battut I., Le Poutre N., Trocherie E., Hecht S., Grandchamp de Raux A., Nicaise JL., Verin X., et al. Use of buserelin to induce ovulation in the cyclic mare. Theriogenology 2001;55:1679-1695.

Becker SE., Johnson AL. Effects of gonadotrophin-releasing hormone infused in a pulsatile or continuous fashion on serum gonadotropin concentrations and ovulation in the mare. J Anim Sci 1992;70:1208-1215.

Berezowski CJ., Stitch KL., Wendt KM., Vest DJ. Clinical comparison of 3 products available to hasten ovulation in cyclic mares. J Equine Vet Sci 2004;24:231-233

Besognet B., Hansen BS., Daels PF. Induction of reproductive function in anestrous mares using a dopamine antagonist. Theriogenology 1997;47:467-480.

Blanchard TL., Varner DD., Scrutchfield WL., Bretzlaff KN., Taylor TS., Martin MT., Elmore RG. Management of Dystocia in Mares: Retained placenta, Metritis, and Laminitis. The Compendium 1990;12:563-569.

Blanchard TL., Varner DD. Therapy for retained placenta in the mare. Vet Med 1993;1:55-59.

Blanchard TL., Brinsko SP., Rigby SL. Effect of deslorelin of hCG administration on reproductive performance in first post partum estrus mares. Theriogenology 2002;58:165-169

Bott RM., Shambley MO., Bailey MT. Induction of ovulation in the mare with the synthetic GnRH analogue Leuprolide. Eq Pract 1996;18:30-33.

Brendemuehl JP. Effect of oxytocin and cloprostenol on luteal formation, function and pregnancy rates in mares. Theriogenology 2002;58:623-626

Bucca S., Fogarty U., Collins A., Small V. Assessment of feto-placental wellbeing in the mare from mid gestation to term: transrectal and transabdominal utrasonographic features. Theriogenology 2005;64:542-557

Camillo F., Pacini M., Panzani D., Vannozzi I., RotaA., and Aria G. Clinical Use of Twice Daily Injections of Buserelin Acetate to Induce Ovulation in the Mare. Vet Res Com 2004;28:169–172

Card C. Post-breeding inflammation and endometrial cytology in mares. Theriogenology 2005;64:580-588

Chevalier-Clément F. Pregnancy loss in the mare. Anim Reprod Sci 1989;20:231-244.

Daels P., Starr M., Kindahl H., Fredriksson G., Hughes JP., Stabenfeldt GH. Effect of Salmonella typhimurium endotoxin on $PGF_{2\alpha}$ release and foetal death in the mare. J Reprod Fertil 1987;Suppl.35:485-492

Daels PF., Stabenfeldt GH., Kindahl H., Hughes JP. Prostaglandin release and luteolysis associated with physiological and pathophysiological conditions of the reproductive cycle of the mare: a review. Equine Vet J 1989;Suppl 8:29-34

Deichsel K., Aurich J. Lactation and lactational effects on metabolism and reproduction in the horse mare. Livestock Prod Sci 2005;98:25–30

Duchamp G., Bour B., Combarnous Y., Palmer E. Alternative solutions to hCG for induction of ovulation in the mare. J Reprod Fertil 1987;Suppl 35:221-228

Edwards JF. Pathologic conditions of the stallion reproductive Tract. Anim Reprod Sci 2008;107:197–207

Evans MJ., Alexander SL., Irvine CHG., Livesey JH., Donald RA. In vitro and in vivo studies of equine prolactin secretion throughout the year. J Reprod Fertil 1991;Suppl 44:27-35.

Giles RC., Donahue JM., Hong CB., Tuttle PA., Petritesmurphy MB., Poonacha KB., et al. Causes of abortion, stillbirth and perinatal death in horses – 3,527 cases. J Am Vet Med Assoc 1993;203:1170–1175.

Ginther OJ., Berfelt DR. Effect of GnRH treatment during the anovulatory season on multiple ovulation rate and on follicular development during the ensuing pregnancy in mares. J Reprod Fertil 1990;88:119-126.

Ginther OJ., Woods BG., Meira C., Beg MA., Bergfelt DR. Hormonal mechanism of follicle deviation as indicated by major versus minor follicular waves during the transition into the anovulatory season in mares. Reproduction 2003;126:653–660

Ginther OJ., Gastal EL., Gastal MO., Beg MA. Dynamics of the Equine Preovulatory Follicle and Periovulatory Hormones: What's New? Review. J Equine Vet Sci 2008a;28:454-460

Ginther OJ., Gastal EL., Gastal MO., Beg MA. Passage of postovulatory follicular fluid into the peritoneal cavity and the effect on concentrations of circulating hormones in mares. Anim Reprod Sci 2008b;107:1–8.

Givens MD., Marley MSD. Infectious causes of embryonic and fetal mortality. Theriogenology 2008;70: 270–285

Grimmert JB., Perkins NR. Human chorionic gonadotrophin (hCG): the effect of dose on ovulation and pregnancy rate in thoroughbred mares experiencing their first ovulation of the breeding season. N Zealand Vet J 2001;49:88-93.

Handler J., Schonlieb S., Hoppen HO., Aurich C. Seasonal effects on attempts to synchronize estrus and ovulation by intravaginal application of progesterone-releasing device (PRID) in mares. Theriogenology 2006;65:1145-1158

Hemberg E., Lundeheim N., Einarsson S. Retrospective study on vulvar conformation in relation to endometrial cytology and fertility in thoroughbred mares. J Vet Med A Physiol Pathol Clin Med. 2005;52:474-7.

Hoffmann C., Ellenberger C., Costa Mattos R., Aupperle H., Dhein S., Stief B., Schoon HA. The equine endometrosis: New insights into the pathogenesis. Anim Reprod Sci 2009;111:261–278

Horteloup MP., Threlfall WR., Funk JA. The early conception factor (ECFTM) lateral flow assay for non-pregnancy determination in the mare. Theriogenology 2005;64:1061–1071

Hurtgen JP. Pathogenesis and treatment of endometritis in the mare: A review. Theriogenology 2006;66:560–566

Irvine CHG., Alexander SL., McKinnon AO. Reproductive hormone profiles in mares during the autumn transition as determined by collection of jugular blood at 6h intervals throughout ovulatory and anovulatory cycles. J Reprod Fertil 2000;118:101-109.

Jacob JC., Gastal EL., Gastal MO., Carvalho GR., Beg MA., Ginther OJ. Temporal relationships and repeatability of follicle diameters and hormone concentrations within individual mares. Reprod Dom Anim 2009;44:92–99

Johnson AL. Pulsatile administration of gonadotrophin-releasing hormone advances ovulation in cyclic mares. Biol Reprod 1986; 35:1123-1130.

Katila T. Sperm – uterine interactions: a review. Animal Reprod Sci 2001:68:267-272

Kenney RM., Doig PA. Equine endometrial biopsy. In: Morrow DA (Ed). Current Therapy in Theriogenology. Philadelphia: WB Saunders. 1986; pg.723-729.

Kenney RM. The aetiology, diagnosis and classification of chronic degenerative endometritis. In: Hughes, J.P. (Ed.), Workshop on Equine Endometritis. Newmarket, UK. Equine Vet J 1992;25:186.

King SS., Roser JF., Jones KL. Follicular Fluid Prolactin and the Periovulatory Prolactin Surge in the Mare. J Equine Vet Sci 2008;28:468-472

Klug E and Jochle W. Advances in synchronizing estrus and ovulation in the mare: a mini review. J Equine Vet Sci 2001;21:474-479

Levy I., Duchamp G. A Single Subcutaneous Administration of Buserelin Induces Ovulation in the Mare: Field Data. Reprod Dom Anim 2007;42:550–554

Logan NL., McCue PM., Alonso MA., Squires EL. Evaluation of three equine FSH superovulation protocols in mares. Anim Reprod Sci 2007;102:48–55

Loomis PR. The equine frozen semen industry. Animal Reprod Sci 2001;68:191-200

Lowis TC., Hyland JH. The effect of an extended artificial photoperiod and gonadotrophin-releasing hormone infusions in inducing fertile oestrus in anoestrous mares. Australian Vet J 1991;68:400-402.

Lu KG. Clinical diagnosis of the cryptorchid stallion. Equine Pract 2005;4:250–256.
Macpherson ML. Treatment strategies for mares with placentitis. Theriogenology 2005;64:528-534
Macpherson ML., Bailey CS. A clinical approach to managing the mare with placentitis. Theriogenology 2008;70:435–440
Malpaux B., Thiery JC., Chemineau P. Melatonin and the seasonal control of reproduction. Reprod Nutr Dev 1999;39:355-366.
Marino E., Threlfall WR., Schwarze RA. Early conception factor lateral flow assays for pregnancy in the mare. Theriogenology 2009;71:877–883
McDonnell AM., Watson ED. The effect of transcervical uterine manipulations on establishment of uterine infection in mares under the influence of progesterone. Theriogenology 1992;38:945–950.
Meyers SA., LeBlanc MM. Induction of parturition: Clinical considerations for successful foalings. Vet Med 1991;86:1117-1121.
Meyers PJ. Using hormones to control cyclicity and ovulation in the broodmare. Vet Med 1991; 11:1106-1111.
Meyers PJ., Bowman T., Blodgett G., Conboy HS., Gimenez T., Reid MP., Taylor BC., et al. Use of the GnRH analogue deslorelin in a slow-release implant to accelerate ovulation in oestrous mares. Vet Rec 1997;140:249-252.
McKinnon AO., Nobelius AM., del Marmol Figueroa ST., Skidmore J., Vasey JR., Trigg TE. Predictable ovulation in mares treated with an implant of the GnRH analogue deslorelin. Equine Vet J 1993;25,321–323.
McKinnon AO., Vasey JR., Lescun TB., Trigg TE. Repeated use of a GnRH analogue deslorelin (Ovuplant) for hastening ovulation in the transitional mare. Eq Vet J 1997;29:153-155.
Morris LH-A and Allen WR. Reproductive efficiency in the Thoroughbred mares in Newmarket. Equine Vet J 2002;34:51-60
Nagy P., Huszenicza G., Juhasz J., Solti L., Kulcsar M. Diagnostic problems associated with ovarian activity in barren and post partum mares early in the breeding season. Reprod Dom Anim 1998a;33:187-192.
Nagy P., Solti L., Kulcsar M., Reiczigel J., Huszenicza G., Abavary KM., Wolfing A. Progesterone determination in equine plasma using different immunoassays. Acta Vet Hung 1998b;46:501-513.
Nagy P., Guillaume D., Daels P. Seasonality in mares. Anim Reprod Sci 2000;60-61:245-262.
Nequin LG., King SS., Roses JF., Soderstrom BL., Carnevale EM., Renaas KG. Uncoupling of equine reproductive axes during transition into anoestrus. Proc 7th Inter Symp Eq Reprod, Pretoria 1998, South Africa, pg. 41.
Newcombe JR., Martinez TA., Peters AR. The effect of the gonadotrophinreleasing hormone analogue, buserelin, on pregnancy rates in horse and pony mares. Theriogenology 2000;55:1619-1631
Newcombe JR., Jochle W., Cuervo-Arango J. Effect of Dose of Cloprostenol on the Interval to Ovulation in the Diestrous Mare: A Retrospective Study. J Equine Vet Sci 2008;28:532-539
Pawlak M., Tischner M. Some observations on the puberty of stallions after long term administration of hCG. Proceedings of the 2nd Meeting of the European Equine Gamete Group. Havemeyer Foundation Monograph 2001;series 5. Loosdracht, the Netherlands, p. 15 (Abstract).
Pycock JF., Newcombe JR. Effect of the GnRH analogue, Buserelin administered in diestrus on pregnancy rates and pregnancy failure in mares. Proc. AAEP 1995;41:268-269.
Pycock JF., Newcombe JR. Assessment of three treatments to remove intrauterine fluid on pregnancy rate in the mare. Vet Rec 1996;138:320-32
Robinson G., Porter MB., Peltier MR., Cleaver BC., Farmerie TA., Wolfe MW.,

Nilson JH., Sharp DC. Regulation of luteinizing hormone and messenger ribonucleic acid by estradiol or gonadotrophin-releasing hormone following pituitary stalk section in ovariectomized pony mares. Biol Reprod Monograph 1995;1:373-383.

Rutten DR., Chaffaux S., Valon M., Deletang F., de Haas V. Progesterone therapies in mares with abnormal oestrous cycles. Vet Rec 1986;119:569-571.

Samper JC., Morris CA. Current methodology for stallion semen cryopreservation: an international survey. Theriogenology 1998;49: 895–904.

Samper JC. Management and fertility of mares bred with frozen semen. Animal Rep Sci 2001;68:219–228

Samper JV. Induction of estrus and ovulation: Why some mares respond and others do not? Theriogenology 2008;70:445-447

Schoon HA., Schoon D., Klug E. Uterusbiopsien als Hilfsmittel fur Diagnose und Prognose von Fertilitatsstorungen der Stute. Pferdeheilkunde 1992;8:355–362.

Shand N., Irvine CHG., Turner JE., Alexander SL. A detailed study of hormonal profiles at the time of luteolysis. Proc of 7th Symp Eq Reprod., Pretoria, South Africa, 1998;pg.71.

Sharp DC., Grubaugh WR., Weithenauer J., Davis SD., Wilcox CJ. Effects of steroid administration on pituitary luteinizing hormone and follicle-stimulating hormone in ovariectomized pony mares in the early spring: pituitary responsiveness to gonadotrophin-releasing hormone and pituitary gonadotrophin content. Biol Reprod 1991;44:983-990.

Silberzahn P., Pouret EJ-M., Zwain I. Androgen and oestrogen response to a single injection of hCG in cryptorchid horses. Equine Vet J 1989;21:126-129.

Squires EL. Progestin. In: McKinnon AO, Voss JL (Eds), Equine Reproduction. Lea and Fabiger, Philadelphia, 1993; pg. 311-318.

Squires EL., Carnevale EM., McCue PM., Bruemmer JE. Embryo technologies in the horse. Theriogenology 2003;59:151-170

Squires EL. Integration of future biotechnologies into the equine industry. Anim Reprod Sci 2005;89:187-198

Squires EL., McCue PM. Superovulation in mares. Anim Reprod Sci 2007;99:1–8

Squires EL. Hormonal Manipulation of the Mare: A Review. J Equine Vet Sci 2008;28:627-634

Stout TAE., Lamming GE., Allen WR. The uterus as a source of oxytocin in cyclic mares. J Reprod Fertil 2000; Suppl. 56:281-287

Stout TAE and Allen WR. Role of prostaglandins in intrauterine migration of the equine conceptus. Reproduction 2001;121:771–775

Stout TEA. Modulating reproductive activity in stallions: a review. Animal Reprod Sci 2005;89:93-103

Troedsson MH., Ababneh MM., Ohlgren AF., Madill S., Vetscher N., Gregas M. Effect of periovulatory prostaglandin F2alpha on pregnancy rates and luteal function in the mare. Theriogenology 2001;55:1897-1899

Vanderwall DK., Juergens TD., Woods GL. Reproductive performance of commercial broodmares after induction of ovulation with hCG or Ovuplant (Deslorelin). J Eq Vet Sci 2001;21:539-542

Vidament M., Dupere A.M., Julienne P., Evain A., Noue P., Palmer, E. Equine frozen semen freezability and fertility results. Theriogenology 1997;48,907–917.

Volkmann D., Zent W., Little T., Riddle T., Durenbereger J., Potenza K., Sibley L., Roser J. Hormone profiles of mares affected by the Mare Reproductive Loss Syndrome. Reprod Dom Anim 2008;43:578–583

Watson ED. Post-breeding endometritis in the mare. Anim Reprod Sci 2000;60-61:221-232

Woods J., Bergfelt, DR., Ginther OJ. Effects of time of insemination relative to ovulation on pregnancy rate and embryonic-loss rate in mares. Equine Vet J1990;22: 41–45.

4 Porcine Reproduction

4.1. Physiology

4.1.1 The oestrous cycle

The oestrous cycle of a non-pregnant sow is represented in Figure 1. The follicular phase lasts 5-6 days (during which the ovarian follicles form, develop and secrete increasing amounts of oestradiol), and culminates in oestrus. This phase is under the control of Follicle Stimulating Hormone (FSH) and Luteinizing Hormone (LH). The luteal phase corresponds to the development of the corpora lutea, which produce progesterone which blocks the secretion of gonadotrophins (FSH, LH). In the sow, the corpus luteum is usually only sensitive to prostaglandin from day 12 of the cycle onwards.
Oestradiol and progesterone exert a negative feedback effect on the secretion of GnRH from the hypothalamus (see Figure 2).

Figure 1 Endocrine profile during the oestrous cycle in the pig

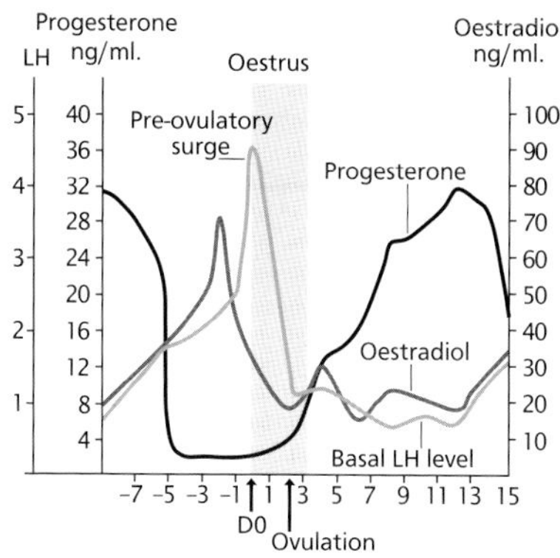

Hormone profile of the oestrous cycle in the pig

Figure 2 Hormonal regulation of reproduction in pigs

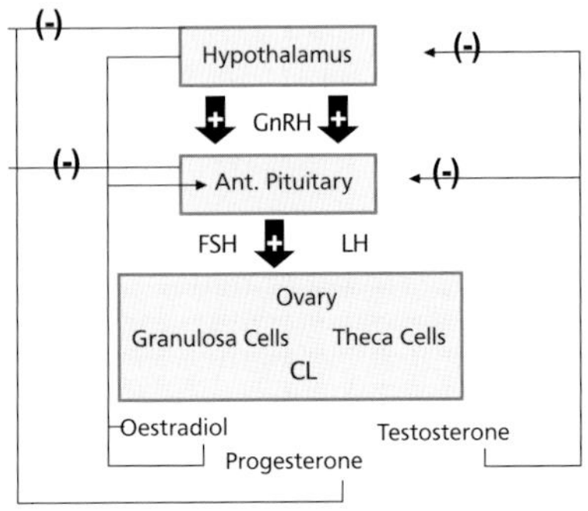

4.1.2 Domestic versus wild pigs

Compared to the wild pig, the domestic pig is much more prolific. In general, the European wild pig produces one litter each year, farrowing between late winter and early spring. The main differences in the reproductive performance of the domestic and the European wild pig are shown in Table 1.

Table 1 Reproductive performance of domestic and wild pigs.

	Number of corpora lutea	**Intra-uterine losses (%)**	**Gestation length (days)**	**Average litter size**	**Number of farrowings/ year**
Domestic pig	15-25	30	114	10-15	Up to 2.5
Wild pig	4-6	13	119	5	1-2

Although there is no real seasonality in the reproduction of the domestic pig, a number of reports have documented reduced fertility during the (late) summer months, a phenomenon that may even be manifested as the 'autumn abortion syndrome' (Almond 1991).

Basically, reproduction in pigs is controlled as discussed in Chapter 1. Gilts usually reach puberty at the age of 6-7 months. The average length of the oestrous cycle is 21 days (range: 18-24 days). The duration of oestrus is 2-3 days, with ovulation occurring during the last third.

Thanks to the introduction of ultrasound, increasing amounts of information are available about the oestrous cycle in pigs. As in other domesticated species, the growing ovarian follicles in pigs undergo the same phases of recruitment and selection leading to the establishment of the dominant follicle(s) and ovulation. The growing antral follicles depend on FSH for their development. The recruitment phase is followed by a decline in FSH due to the negative feedback exerted by oestradiol, and inhibition of the recruited follicles to below the threshold for further follicular selection. Thereafter, LH supports the further development of the dominant follicle (Lucy 2001; Knox 2005).

Many reports have indicated that the time between the onset of oestrus and ovulation is relatively stable in sows - 37.0-40.6 hours. Similarly, both the interval between the peak oestradiol levels and peak of the pre-ovulatory LH (10.6-12.6 hours), and that between the LH peak and ovulation (30.0-37.1 hours) vary little between individuals (Madej et al., 2005).

Table 2 Ovarian and oestrous cycle characteristics in pigs

Characteristic	Average value in pig
Ovulation rate	15-25
Length of follicular phase (days)	4-7
Diameter of ovulatory follicle (mm)	8-10
Maximum follicle diameter during luteal phase (mm)	5-6
Diameter from which follicle is gonadotrophin-dependent (mm)	3-4
Follicular diameter at which granulosa cells acquire LH receptors (mm)	5-6

Fertilization takes place in the region of transition from the ampulla into the oviductal isthmus. Zygotes descend into the uterus approximately 46 hours after fertilization and remain in the upper part of the uterine horns for 2-3 days. Up to day 13 after fertilization, blastocysts remain free and, until implantation occurs, they continue to migrate throughout the uterine lumen. Implantation in pigs takes place from 13 to 14 days after fertilization.

The first 2-3 weeks after fertilization are especially critical for the survival and further development of porcine embryos. It has been postulated that this is the period during which maternal recognition of pregnancy takes place, and certain factors are generated which ensure the maintenance of luteal function. The products of this interaction between mother and embryo are currently considered to be important in influencing luteal function, through the modulation of LH secretion, for the maintenance of early pregnancy (Peltoniemi et al., 2000). In the pig, oestrogens derived from the conceptus (days 11 and 13 of pregnancy) seem to be crucial in the maternal recognition of pregnancy.

These oestrogens stimulate the signalling mechanisms which result in the orientation of the prostaglandin $F_{2\alpha}$ ($PGF_{2\alpha}$) secretion towards the uterine lumen, where it is sequestered away from the corpora lutea, thus preventing luteolysis (Krzymowski and Stefanczyk-Krzymowska 2002). Results of recent research in this field suggest that oestrogens also stimulate an increase in the PGE_2 secretion by the uterus, which protects the corpus luteum from the luteolytic actions of $PGF_{2\alpha}$. Furthermore, oestrogens appear to have a direct luteotrophic effect exercised via the maintenance of the LH receptors in the luteal cells (Ziecik 2002). Embryonic oestrogens are also believed to be an important factor in influencing the functional transformation of the endometrium to a state capable of supporting the implantation of the blastocyst and its further development.

In pigs, the maintenance of pregnancy seems to depend primarily on the level of progesterone. The main sources of progesterone throughout gestation are the corpora lutea. A minimum serum progesterone of 6 ng/ml is required to maintain pregnancy.

It has also been found that there is a threshold level for oestrogenic signals generated by the growing embryos. This

hypothesis is based on the fact that, 14-15 days after fertilization, at least four viable embryos are needed in the uterine lumen for the maintenance of CL secretion. This suggests the need for the generation of a certain intensity of embryonic signal.
The first oestrogenic signal from the embryo takes place approximately 11-13 days after fertilization (Findlay et al., 1993). The second signal, most probably around day 18 of pregnancy, is a prerequisite for the maintenance of CL activity beyond day 30 of pregnancy (Pusateri et al., 1996).

In pigs, prostaglandins do not affect the developing CL until day 12 of the oestrous cycle. From then until parturition, prostaglandins can be used for the induction of abortion or parturition.
In lactating sows, the occurrence of oestrus and ovulation are inhibited by low plasma levels and a low frequency of LH pulses. Weaning is followed closely by an increase in pulse frequency which, in turn, stimulates pre-ovulatory follicular development followed by oestrus and ovulation within 4-8 days. FSH has a role in regulating the number of ovarian follicles that mature at weaning, and thus affects the ovulation rate.

4.2 Reproductive management of sow herds

4.2.1 Reproductive parameters

It is important to realise that the expression of any reproductive trait depends on both the genetic background of the pig and its environment.
Overall herd performance is usually expressed as the number of piglets weaned or sold per sow per year. It is therefore important to define a 'sow'. Some call a gilt, once mated, a sow. Others class an animal after its first litter as a sow. This can easily result in a difference of 3-4 piglets quoted as weaned per 'sow' per year. In Fig.3 is an overview of the reproduction parameters integral to herd performance.

Figure 3 Determinants of the number of piglets born per sow per year

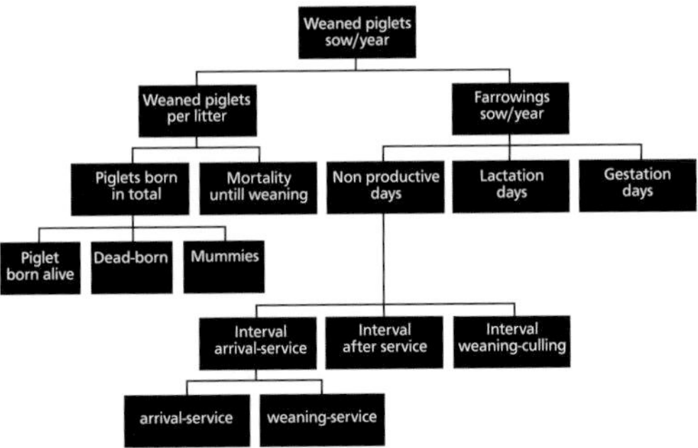

Schukken et al. (1992) concluded that the optimum economic age at first breeding was 200-220 days. They found that the increase in litter size in gilts bred later was outweighed by a shorter expected time spent in the herd. Nowadays, however, the tendency is to let the replacement gilts mature for longer, and mate or inseminate them significantly later, i.e. between 220 and 250 days. Breeding gilts later has a positive effect on their longevity as well as on the length of their reproductive life.

The production targets for a sow unit should be based on past performance and on published data from other herds of the same type. Because the net economic value of each pig reared is high (Dijkhuizen 1989), herd performance has to be re-assessed periodically. Culling rate must be included in any assessment because of the negative effect a high rate will have on number of litters per sow per year, number of pigs weaned per sow per year, and cost per weaned pig (Stein et al., 1990).
Reproductive failure is the commonest reason for culling, and compared with other reasons, it accounts for the longest interval between farrowing and removal from the herd. This means that it is also the main cause of non-productive sow days. The cost per sow (empty or non-productive) may easily reach US$3 per day.

Table 3 A guide to reference standards for reproductive parameters and the limits above or below which active control measures may be necessary

Parameter	Reference standard	Limiting values
Age at first service	210-230 days	250 days
Weaning-to-service interval	6 days	> 10 days
Regular returns to oestrus (21 ± 3 days)	10%	> 20%
Irregular returns	3%	> 6%
Abortions	1%	> 2.5%
Failures to farrow (detected at term)	1%	> 2%
Farrowing rate	90%	80%
Pigs born alive per litter (gilts)	9.5-12.5	< 9.5
Pigs born alive per litter (sows)	10.5-14.0	< 10.5
Pigs born dead (stillborn)	5%	> 7.5%
Pigs born mummified	1.5%	> 3.0%
Farrowings/sow/year	2.35	< 2.1

4.2.2 Pregnancy diagnosis

Many techniques for pregnancy diagnosis have been developed in pigs. Non-return to oestrus, external physical signs (such as enlargement of the ventral abdomen and udder), ultrasound (Amode, Doppler and Real-time), echography, blood progesterone and oestrone sulphate, can all be used. Because the aim of pregnancy testing is to reduce the number of non-productive days, the sensitivity (accuracy of detecting pregnancy) of such tests is less important than their specificity (accuracy of detecting nonpregnant sows). In general, the sensitivity of the existing tests is better than their specificity. A high degree of sensitivity is particularly important when pregnant animals are to be sold.

Ultrasound equipment, utilizing the *Doppler effect*, allows any liquid movement to be identified, such as blood flow in the middle uterine artery, umbilical arteries or the foetal heart.
A-mode ultrasound apparatus converts the returning echo signal into an audible tone or a green light. Pregnancy is taken to be confirmed when the sound waves reflect a uterus filled with

foetal fluid. False positive results are mainly associated with echoes from other fluid-filled structures such as the urinary bladder or from a uterus filled with pathological fluid, e.g. as in pyometra.
Both these methods can be used by non-veterinary professionals as a part of routine herd management.
Real time (B-mode) ultrasonography produces a two-dimensional real-time image of scanned tissues and structures on screen. The B-mode scanners are useful in the management of reproduction because they made it is possible to diagnose pregnancy at >21 days post mating/AI (using a transabdominal probe), to confirm pregnancy between 42 and 63 days post mating/AI, as well as to investigate ovarian and uterine problems.
Ultrasonography has a clinical value in diagnosing pregnancy failure and early embryonic death leading to either foetal mummification or partial embryonic decomposition.
However, the use of ultrasound to diagnose reproductive disorders in pigs requires much more skill and experience than routine pregnancy diagnosis. Ultrasonographic detection of pregnancy in pigs is usually carried out at 30-45 days of gestation with a reported 90-95% accuracy. The sow or gilt is examined in a standing position with the probe placed near the 2nd teat from the rear and pointing towards the middle of the back. Pregnancy can be detected as early as day 16-19 of gestation using a rectal probe. Kauffold and Althouse (2007) published an overview of the use of B-mode ultrasonography in female pigs.

Induction with gonadotrophins offers another feasible and relatively inexpensive method of pregnancy diagnosis in pigs. A combination of pregnant mare serum gonadotrophin/equine chorionic gonadotrophin (PMSG/eCG) and human chorionic gonadotrophin (hCG) (e.g. PG 600®) has been used between 21 and 80 days of pregnancy, predominantly in order to detect non-pregnant females so they can be submitted
again for mating or insemination. In pregnant sows, the ovaries are not responsive to exogenous gonadotrophins, so no signs of oestrus are observed after PG 600® administration. However, non-pregnant animals can respond to the gonadotrophin stimulus and will show oestrus. This allows for a rapid re-introduction of such females to mating and fewer so-called 'empty' days.

4.2.3 Oestrus and oestrus detection

Oestrus is the period in which a mature boar can evoke a 'standing reflex' in a gilt or sow. There is enormous variation between sows in the duration of oestrus (36-96 hours). Oestrus is preceded by a period of 1-2 days in which there is an increasing reddening and swelling of the vulva, which reaches a peak at the beginning of oestrus.

Oestrus can be divided into three phases (see Figure 1, Chapter 4.2.4). During the first and last of these, only the boar can induce a standing reflex. With no boar present, a handler can produce a standing reflex (the 'back pressure' test) during the middle phase. The use of a synthetic boar aerosol improves the response to this test.

A gilt or sow in oestrus behaves differently to those not in oestrus, thus:

- restlessness during feeding
- not settling down after feeding
- frequently voiding small quantities of urine
- cocking the ears after sniffing the vulva of other animals or smelling the odour of the boar.

Ovulation takes place during the last third of oestrus. Several workers have measured breed differences in the age at puberty, weaning-to-oestrus interval, and the percentage of sows returning to oestrus within 10 days of weaning. According to these criteria, hybrids perform better than purebred sows. However, oestrus activity is also influenced by a number of other factors, such as social environment and nutrition. The boar stimulates the sow sexually before mating. This process involves pheromonal, auditory, visual and tactile stimuli, all of which are known to affect the release of pituitary oxytocin in sows and gilts (Madej et al., 2005). Langendijk et al. (2003) reported that the presence of the boar induced the release of oxytocin and clearly increased the myometrial activity in sows. The effects of boar contact also include follicular growth, leading to the expression of oestrus and ovulation in more primiparous sows (Langendijk et al., 2000). Salivary pheromones released by the submaxillary glands of boars over 10 months old also stimulate oestrus and oestrus behaviour. Pharmaceutical products containing porcine pheromones are available (e.g. SOA Spray®) and can be used to enhance oestrus expression in sows, leading to improved heat detection rates.

It is now well recognised that both mating and artificial insemination have a profound effect on the events associated with oestrus in pigs, and result in a reduction of the interval between oestrus and ovulation by up to 14 hours in gilts and sows.

In practice, the so-called 'transport stress-induced oestrus' in gilts is observed at about 6 months of age. This results in a high oestrus rate (up to 70%) in the first week following transportation, peaking at day 4-6. The maximum effect of this 'transport stress' can be expected immediately after transport, if there is boar contact, regrouping, etc. (Cole et al., 1982; Eliasson et al., 1991; Signoret et al., 1990).

Housing female pigs in oestrus in the same pens as pre-pubertal gilts, or recently weaned sows, also has a positive effect (Pearce 1992). Scientific opinion about the effects on reproductive performance of the individual or group housing of pigs is equivocal. One reason for this may be that the design of the house, rather than the system itself, is an important determinant of the physiological response of female pigs (Barnet et al., 1991). It has also been demonstrated that if a stock-person's behaviour induces fear in the sows, it can have a significant and negative affect on their reproductive performance (Meunier-Salyn et al., 1990).

There have often been conflicting results from studies of the influence of nutrition on the onset of oestrus. This may be because of differences in the interactions between breed, boar and season, for example. The nutritional effect on the onset of puberty is possibly mediated through its effect on growth rate, body composition, etc., which is supported by a Swedish study involving 547 Swedish Yorkshire gilts. The gilts were kept under the same management conditions and fed according to the standard regime for pigs for slaughter. The results showed that gilts with a high growth rate attain puberty earlier, but there was no influence of growth rate on the signs of oestrus displayed at puberty. Animals with a low back-fat thickness at 90 kg body weight show a less intense and shorter duration of reddening and swelling of the vulva at their first oestrus. The animals reached puberty at an average age of 210.9 ± 19.8 days and body-weight of 118.8 ± 14.8 kg, but about 10% of them did not reach puberty until 260 days of age (Eliasson et al., 1991).

Nutritional deficiencies during the pre-follicular phase are known to have several effects on reproduction in pigs. Inadequate feeding during lactation may negatively affect subsequent weaning-to-oestrus interval, ovulation rate and embryo survival (Hazeleger et al., 2005). The effects of negative energy balance on reproduction in pigs seem to be related to the suppressive effects of a low level of feeding on the frequency and amplitude of LH pulses and follicular development, and it is suggested that they are mediated by changes in insulin levels (Cox et al., 1997). The results reported by Clowes et al. (2003) show that the poorest litter growth rate during lactation, and the lowest ovarian development, were observed in animals that were smaller initially, and mobilized the most body protein during lactation. A larger body mass at parturition ensured a better litter growth rate, and was associated with improved follicular development.

In primiparous sows, oestrus rates within 10 days of weaning are significantly lower than in multiparous sows. Weaning after a lactation of less than 14 days, or more than 41 days, has a negative effect on the occurrence of oestrus.

Early weaning

After parturition, complete involution of the uterus takes about 3 weeks. This is one of the reasons that weaning piglets at 17-25 days of age is considered in Europe as being most profitable. In the United States, however, a programme called the Early Segregated Weaning System is popular, in which piglets are weaned as early as 12-14 days of age. This system is aimed primarily at reducing the possible transmission of various infectious diseases from the sows to their progeny, once the piglets have become susceptible (as maternal immunity wanes).

In spite of the clear health advantages, early weaning systems can have a profound effect on sow reproductive performance, and have generated much controversy with respect to animal welfare. Numerous reports indicate that the early weaning of sows results in extended weaning-to-oestrus intervals, reduced conception and farrowing rates and smaller litter sizes (Koutsotheodoros et al., 1998). Moreover, there are indications that weaning piglets between 15 and 20 days old may impact significantly on their growth rate during the nursery stage (Smith et al., 2007).

The reduction of subsequent litter size in the early weaned sow is of greatest significance because it may well offset any advantage gained by reducing the length of lactation. This reduction in subsequent litter size is clearly due to a decrease in the early embryonic survival following early weaning, with most of the embryo losses occurring at or around implantation. It has been suggested that a farrowing to breeding interval of at least 20 days is required, to allow for embryo development, given that the uterus has completely recovered both morphologically, and histologically, by at least three weeks post partum. Weaning at earlier than 21 days is not allowed in Europe.

4.2.4 Timing of mating and artificial insemination

It has been shown repeatedly that the timing of mating or artificial insemination (AI) influences fertility in terms of litter size and pregnancy rate, and a 'fertility curve' can be constructed (see Figure 4). Peak fertility only occurs after mating or AI in the middle of oestrus. Ovulation takes place approximately two thirds into the oestrus period, with the optimal timing for insemination being 0-8 hours before ovulation.

Figure 4 Aspect of the vulva, sexual behaviour of the sow and fertility

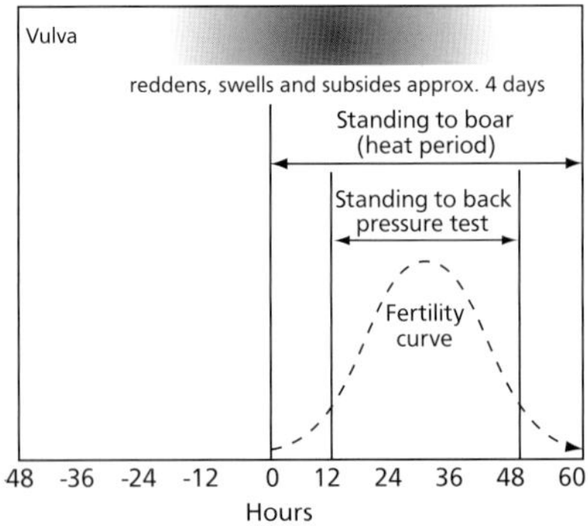

Table 4 lists the physical signs to consider in choosing the optimum time to mate sows

Table 4 Timing of mating and AI.

Too early	- vulva heavily red and swollen - hardly any mucus on vaginal mucosa - negative back pressure test; standing reflex only when boar present
Ideal	- vulva moderately red and swollen - vaginal mucosa with mucus - positive back pressure test
Too late	- no redness or swelling of vulva - 'sticky' vaginal mucosa - negative back pressure test; standing reflex only when boar present

Repeat mating or AI is only necessary in animals still showing a positive back pressure test 24 hours after the first.

Development of artificial insemination in pigs

The use of artificial insemination in the pig industry has increased dramatically over the last 25 years, all round the world. Singleton (2001) indicated that the current use of AI in the US accounts for about 60% of all matings, as compared to less than 5% in 1990. This progress has definitely been stimulated by the pressure for genetic improvement in pigs. Moreover, the structure of the pork industry in many countries has altered. Breeding and farrowing units have become larger and more specialized, and AI technology has become more feasible and cost effective. The vast majority of semen is used fresh and is stored at room temperature. Frozen/thawed semen is available on a limited basis. Because of the poorer results with frozen/thawed semen compared to fresh, its use has been limited to specialized breeding programmes, or for export purposes. The efficacy of insemination with fresh or frozen/thawed semen is still not consistent enough for it to be feasible to opt for a single fixed time insemination. The typical female receives about 2.2 doses of fresh semen per mating. More doses are needed to obtain comparable results with frozen semen.

The interval between AI and ovulation is a major factor

affecting fertility whether using fresh or frozen semen. Bolarín et al. (2006) proposed that the interval from insemination to ovulation is the major explanation for the differences in fertility between farms using frozen semen. Insemination must be close to ovulation to achieve acceptable fertility especially with frozen semen, because of the limited life span of thawed spermatozoa. In this case, the optimum interval between AI and ovulation has been determined to be from 0 to 8 hours.
There is a clear need for the development of tailor-made, clear and simple, synchronization systems for oestrus and ovulation in pigs, which would allow for single, fixed time insemination, leading to higher pregnancy rates and larger litter sizes.

4.3 Control of oestrus

In addition to adjustments in general management and nutrition, the pharmacological control of oestrus is now a well-established method by which to address the contribution to poor reproductive performance (i.e. more non-productive days, fewer piglets/sow/year) of sows that fail to return to oestrus and be served within a week of weaning, and replacement gilts exhibiting delayed puberty (i.e. all the problems associated with larger pools of gilts).

The control of oestrus is therefore aimed at:
- Optimizing the number of piglets weaned per sow per year.
- Reducing the number of non-productive days.

These can only be achieved with an efficient identification system for sows and boars, and a recording scheme capable of regular periodic analysis. Technical results have to be compared with the herd targets, historical performance figures, and those of similar herds.
At present, a number of natural and synthetic hormones are used for controlling and/or optimizing reproductive performance. Both progestagens and gonadotrophins can be used to induce or synchronize normal fertile oestrus.

Progestagens

In cyclic gilts and sows, progestagens can be used to synchronize oestrus. Oral treatment (gilts for 18 days, sows for 5-17 days) leads to oestrus 5-6 days after the cessation of treatment. One of the available preparations, Regumate Porcine®/FolliPlan®, contains altrenogest, a potent synthetic progestagen.

The inhibitory effect of altrenogest on the pituitary gland, suppresses the release of gonadotrophins during the treatment period. Once the treatment is withdrawn, the inhibitory effect is removed, and the gonadotrophins stimulate the rapid and synchronous growth of a new follicular wave, leading to ovulation (Wood et al., 1992; Kauffold et al., 2000). Regumate®/FolliPlan® itself is usually given orally for 18 consecutive days, after which treated animals should be observed for signs of oestrus between 4 and 6 days. The system can be used in both cyclic gilts and multiparous sows.

Management of oestrus in replacement gilts with progestagens

Oestrus synchronization with Regumate®/FolliPlan® is especially suitable for replacement gilts, as it enables the producer to adjust the timing of their oestrus to that of the rest of the herd. To achieve this, the start of treatment should be adjusted so that the last dose of Regumate®/FolliPlan® is given to replacement gilts on the same day as the sows are weaned. This synchronization is especially important when all in-all out regimes are in operation e.g. with batch production.

Progestagens should not be given to pregnant animals, or to gilts before puberty.

Figure 5 presents one possible treatment regimen for the introduction of replacement gilts into a herd breeding programme.

Figure 5 Treatment of replacement gilts with Regumate®/FolliPlan®

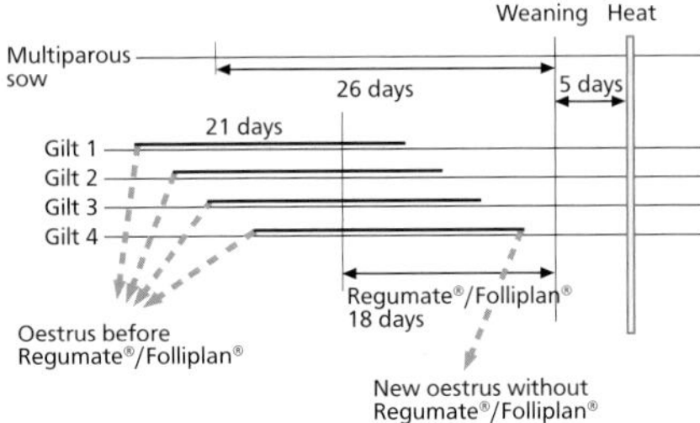

Gonadotrophins

In animals which are not cycling, gonadotrophins have to be used. They are safe in all animals and have no withdrawal time. For years, the combination of PMSG/eCG and hCG (e.g. PG 600®) has proven to be very effective, and easier to use, than two separate injections of PMSG/eCG and hCG (Bates et al., 1991; Knox et al., 2001).

The combined product can be used, routinely, either in pre-pubertal gilts (about 6 months of age) to reduce the number of days between final selection and first spontaneous oestrus, or in sows on the day of weaning. It may be that treatment is only advisable for sows during certain periods e.g. to cope with summer infertility, or for certain groups e.g., primiparous sows in which return to oestrus rates (by <10 days post weaning) are low.

Individual treatment with PG 600® can be given to anoestrus gilts (>7 months) or to sows 8-10 days after weaning. In both cases, oestrus detection must be of an adequate standard, to minimize the risk of treating cyclic animals (which will not respond to treatment if in the luteal phase).

To ensure that no active luteal tissue is present at the time of gonadotrophin treatment (being administered to animals later than 10-14 days after weaning), $PGF_{2\alpha}$ may be given 24-48 hours beforehand. However, care should be always taken over proper identification, to avoid treating pregnant animals and sows with a corpus luteum younger than 12 days.

Individual treatment can also be given to animals with a negative ultrasonic pregnancy test result as an extra check, to avoid the risk of culling any sows falsely diagnosed as non-pregnant. True negatives will respond with oestrus within 3-7 days of treatment, as usual.
In the case of weakly expressed oestrus (in natural as well as induced heats) the use of synthetic boar odour aerosol (SOA Spray®) serves to stimulate the signs of oestrus.
PMSG and hCG are sometimes used separately in oestrus and ovulation synchronization in sows. But although the system can be effective, it requires the precise timing of treatments, and is certainly labour intensive.

Figure 6 Example of the use of PMSG and hCG in ovulation synchronization with fixed time insemination in gilts and sows

(adapted from Schnurrbusch and Huhn 1994)

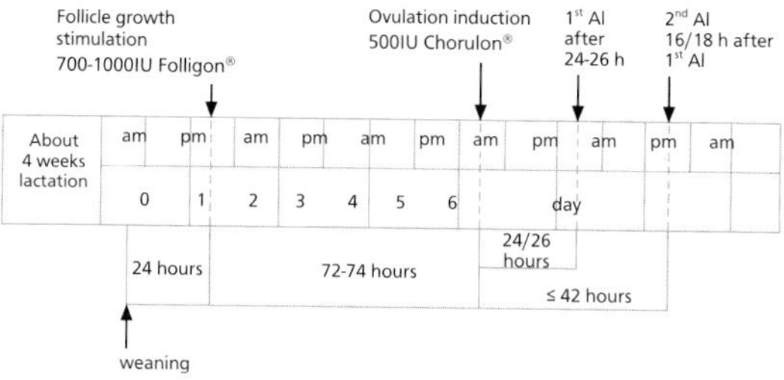

Progestagens/Gonadotrophins
The combination of progestagen treatment followed by stimulation of follicular growth with gonadotrophins has been reported to lead to precise synchrony and a high fertility rate to the induced oestrus. Females can receive PG 600® approximately 24 after the standard 18-day treatment with Regumate®/FolliPlan®. Alternatively, as proposed by Hühn et al. (2000) 800 IU of PMSG/eCG (Folligon®) can be administered 24 hours after the last dose of Regumate®/FolliPlan®.

Management of oestrus in early weaning systems

The adverse effects of early weaning on subsequent fertility and fecundity may be alleviated by allowing a longer interval between weaning and conception. A possible way of achieving this is treatment of the early-weaned sow with a progestagen, to inhibit oestrus for several days after weaning.

In a study reported by Koutsotheodoros et al. (1998), altrenogest (Regumate®/FolliPlan®) was used in sows weaned 12 days post partum. This resulted in excellent synchronization, with 97% of treated sows exhibiting oestrus 5-7 days after the end of treatment, and a significantly increased ovulation rate in the Regumate®/FolliPlan® treated sows compared with both untreated early weaned sows, and with sows weaned at the standard time. These authors concluded that early weaned sows, treated with Regumate®/Folliplan® over a sufficient period post weaning, led to increased ovulation rate and embryo survival, possibly due to a nutritionally-mediated maximal development of the pre-ovulatory follicle, and hence optimal maturation of the oocyte.

Gonadotrophin releasing hormone (GnRH)

GnRH analogues, alone or in combination with progestagens (Regumate®/FolliPlan®), have been administered to sows at oestrus to induce ovulation, with variable success.

Fixed insemination systems have used GnRH mainly to induce ovulation. Fig.7 shows one of these systems used with considerable success in the past on large multiplying farms in Eastern Germany.

Unfortunately only a few products on the market are licensed for use in pigs, with established dosage and administration regimes.

Figure 7 Oestrus and Ovulation synchronization in gilts for fixed time insemination
(Adapted from Schnurrbusch and Huhn 1994)

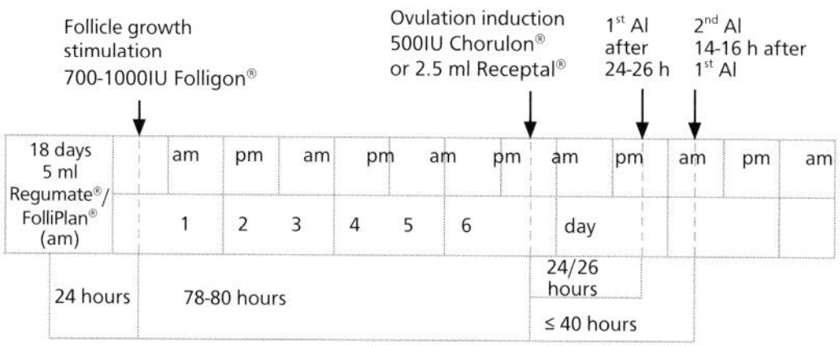

4.4 Reproductive disorders

Reproductive failure accounts for the highest proportion of sows culled, varying from 25-40% (Stein et al., 1990).
The reasons for culling in this category are:

- Anoestrus
- Repeat breeding and seasonal sub(in)fertility
- Barren sows (negative at pregnancy testing)
- Abortion
- Poor mothering ability

4.4.1 Anoestrus

A gilt or sow in anoestrus may have active, inactive or cystic ovaries. In a controlled study in gilts (Eliasson et al., 1991), it appeared that only 2-3% of the animals ovulated in the absence of oestrus symptoms, and 13-14% had weak oestrus signs (i.e. absence of standing oestrus). In a slaughterhouse survey of culled sows, it was found that the overall prevalence of inactive ovaries was approximately 14-21%, and that of cystic ovaries, 6%. Inactive ovaries were most frequently found in young animals, while cystic ovaries were distributed equally between all age groups (Geudeke 1992). Not all cysts cause anoestrus, it depends on the number and type of cysts. Only large numbers (>7) of persistent, follicular thecal cysts lead to anoestrus (Schnurrbusch et al., 1991).

Delayed puberty

Delayed puberty in gilts can be a real problem, especially in herds with a high replacement rate. Breed, nutritional status, stress, housing and social interactions, as well as climatic conditions, can contribute to a delay in puberty in pigs.

Induction of the first oestrus in pre-pubertal gilts can be adopted routinely as prophylaxis, or used therapeutically in females already exhibiting delayed puberty. Biological methods are sometimes used to promote puberty in gilts. Although their efficacy is variable, they should not be forgotten, as they can be used prior to, or concurrently with, pharmacological treatment, to improve the overall success of induction. The most commonly used methods include so-called protein/energy flushing, and vitamin A, E and folic acid supplementation (Beltranema et al., 1991; Cosgrove and Foxcroft 1996). Puberty in gilts can also be hastened by the introduction of a boar, by housing the gilts with cyclic sows, and by improvements in housing (Dyck 1989). The golden rule is to correct any existing feeding and housing deficiencies before undertaking any pharmacological treatment.

Additional care should be taken not to include gilts younger than 210 days or with a body weight less than 105 kg. Any attempt to induce puberty in gilts too young or under weight can lead to a complete lack of response, or to very small litters. What is more, it is well known that gilts giving birth when too young can exhibit an inadequate maternal instinct and reduced milk production.

Puberty and first oestrus can be induced with gonadotrophins (e.g. PG 600®); gilts should be observed for oestrus signs 3-6 days after the treatment.

4.4.2 Repeat breeding

The length of the oestrous cycle in the sow is generally assumed to be 21±3 days. Sows returning to oestrus and failing to conceive within this period are classified as regular returns. Another group, about a quarter of those returning at the normal time, return at approximately 25 days. This is probably due to early embryonic loss, which is quite common on farms with no other reproductive problem.

From day 31 of pregnancy until parturition, idiopathic foetal death is rare, so late returns to oestrus are abnormal. If they do occur, they are generally caused by infections (Aujeszky's Disease, Porcine Parvo Virus, Leptospirosis, Erysipelas, Porcine Reproductive Respiratory Virus). See also Table 5.

Seasonal anoestrus/seasonal infertility

In spite of the innate ability to produce litters throughout the year, the domestic sow exhibits reduced fertility in late summer and early autumn, which coincides with the seasonal reproductive inactivity in European wild boar. This phenomenon is sometimes called seasonal anoestrus, although it is very seldom represented by a complete cessation of reproductive activity. Manifestations of this seasonal infertility or decreased fertility, include reduced farrowing rate in otherwise prolific females (Xu et al., 1994; Peltoniemi et al., 1999), delayed puberty in gilts (Peltoniemi et al., 1999), prolonged weaning-to-oestrus intervals (Prunier et al., 1996; Peltoniemi et al., 1999), and possibly a reduced litter size during the late summer and early autumn months.

An overview cited by Dawson at al. (1998) demonstrated that returns to service indicated significantly higher total early embryonic losses between July and September. Litter sizes were also lower by about 0.5 piglets per litter, for sows served between August and October.

Autumn abortion syndrome (AAS) results in an additional 3% to 5% pregnancy loss beyond 30 days gestation, leading to an increase in the number of sows failing to farrow and precluding the achievement of full production capacity (Holyoake 2005).

Reduced concentrations of progesterone have been reported in sows during the autumn compared with other times of the year. It is therefore plausible that lower progesterone concentrations associated with shorter day length may increase the susceptibility of pregnant females to late pregnancy loss.

A study by Bertoldo et al. (2009) identified age at first service, parity, lactation length, number of piglets weaned per litter, and weaning-to-service interval as risk factors for late pregnancy losses during the period of seasonal infertility, highlighting the multifactorial nature of the seasonal infertility problem.

The effect of season and temperature on reproductive performance in pigs has become especially important in countries where there has been a growing trend towards keeping breeding sows outdoors (UK, Spain) and therefore more exposed to natural changes in photoperiod and ambient temperature.

Treatment with gonadotrophins (e.g. PG 600®) can be used to alleviate the negative seasonal influence, especially at weaning.

Embryonic and foetal mortality

Foetal losses and pre-weaning mortality are amongst the most important causes of loss in commercial swine herds (Dial et al., 1992). Foetal losses (mummified foetuses and stillborns) can vary from 5 to 15% (Van der Lende 2000). Several factors have been associated with stillbirth, such as infectious diseases, gestation length, parity, litter size, duration of farrowing, interval between births, birth weight, dystocia, stress due to high environmental temperatures or transfer to the farrowing house, human interference at parturition, body condition score and nutritional deficiencies.

4.4.3 Barren sows

The management of the sow during the post service period is crucial, if the breeding efficiency of a herd is to be optimized. Pregnancy testing at about one month after service is common practice on many commercial farms. Amongst those culled as reproductive failures, up to 45% may be removed because of a negative pregnancy test (Stein et al., 1990). All pregnancy tests, however, produce occasional errors. False negative results in pregnant sows are particularly costly if the sows are culled as a consequence.

4.4.4 Abortion

Abortions account for approximately 10% of all sows culled for reasons of reproductive failure. Only a small proportion can be positively linked to infection, but this is without doubt partly due to the unavailability of adequate diagnostic samples, and the fact that serology is often unsuitable for diagnostic purposes. The main infectious causes of abortion in pigs include: leptospirosis, brucellosis, erysipelas, parvovirosis, swine influenza, Auyeszky 's disease, classical swine fever and PRRS.

Table 5 lists the most common infectious causes of reproductive failure and abortion in sows.

Table 5 Infectious causes of infertility and abortion in domestic animals (Adapted from Givens 2008)

Bacterial	*Brucella suis* *Erysipelothrix rhusiopathiae* *Leptospira pomona* *Streptococcus suis* *Chlamydia spp.* *Actinobacillus* *Mycoplasma suis*
Protozoan	*Toxoplasma gondii*
Viral	Porcine parvovirus Porcine enterovirus and teschovirus Pseudorabies (Aujeszky's disease) virus Classical Swine Fever virus Porcine Reproductive and Respiratory Syndrome (PRRS) virus Encephalomyocarditis virus Porcine cytomegalovirus Rubulavirus Menangle virus Porcine circovirus type 2 Japanese encephalitis virus African Swine Fever virus

Leptospirosis

Leptospirosis is caused by gram-negative spirochetes of the genus Leptospira. The organisms are excreted in the urine and transmission between animals occurs through contact between contaminated urine and oral, nasal or ocular mucosa. Pigs are considered to be the maintenance hosts for serogroups *Pomona*, *Australis* and *Tarassovi*, whereas incidental infections may occur with strains of the *Canicola*, *Icterohaemorrhagiae*, and *Grippotyphosa* serogroups. Chronic leptospirosis may be associated with signs of reproductive disorders such as abortions, stillbirths, infertility, and the birth of weak piglets. It should be borne in mind that leptospirosis is an important occupational zoonosis for farmers and abattoir staff in contact with pigs.

Diagnosis is based on the demonstration of leptospires in foetal tissues or stomach contents. Vaccination with a multivalent vaccine every 6 months is practised in some regions and helps prevent the disease.

Erysipelas

Erysipelas is caused by a gram-positive bacterium, *Erysipelothrix rhusiopathiae*, which is present in the pig industry throughout the world and is transmitted mainly via the oronasal route. The main consequences of infection include abortion, fever, diamond-shaped skin lesions, arthritis, vegetative endocarditis, and sudden death. Abortion can occur at any stage of gestation. Mummification of foetuses and embryo resorption can occur. The disease is zoonotic; the bacteria cause erysipeloid in humans.

Diagnosis of erysipelas is most commonly made on the typical diamond-shaped skin lesions. Serology can prove unreliable, although a rising titre in an agglutination test (with controls) is helpful, as is the complement fixation test. An ELISA has been developed and is considered reliable for chronic infections on a herd basis. *E rhusiopathiae* can be isolated readily on blood agar plates from spleen, kidney, and the long bones of acutely sick animals (and from the tonsils and other lymph nodes of many apparently healthy ones).

In most countries, regular vaccination with mono- or polyvalent vaccines is part of routine herd management (e.g. Porcilis® Ery, Porcilis® Ery+Parvo).

Porcine Reproductive and Respiratory Syndrome (PRRS)

PRRS virus can be shed in nasal secretions, faeces and urine. The infection spreads by direct contact with infected animals, as well as through oral and aerosol transmission. Experimental transmission of the PRRS virus has been demonstrated in semen. Additionally, the virus can be transmitted transplacentally, most commonly in the last trimester of pregnancy. During the initial phase of the disease, reproductive signs include abortions and irregular returns to oestrus, while later infections may result in the birth of litters with a combination of normal or weak piglets and stillborn, autolytic, or mummified foetuses.

As not all foetuses are necessarily infected, multiple foetuses should be sampled for diagnostic purposes. Viral antigen can be found most consistently in the foetal thymus and in fluid collected from the foetal thoracic cavity. PCR testing of pooled thoracic fluid from 3-5 foetuses is the most reliable means of diagnosis.

Herd management is important in the control and prevention of PRRS. Inactivated and modified live virus vaccines are available (e.g. Porcilis® PRRS).

Parvovirosis

Porcine parvovirus is widespread and transmitted oronasally and transplacentally. Infection at 10–30 days of gestation results in resorption of embryos and irregular returns to oestrus. Infection at 30–70 days can cause mummification, whereas if the infection takes place after 70 days of gestation, most of the foetuses are capable of an immune response and elimination of the virus, and are healthy at birth. Other clinical signs of porcine parvovirosis may include infertility, stillbirth, neonatal death, and reduced neonatal vitality. It is important to note that during transplacental infection part of a litter might become infected, with subsequent spread of the virus in utero to the litter mates. In this way, a combination of resorption, mummification, and stillbirth can all occur within a single litter.

Diagnosis of parvovirosis is usually made using immunofluorescence assay (IFAT) or by virus isolation from samples of lung tissue from mummified foetuses, or by the demonstration of precolostral antibodies in stillborn pigs.

Monovalent inactivated vaccines are available (e.g. Porcilis® Parvo), as well as polyvalent combinations (e.g. Porcilis® Ery+Parvo).

Pseudorabies/Aujeszky's disease

Pseudorabies or Aujeszky's disease is caused by an alpha herpesvirus of which pigs are the only natural host. Other domestic species (cattle, sheep, goats, dogs, and cats) can become infected, usually fatally. Transmission of the infection in pig herds occurs primarily through direct contact with nasal and oral secretions, but also through aerosols, venereally, or transplacentally. As with other herpesviruses, Pseudorabies can become established as a latent infection.

Infection during the first trimester results in resorption and a return to oestrus, whereas infection during the second and third trimester results in abortion, stillbirth, or the birth of weak piglets.

Diagnosis is by virus isolation or fluorescent antibody staining. Gene-deleted vaccines are available which allow the differentiation of vaccinated from naturally infected pigs by serology (e.g. Porcilis® Aujeszky).

Classical Swine Fever

Classical Swine Fever, previously known as Hog Cholera, is caused by a pestivirus.

Transplacental infection can take place at any stage of gestation causing abortion, foetal mummification and stillbirth. Infection at 50–70 days of gestation can result in the birth of persistently viraemic piglets. Fluorescent antibody staining and virus isolation are used for diagnosis.

Both inactivated and modified live vaccines are available, but their use is subject to strict regulations which vary between different nations.

Adequate control of the infectious diseases which impact on reproductive efficacy should be a basic element in comprehensive reproduction management systems in breeding herds. Biosecurity measures should be observed throughout the whole production process, but the appropriate and secure disposal of aborted/stillborn foetuses and foetal membranes is especially important, and the isolation of aborting sows is crucial. Carefully planned prophylactic vaccination programs form an indispensable element of management, which need to be matched to the prevalent epizootic situation on the farm and the surrounding area. For some diseases, (e.g. Aujeszky's Disease, Classical Swine Fever) compulsory national measures are in place.

Early embryo mortality

Reduced litter size due to early embryonic loss is a major limitation on the profitability of pig production. The ovulation rate in pigs is often 30 to 40% higher than litter size at farrowing. As 90-95% of the ova are fertilized, most of the losses are thus due to prenatal mortality, which occurs mainly during the embryonic phase, before day 30 of gestation.

To some extent, the phenomenon of early embryonic mortality is a natural mechanism. It has been suggested that sows seem to be able to ensure the development to term of only a limited number of foetuses. Uterine capacity limits litter size and foetal development, even in sows with a conventional fecundity. Limitation of uterine space available to the developing embryos and competition between embryos for biochemical factors or nutrients have been suggested as mechanisms. Asynchrony in the development rate between embryos was also suggested as a potential factor contributing to embryonic losses (Pope et al., 1990).

Factors which can contribute to early embryonic loss in pigs include housing and social stress (Gordon 1997), nutrition (Dziuk 1992) and seasonal influences (Peltoniemi et al., 2000).

4.5 Induction of parturition

(Gordon 1997).

If a high survival rate of neonatal piglets is to be achieved, control around the time of parturition is essential. This can be facilitated by induction of parturition and the careful treatment of the sow after farrowing.
The entire process of parturition takes 2-5 hours, with piglets being delivered at about 15 minute intervals. Farrowing occurs slightly more frequently in the late afternoon and at night. The placentae are delivered either after the emptying of one uterine horn or within 4 hours of the last piglet being delivered. Primiparous sows often need more assistance at delivery than multiparous ones.
Litter sizes may vary enormously, from 1 to 19 piglets. Most stillborn piglets have died during parturition itself. Births lasting more than 6 hours result in higher rates of stillbirth. There is not only variation in numbers between litters, there can also be an enormous variation in birth weight within litters. There is a very close relationship between birth weight and piglet survival.

Over the last few years, various analogues of $PGF_{2\alpha}$ have been used successfully to induce and synchronize farrowing in sows (Alexopulous et al., 1992; Gielent et al., 1992; Leike and Huhn 1992; Cameron et al., 2000).
Parturition can be induced by treating sows with prostaglandins (e.g. Planate®, Estrumate®) 2 days before the expected farrowing date. In farrowings induced with prostaglandin $F_{2\alpha}$ analogues, the majority of sows start labour between 20 and 30 hours after injection.

Figure 8 Distribution of farrowing after induction with cloprostenol racemate

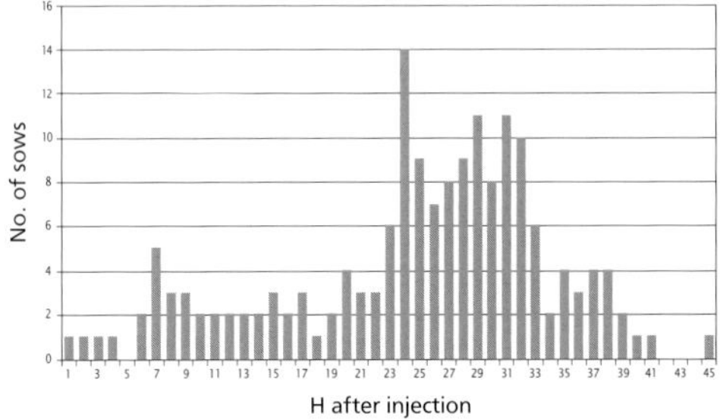

Farrowing may also be synchronized with an injection of oxytocin 20 - 24 hours after prostaglandin treatment (Clark et al., 2002). Induction facilitates supervision at farrowing, and improves the possibilities for cross-fostering soon after birth. Cross-fostering not only allows the creation of litters of equal numbers, but also of litters with piglets of more uniform body weights. If the interval between the births of two piglets is prolonged (e.g. >20 minutes), or when farrowing takes too long overall (e.g. >5 hours), parturition can be accelerated using oxytocin, which can also be used to improve uterine involution and milk let-down.

Administration of prostaglandins after parturition

In sows, the endometrial regeneration after farrowing takes approximately 18 days.

Inadequate recuperation after a previous pregnancy is believed to contribute to an extended weaning to service interval and decreased conception and consequently farrowing rates, especially in early weaning systems. Moreover, uterine disorders such as endometritris and metritis-mastitis-agalactia (MMA) syndrome are associated with reduced fertility, losses of piglets and even sow mortality.

Over the last five years, it has been postulated that the administration of prostaglandin $F_{2\alpha}$ shortly after farrowing may have a beneficial effect on reproductive performance.

The mechanism by which prostaglandin administration might alter the association between the lactation length and subsequent litter size and uterine health has been suggested to be:

- a direct effect of prostaglandin on the uterus and the hastening of endometrial repair
- the induction of luteolysis of corpora lutea

In some studies, a considerable number of older sows (7.9%) were found to have elevated progesterone concentrations after farrowing (Elbers et al., 1994). It has been postulated that some, especially older, sows can maintain partially active luteal tissue even after farrowing. Bearing in mind the immunosuppressive effect of progesterone on the uterine defence mechanisms (Lewis et al., 2004) elimination of the luteal tissue after farrowing should favour uterine involution.
However, the results of field studies reported over the last few years conflict with other trials showing a clear benefit in terms of the weaning to conception interval and conception rates (Izeta-Mayorga et al., 2000; Prieto et al., 2002), and yet others showing such effects only in certain age groups (Koketsu et al., 2002).
There are some indications that herds with a high incidence of vulval discharge may benefit from this use of prostaglandins (Lopez et al., 2009).

4.6 The boar

Boar management
The technical performance of a sow unit depends to a large extent on boar management.
As with the male of other domesticated animals, reproductive efficiency in the boar can be influenced by many environmental and management factors such as:

- *Temperature*
  High ambient temperature is widely recognised as reducing sperm production in boars. It has also been shown, in many trials, to have a negative effect on semen quality, as measured by reduced sperm motility and the proportion of normal spermatozoa (Kunavongkrit et al., 2005). Apart from a direct influence on testicular function, high ambient temperatures may cause pigs to eat less and the resultant nutritional imbalance, especially reduced protein intake, can affect semen quality (Rinaldo et al., 2000).

- *Photoperiod*
  Claus et al. (1985) reported that light or photoperiod could influence sperm quality and libido in boars. It has also been noted that short day length stimulates the pubertal maturation of spermatogenesis (Andersson 2000). Artificially adjusting the day length, or administering exogenous melatonin, may have a positive effect on reproductive performance in boars during problem months.
- *Nutrition*
  Proper nutrition and adequate body condition are essential for the boar's reproductive performance. Feed containing 14% protein and 70% energy fed at 3–4 kg per day, depending on body weight and condition, has been widely recommended for boars. These figures may be adjusted and modified according to the breed and line specificity of the boar. Factors such as temperature and social interactions may negatively influence feed intake and lead to decreased sperm quality.
- *Housing*
  Confining boars and/or forcing them into social hierarchies can influence their sexual behaviour, and occasionally can have more profound effects, on sperm production and quality. The reproductive efficiency of breeding herds can be improved by adapting the management of boars to optimize their sperm production. The effective management of the boar's environment is important in overcoming heat stress, high humidity or unfavourably low temperatures and changing photoperiods, as well as problems of feed intake.

Some guidelines for the management of the breeding boar are given in Table 6.

Table 6 Some guidelines for boar management.

Boar: sow ratio	approximately 1:25
Minimum age for breeding	7.5 months
Mating frequency	boars < 9 months, not more than 3 times per week boars > 9 months, not more than 5 times per week
Semen quality	regular investigation is recommended. In addition, it should always be carried out 3-5 weeks after a period of pyrexia

Do not use two boars for the double mating of a sow, as a low fertility in one of them may be masked by the other. All natural matings should be supervised and mating records should be kept for each boar.

AI and semen quality

The use of AI with high quality ejaculates reduces the number of boars required. One boar can produce up to 1300-1600 AI doses of semen annually. Sperm production can easily fluctuate as much as 25-30%, so regular quality assessment is essential. Table 7 shows a number of parameters which can be used to assess the quality of semen.

Table 7 Parameters for evaluating semen quality.

Volume (without gel mass)	>100 ml
Motility at time of collection	>65%
Concentration	>100 x 10^3 sperm cells/ml
Abnormal sperm cells	<20%

One AI dose should contain at least 2 x 10^9 motile sperm cells with a minimum volume of 80 ml. Tail abnormalities of spermatozoa are considered to be less important than abnormalities of the head.

Conservation of boar semen and artificial insemination

The key to the widespread application of AI worldwide is the ability to store semen extended in buffers, for up to a week at near room temperature. Many extenders have been developed over the years, increasing storage time from 3 days to 5–7 days.

Frozen semen has been used primarily for export and in specific genetics programmes. In spite of the availability of freezing technology, frozen semen is not widely used in commercial pig production, mainly because it is not as cost effective as fresh semen.

The fertility results currently obtained with frozen–thawed boar semen are quite satisfactory (Thilmant 1997; Eriksson et al., 2002). Under ideal conditions, these can approach those obtained with fresh semen. However, it seems that frozen boar semen does not yet have the quality needed to achieve adequate results under the broad range of conditions encountered in the field.

In contrast to cattle breeding, sexed sperm is not yet available for use in commercial breeding operations, although the technology for sexing the semen is well enough established.

In the last few years, numerous reports have appeared indicating that the addition of prostaglandin analogues to semen has beneficial effects. Waberski (1997) as well as Horvat and Bilkei (2003) indicated that this process increased the chance of spermatozoa reaching the site of fertilization, and can result in increased conception and farrowing rates. In a recently reported study by Kos and Bilkei (2004), conception and farrowing rates, as well as regular returns to oestrus, were favourably affected by the supplementation of semen with $PGF_{2\alpha}$. The total number of piglets born and piglets weaned per sow per year were increased by using prostaglandin supplemented semen.

Biotechnology in pigs

The implementation of methods for long-term embryo preservation and transfer in pigs would provide a means for the effective use of the world's most valuable genetic resources, on a global basis, while enhancing genetic improvement programmes. Moreover, embryo transfer would facilitate the transfer of improved genetic potential around the world, while minimizing the risk of disease transmission. The USDA Swine Embryo Cryopreservation Technology provides a non-invasive method of freezing all stages of pre-implantation pig embryos, from zygotes to hatched blastocysts, and has been reported to result in live, healthy piglets that grow normally and are of excellent fecundity (Gerrits et al., 2005).

4.7 References

Alexopoulos C., Saratsis Ph., Samouilidis S., Saoulidis K., Brozos Ch., Kyriakis SC. The effect of cloprostenol alone or with oxytocin on induction of parturition, litter characteristics and subsequent fertility of the sow. Reprod Dom Anim 1998;33:83-88.

Almond GA. Seasonal infertility in Domestic Swine. AASP Newsletter, 1991;3:1-5.

Andersson H. Photoperiodism in pigs: studies on timing of male puberty and melatonin. Thesis, Swedish University Agricultural Science, vol. 90. Uppsala, Sweden; 2000. p. 46.

Barnet JL., Hemsworth PH. The effects of individual and group housing on sexual behaviour and pregnancy in pigs. Anim Reprod Sci 1991;25:265-73.

Bates RO., Day BN., Britt JH., Clark LK., Brauer MA. Reproductive performance of sows treated with a combination of pregnant mare's serum gonadotropin and human chorionic gonadotropin at weaning in the summer. J Anim Sci 1991;69:894-898

Beltranena E., Foxcroft GR., Aherne FX., Kirkwood RN. Endocrinology of nutritional flushing in gilts. Can J Anim Sci 1991;71:1063-1071

Bertoldo M., Grupen CG., Thomson PC., Evans G., Holyoake PK. Identification of sow-specific risk factors for late pregnancy loss during the seasonal infertility period in pigs. Theriogenology 2009; in press

Bolarin A., Roca J., Rodriguez-Martinez H., Hernandez M., Vazquez JM., Martinez EA. Dissimilarities in sows' ovarian status at the insemination time could explain differences in fertility between farms when frozen-thawed semen is used. Theriogenology 2006;65: 669–680

Cameron RDA., Kieran PJ., Martin I. The efficacy of inducing batch farrowing and the impact on sow behaviour of the prostaglandins cloprostenol and dinoprost. Proceedings of 16th IPVSC, Melbourne, Australia 2000: p. 386

Clark MH., Bilkei G. Multiple oxytocin application increases the predictability of prostaglandin induced farrowing in swine. Dtsch Tierarztl Wochenschr. 2002;109:489-90.

Claus R., Weiler U, Wagner H-G. Photoperiodic influences on reproduction of domestic boars. II. Light influences on semen charecteristics and libido. J Vet Med Series A 1985;32:99–109.

Clowes EJ., Aherne FX., Schaefer AL., Foxcroft GR., Baracos VE. Parturition body size and body protein loss during lactation influence performance during lactation and ovarian function at weaning in first-parity sows. J. Anim. Sci. 2003;81:1517–1528

Cole DJA., Foxcroft GR. Control of Pig Reproduction. London: Butterworth, 1982.

Cosgrove JR., Foxcroft GR. Nutrition and reproduction in the pig: ovarian aetiology. Anim Reprod Sci 1996;42:131-141

Cox NM. Control of follicular development and ovulation rate in pigs. J Reprod Fertil 1997;Suppl 52:31–46.

Dawson A., Pitt R., Peters AR. Seasonality and reproduction. In Progress in Pig Science. Eds J . Wiseman, MA. Varley, J.P. Chadwick. Nottingham 1998, Nottingham University Press, pp. 327-342

Dial GD., Marsh WE., Polson DD., Vaillancourt JP. Reproductive failure: differential diagnosis. In: Leman, A.D., Straw, B.E., Mengeling, W.L., D'Allaire, S., Taylor, D.J. (Eds.), Diseases of Swine, seventh ed. Iowa State University Press 1992, Ames, IA, pp. 88–137.

Dijkhuizen AA. Economic aspects of common health and fertility problems for the individual pig producer: an overview. The Vet Quart 1989;11:116-24.

Dyck GW. Influence of sire, dietary intake and housing facilities on the attainment of puberty in crossbred gilts. Can J Anim Sci 1989; 69: 939-946

Dziuk PJ. Embryonic development and fetal growth. Anim. Reprod. Sci. 1992;28:299-308

Eliasson L., Rydhmer L., Emarsson S., Andersson K. Relationships between puberty and production traits in the gilt.
a. Age at puberty. Anim Reprod Sci 1991;25:143-54.
b. Oestrus symptoms at puberty. Anim Reprod Sci 1991;25:255-64.

Eriksson BM., Petersson H., Rodriguez-Martinez H. Field fertility with exported boar semen frozen in the new flatpack container. Theriogenology 2002;58:1065–79.

Findlay JK. Physiology of the uterus and implantation. In: Batterham, ES (Ed.) Manipulating Pig Production IV. Australasian Pig Science Association, Attwood, Victoria, Australia 1993, pp. 235-244

Gerrits RJ., Lunney JK., Johnson LA., Pursel VG., Kraeling RR., Rohrer GA., Dobrinsky JR. Perspectives for artificial insemination and genomics to improve global swine populations. Theriogenology 2005;63:283-299

Geudeke MJ. The use of slaughterhouse information in monitoring systems for herd health control in sows [Thesis]. Utrecht: 1992.

Gielen j Th., Egger W., van de Kamp J. Induction of a synchronised farrowing in sows and gilts with luprostiol. Proc 12th Inter Cong Anim Reprod, The Hague, The Netherlands 1992, vol 2, pp.849-853

Givens MD., Marley MSD. Infectious causes of embryonic and fetal mortality. Theriogenology 2008;70: 270–285

Gordon I, Controlled reproduction in pigs, 1997, CAB International U.K. ISBN 085991165.

Hazeleger W., Soede NM., Kemp B. The effect of feeding strategy during the pre-follicular phase on subsequent follicular development in pigs. Dom Anim Endocrinol 2005;29:362-370

Holyoake T. What dowe know of pregnancy loss during seasonal infertility? Proceedings of the Australian Association of Pig Veterinarians Gold Coast, Australia, 2005; 13-17. Australian Association of Pig Veterinarians, The University of Sydney.

Horvat G., Bilkei G. Exogenous prostaglandin F2a at time of ovulation improves reproductive efficiency in repeat breeder sows. Theriogenology 2003;59:1479-1484

Hunter MG., Robinson RS., Mann GE., Webb R. Endocrine and paracrine control of follicular development and ovulation rate in farm species. Animal Reprod Sci 2004;82–83:461–477

Hühn U., Wähner M. Biotechnical integration of gilts and sows in herds with farrowing systems. 14th ICAR, Stockholm 2000, Abstracts, Vol 2: p. 56

Izeta-Mayorga J., Ramos R., Galicia J. Comparison of two different prostaglandins (dinoprosta and cloprostenol) used 24 hours post partum in sows. Proc 16th IPVS Congress, Melbourne, Australia, 2000:

Kauffold J., Rautenberg T., Richter A., Sobiraj A. Estrus synchronisation and rebreeding of failed female swine. Proc 16th IPVSC, Melbourne, Australia 2000, p. 384

Kauffold J and Althouse GC. update on the use of B-mode ultrasonography in female pig reproduction. Theriogenology 2007;67: 901–911

Knox RV., Rodriguez-Zas SL., Miller GM., Willenburg KL., Robb JA. Administration of PG 600 to sows at weaning and the time of ovulation as determined by transrectal ultrasound. J Anim Sci 2001;79:796-802

Knox RV. Recruitment and selection of ovarian follicles for determination of ovulation rate in the pig. Domestic Animal Endocrinology 2005;29:385–397

Koketsu Y., Dial GD. Administration of prostaglandin $F_{2\alpha}$ after farrowing alters the association between lactation length and subsequent litter size in mid and old parity sows. Theriogenology 2002;57:837-843

Kos M., Bilkei G. Prostaglandin $F_{2\alpha}$ supplemented semen improves reproductive performance in artificially inseminated sows. Animal Reprod Sci 2004;80:113-120

Koutsotheodoros F., Hughes PE., Parr RA., Dunshea FR., Fry RC., Tilton JE. The effects of post-weaning progestagen treatment (Regumate) of earlyweaned primiparous sows on subsequent reproductive performance. Animal Reproduction Science 1998;52:71–79

Krzymowski T., Stefanczyk-Krzymowska S., Uterine blood supply as a main factor involved in the regulation of the estrous cycle – a new theory. Reprod Biol 2002;2: 93–114.

Kunavongkrit A., Suriyasomboon A., Lundeheim N., Heard TW., Einarsson S. Management and sperm production of boars under differing environmental conditions. Theriogenology 2005;63:657–667

Langendijk P., van den Brand H., Soede NM., Kemp B. Effect of boar contact on follicular development and on estrus expression after weaning in primiparous sows. Theriogenology 2000;54:1295–303

Langendijk P., Bouwman EG., Schams D., Soede NM., Kemp B. Effects of different stimuli on oxytocin release, uterine activity and receptive behaviour in estrous sows. Theriogenology 2003;59:849–61.

Leike J., Huhn U. The synchronisation of sow parturition using a combined treatment regimen of cloprostenol Jenapharm and depotocin Spofa. Berl Munch Tierarztl Wochenschr 1992;105:345-349

Lende van der T. Embryonic and fetal mortality in swine: causes, consequences and how to prevent these losses. In: Proceedings of the 7th Simpósio Internacional de Reproducao e Inseminacao Artificial em Suinos, Foz do Iguacu, Brazil 2000, pp. 243–252

Lewis GS. Steroidal regulation of uterine immune defenses. Anim Reprod Sci 2004; 82–83: 281–294

Lopez JV., Ptaszynska MP., Gonzales M and Martens M R T M. Beneficial effects on the reproductive performance of sows of administering prostaglandin analogues after farrowing the Veterinary Record 2009;164:807-809

Lucy MC., Liu J., Boyd CK., Bracken CJ. Ovarian follicular growth in sows. Reproduction 2001;Suppl.58:31–45.

Madej A., Lang A., Brandt Y., Kindahl H., Madsen MT., Einarsson S. Factors regulating ovarian funstion in pigs. Dom Anim Endocrinol 2005;29:347-361

Meunier-Saiyn MC., Dantzer R. Behaviour environment relationships in pigs: importance for the design of housing and management systems in intensive husbandry. Pig News and Info 1990;11:507-14.

Peltoniemi OAT., Heinonen M., Leppävuori A., Love RJ. Seasonal effects on reproduction in the domestic sow – a herd record study. Acta Vet Scand 1999a;40:133-144

Peltoniemi OAT., Love RJ., Heinonen M., Tuovinen V., Saloniemi H. Seasonal and management effects on fertility of the sow: a descriptive study. Anim Reprod Sci 1999b;55:47-61

Peltoniemi OAT., Tast A., Love RJ. Factors effecting reproduction in the pig: seasonal effects and restricted feeding of the pregnant gilt and sow. Anim reprod Sci 2000;60-61:173-184

Pearce GP. Contact with oestrus female pigs stimulates and synchronizes puberty in gilts. Vet Rec 1992;130:318-23.
Pope WF., Xie S. Broermann DM, Nephew KP. Causes and consequences of early embryonic diversity in pigs. J Reprod Fertil 1990; Suppl 40:251-260
Prieto C., Lopez JV., Martens MR. Effect of postpartum luprostiol (Prosolvin) treatment on sow performance. Proc 17th IPVS Congress, Iowa, USA, 2002; Vol 2:676
Prunier A., Quesnel H., Messias de Braganca M., Kermabon AY. Environmental and seasonal influences on the return-to-oestrus after weaning in primiparous sows: a review. Lives Prod Sci 1996; 45: 103-110
Pusateri AE., Smith JM., Smith JW., Thomford PJ., Diekman MA. Maternal recognition of pregnancy in swine: I. Minimal requirement for exogenous estradiol-17 beta to induce either short or long pseudopregnancy in cycling gilts. Biol Reprod 1996;55:582-589
Rinaldo D., Dividich JL., Noblet J. Adverse effects of tropical climate on voluntary feed intake and performance of growing pigs. Livest Prod Sci 2000;66:223–34.
Schnurrbusch U., Scharfe S. Zum Vorkommen verschiedener Formen der Ovarialzysten des Schweines unter besonderer Bercksichtigung ihres Einfluses auf den Zyklusverlauf TierŠrztl Prax 1991;19:635-43.
Schnurrbusch U and Huhn U. Fortpflanzungstereurung beim weiblichen Dchwein. Gustav Fischer Verlag, Jena, Stuttgart 1994.
Schukken YH., Buurman J., Huirne RBM., Willemse AH., Vernooy JCM., Broek J van den., Verheyden IHM. Epidemiological evaluation of fertility management in swine herds. Anim Reprod Sci 1992;28:45-50.
Signoret JP., Martinat-Botte F., Bariteau F., Fergerit Y., Macar C., Moreau A., Terqui M. Control of oestrus in gilts. I. Management induced puberty. Anim Reprod Sci 1990;22:221-25.
Singleton WL. state of the art in artificial insemination of pigs in the united states. Theriogenology 2001;56:1305-1310
Smith AL., Stalder KJ., Serenius TV., Baas TJ., Mabry JW. Effect of weaning age on nursery pig and sow reproductive performance. J Swine Health Prod. 2008;16:131–137.
Stein TE., Dijkhuizen A., D'Allaire S., Morris S. Sow culling and mortality in commercial swine breeding herds. Prev Vet Med 1990;9:85-94.
Thilmant P. Congelation du sperme de verrat en paillettes de 0.5 ml. Resultats sur le terrain. Ann Med Vet 1997;141:457–62.
Waberski D. Effects of semen components on ovulation and fertilisation. J Reprod Fertil 1997; Suppl 52:105-109
Wood CM., Kornegay ET., Shipley CF. Efficacy of altrenogest in synchronizing estrus in two swine breeding programs and effects on subsequent reproductive performance of sows. J Anim Sci 1992;70:1357-1364
Xue JL., Dial GD., Marsh WE., Davies PR. Multiple manifestations of season on reproductive performance of commercial swine. J A V M A 1994;204:1486-1489
Ziecik AJ., Old, new and newest concepts of inhibition of luteolysis during early pregnancy in pig. Dom Anim Endocrinol 2002;23:265–275.

5 Ovine Reproduction

5.1 Physiology

5.1.1 Seasonality of sexual and ovarian activity

One of the most important features of ovine reproduction is seasonality, though this is not exclusive to sheep, of course. Reproduction follows a seasonal pattern in ewes, i.e. alternating periods of anoestrus and sexual activity. In temperate regions, seasonality is regulated by the photoperiod, or daylight length (reducing daylight length stimulates sexual activity, and increasing daylight length induces anoestrus). Sheep are therefore categorized as 'short day' breeders.

Ewes are able to 'monitor' changes in the daily photoperiod by the circadian secretion of melatonin from the pineal gland. Melatonin output is regulated by photoperiod and elevated concentrations are found in blood only during the hours of darkness (O'Callaghan 1994; Rosa et al., 2003). The characteristics of the circadian pattern of melatonin secretion vary with changes in the light-dark cycle throughout the year, enabling the animal to 'recognise' the changes in the light/dark ratio. Melatonin has a profound effect on the secretion of gonadotrophin-releasing hormone (GnRH) from the hypothalamus, which modulates the release of pituitary gonadotrophins, and these, in turn, control seasonal reproductive activity.

While the photoperiod is the main determinant of seasonality, other factors can influence reproductive patterns, such as genetics (some breeds being sensitive to daylight variation), management practices (e.g. the ram effect; see 5.3.2) and social interactions (Henderson and Robinson 2000).

The length of the breeding season varies between breeds. Dorset Horn ewes are theoretically capable of lambing at any time of the year, although an 8-month breeding season might be expected within a particular flock (Henderson and Robinson, 2000). Mountain breeds, such as the Scottish Blackface, Swaledale, Welsh Mountain and Cheviot, exhibit much shorter

seasons of approximately 4 months. Crossbreeds (Greyface and Mule) are often characterized by only a moderate duration of reproductive activity. Despite these variations, there is a peak of fertility in late autumn (October-November) for most of the breeds in the northern hemisphere. Therefore, the highest lambing rates are recorded in late March and April. Breeds from the intermediate latitudes, such as the Australian Merino and Mediterranean breeds, have a short anoestrus during which a proportion of ewes ovulate spontaneously. In tropical and subtropical environments, ewes are either completely non-seasonal or intermittently polyoestrus, with the availability and quality of food dictating sexual activity.
Yearling ewes and ewe lambs have a shorter breeding season than older ewes.

During the non-breeding season (anoestrus), oestrous cycles as such are not observed. Although the behavioural signs of oestrus and ovulation are absent, dynamic changes in ovarian follicular growth and regression nevertheless occur throughout the non-breeding season. Anoestrus is due to the failure of antral follicles to proceed to growth and maturation, which normally happens in the pre-ovulatory phase of the oestrous cycle (O'Callaghan 1994). However, the further development of these follicles can be stimulated artificially, which allows for breeding during anoestrus or the transition periods.
Seasonality not only affects the mature animal, it can also influence the age of onset of puberty. Although genetics plays a major part in determining age at puberty, the season in which birth takes place (i.e. the photoperiod at that time) can either advance or delay puberty for several months. Oestrus activity ceases with pregnancy and is not resumed for some time after lambing, due to so-called 'post partum anoestrus', also known as 'lactational anoestrus'. The length of this period varies with breed, management practices and the date of parturition, since seasonal and post partum anoestrus may overlap in some instances. Post partum anoestrus is mainly due to the 'anti-gonadotrophic' effect of the sucking lamb, so it normally ends shortly after weaning.
But even when not suckling lambs (e.g. when lambs are reared on milk replacer), the ewes' immediate post partum period is mostly spent in anoestrus.

Whilst rams are able to mate at any time of the year, both the lack of libido and the lower quality and quantity of the ejaculate during the non-breeding season, can reduce the efficiency of out-of-season breeding (Henderson and Robinson 2000).

It is well known that, independent of seasonal influences, nutrition affects many aspects of reproductive performance in sheep, e.g. age at puberty in both sexes, fertility, ovulation rate, embryo survival, parturition to re-breeding interval, testicular growth and production of spermatozoa (Rosa et al., 2003). Lactation length can also affect the breeding season. Under normal conditions, in highly seasonal breeds, birth occurs during seasonal anoestrus and therefore there is no obvious lactational anoestrus. When the ewes are induced to breed during seasonal anoestrus, however, they lamb during the usual breeding season and the resumption of ovarian activity is known to be delayed in lactating animals.

Influence of high ambient temperatures on reproductive function in sheep
Marai et al. (2007) recently reviewed the impact of high ambient temperatures on various physiological features in sheep. They concluded that exposure to high temperatures evokes a series of drastic functional changes which include reduction in feed intake and conversion, disturbances of water, protein, energy metabolism, and interference with mineral balances, enzyme-controlled reactions, hormonal secretions and blood metabolites.
Such changes result in an impairment of production and reproductive performance. The effect of heat stress is aggravated when accompanied by high humidity.
These data highlight that ambient temperature should be taken into consideration both when planning breeding programs, as well as when evaluating their results.

5.1.2 The oestrous cycle

Non-pregnant females separated from the ram, or failing to conceive after mating, have alternate periods of anoestrus and sexual activity. The latter are characterized by a succession of regular oestrous cycles.

The length of the oestrous cycle is 16-17 days, with a range of 14-19 days. However, in the transition period between anoestrus and sexual activity (end of summer), short cycles of less than 12 days are quite common. The first ovulations of the season are often not accompanied by oestrus behaviour (known as 'silent oestrus' or 'silent heat').

As in other species, the oestrous cycle can be divided into two phases: the follicular phase of 3-4 days and the luteal phase lasting about 13 days.
A wave-like pattern of follicular growth has been recorded in sheep, similar to that observed in cattle, with two to four waves per cycle being the most common (Evans 2003). In general, follicle waves are preceded by a transient increase in FSH concentrations, and a hierarchy is established among the follicles of a wave in respect of their diameter and the oestradiol concentration in the follicular fluid. There is no consensus as to whether or not an absolutely dominant follicle develops during each wave.
Follicular growth continues even during periods of anoestrus supported by FSH fluctuations, but this does not lead to ovulation.

The duration of oestrus varies with age, breed and season, ranging between 18 and 72 hours, with an average of 36 hours. In mature ewes of most British breeds, oestrus lasts 30 hours on average, while in lambs it is at least 10 hours shorter. In Merino ewes, heat may even last up to 48 hours. Ovulation is spontaneous and takes place approximately 20-40 hours after the beginning of oestrus (Henderson and Robinson 2000). As in other species, the overt signs of oestrus result from elevated concentrations of circulating oestrogen which reach a peak just before the onset of oestrus proper, and immediately prior to the luteinizing hormone (LH) surge.
Oestrus in the ewe is a less obvious event than in other ruminants. The vulva of ewes in heat is slightly swollen and congested, and a limited discharge of clear mucus can often be noticed. If a ram is present, ewes in oestrus will seek him out and may display tail-wagging and nuzzle his scrotum. Simultaneously the ram will 'test' the receptivity of ewes in his group by pawing with a forefoot, by rubbing his head along the ewe's flank and

by nibbling her wool. A non-receptive ewe will move away, while one which is fully in heat will stand to be mounted.
But in the absence of a ram, or when only an inexperienced ram is present, oestrus can often go undetected.

Ovulation rate (number of eggs released at ovulation) is influenced by a number of factors, including breed, age, reproductive status (dry or lactating), season of the year, nutritional status and the body condition of the ewe. At the beginning of the breeding season, ovulation rates are usually lower, and oestrus is generally shorter, less intensely demonstrated and of lower fertility.
Fertilization takes place in the fallopian ampulla, approximately 25-31 hours after the first signs of oestrus, with zygotes descending into the uterus 60-65 hours later. Until day 15 after fertilization, ovine embryos migrate throughout the uterine lumen.

The luteal phase is characterized by the maturation of the corpus luteum and elevated levels of circulating progesterone which reach a peak at about 6 days after ovulation. The luteolytic mechanism is similar to that of the cow, with an increase in the numbers of oxytocin receptors, up-regulated by increasing concentrations of oestradiol produced by the pre-ovulatory follicle of the next wave. Stimulation of the oxytocin receptors triggers the release of $PGF_{2\alpha}$ and both the functional and the structural demise of the corpus luteum (Mann and Lamming 1995). The luteal phase following the first ovulation of a breeding season is usually shorter in duration.

The gestation period in sheep is about 5 months, 145-152 days on average. Its length varies mainly with breed, parity and litter size.
Prior to the maternal recognition of pregnancy, the cyclical corpus luteum in the ovary is the only source of progesterone. The corpus luteum of pregnancy continues to be the predominant source between 13 and 55 days post fertilization in sheep, whereas the placental production of progesterone is sufficient to maintain pregnancy from 55 days of gestation onwards (Sammin et al., 2009).

Similar mechanisms to those in cattle for the recognition and maintenance of pregnancy have been defined in sheep. Briefly, the production of interferon tau by trophoblasts between 8 and 21 days post conception, exerts a local action on the endometrium which blocks the pulsatile secretion of $PGF_{2\alpha}$ thus prolonging the lifespan of the corpus luteum.

5.2 Flock reproduction management

5.2.1 Introduction

Low productivity is a feature of traditional extensive systems of sheep production. The seasonal nature of production reduces the economic viability of the traditional flock. Therefore, more modern management systems must be associated with various levels of intensification, the success of which are determined to a large extent by the efficiency of reproductive management.

Reproduction may be managed for various reasons:

1. **Improvement in productivity of the flock**
   - general improvement of fertility
   - increased prolificacy
   - increased number of lambings per year
2. **Planned reproduction**
   - seasonal demands: meat breeds to cater for periods when price or demand is highest
   - introduction of ewe lambs to the flock
   - sustained milk production, ensuring production in periods when the milk price is high
   - labour efficiency
   - in specific conditions: extensive, small scale production
   - sustained supply for the community/family with milk and meat
3. **Use of Artificial Insemination**
   - genetic improvement
   - scrapie control measures: use of rams with scrapie resistant genotypes
   - maximising the use of the best rams
   - reduction of the number of rams needed within the flock
   - reduction in the spread of infectious disease

Table 1 presents the basic parameters used to evaluate reproductive efficiency in sheep flocks.

Table 1 Definitions of reproductive parameters frequently used in ovine reproduction.

Fertility	= Number of ewes lambing / Number of ewes exposed to the ram or artificially inseminated	x100
Prolificacy	= Number of lambs born (dead and alive) / Number of ewes lambing	x100
Fecundity	= Number of lambs born (dead and alive) / Number of ewes exposed to the ram or artificially inseminated	x100

Fertility, the proportion of ewes lambing of all those exposed to the ram during a defined period (usually expressed as a percentage) varies with breed, season, age, nutritional status, breeding management and farm conditions. An average figure of 70 to 80% following natural mating is considered normal to good for autumn breeding, and good to very good for spring breeding.
Artificial insemination (AI) produces poorer results than these. Prolificacy (the number of lambs born per lambing ewe), usually expressed as a percentage, varies widely according to the same factors as for fertility. The Merino is recognised as a breed of low prolificacy, commonly 110 – 120%, while the Romanoff breed frequently reaches levels of 350%. Fecundity represents the number of lambs born per ewe mated, during a defined period.

5.2.2 Pregnancy diagnosis

Pregnancy diagnosis can help to increase reproductive efficiency. Amongst other benefits are the early re-mating of non-pregnant ewes, and the supplementary feeding of those which are pregnant. Moreover the ability to predict the number of foetuses allows more appropriate nutritional management of the ewes in late gestation aimed at preventing pregnancy toxaemia, minimizing pre-lambing feeding costs, optimizing birth weights, viability and weaning weights of lambs and reducing the incidence of dystocia.

Of the various methods of pregnancy diagnosis in sheep, ultrasound scanning is the most accurate and reliable.
A-mode ultrasound (Amplitude-depth or echo-pulse) can be used. It is a quick, convenient and simple technique, but it cannot predict foetal numbers and the viability of the foetus. Real-time B-mode ultrasonic scanning of the uterus in sheep is very much more common. When performed by a skilled operator, it offers an accurate, rapid, safe and practical means for diagnosing pregnancy, determination of foetal numbers and estimation of gestational age.
For transabdominal pregnancy diagnosis the probe of the ultrasound scanner is applied flat against the bare area of the right flank, 2 to 3 inches forward of the right teat. Good contact between the ultrasound probe and the skin is essential, so the area should be cleaned adequately before the examination, and the application of ultrasound gel is very helpful.

The optimum time for transabdominal or transrectal ultrasonography in sheep ranges from 25 to 100 days of gestation. Real-time ultrasound can detect pregnancy as early as 23 days of gestation using a rectal probe, and by 40 days using external trans-abdominal scanning. The number of foetuses can be counted accurately from about 45 to 100 days of pregnancy.
After 100 days it becomes more difficult to count accurately, so scanning is normally undertaken between the 12th and 13th weeks after the rams are introduced to the ewes.

Possible causes for diagnostic errors include:

- Incorrect probe placement – misdirection of the beam towards the urinary bladder
- Pockets of gas accumulated in the intestines interpreted wrongly as embryonic vesicles
- Ewes in oestrus occasionally accumulate enough uterine fluid to cause the uterus to sink to the bottom of abdominal cavity making accurate examination difficult

Doppler and amplitude-depth (A-mode) ultrasound are cheaper alternatives during the second half of gestation.

Other methods
The use of the oestrone sulphate assay can detect pregnancy accurately in ewes from day 30 to 35.
Detection of specific pregnancy-associated proteins is possible in pregnant sheep. Both Pregnancy-Specific Protein B (PSPB) and Ovine Pregnancy-Associated Glycoproteins (oPAGs) can be used. These methods however are still limited in availability under field conditions and cannot be used to detect the number of foetuses.

5.2.3 Oestrus detection

Oestrus is not generally well expressed in sheep, especially in the absence of rams; the most obvious sign is standing to be mounted by a ram. While oestrus detection is of no importance in natural mating, it is vital for the success of AI or 'hand mating' (see 5.2.4) as these can only be successfully performed at a fixed time in relation to ovulation or to the onset of oestrus.
For ewes managed in flocks, the most common methods of oestrus detection are the use of entire, 'aproned' rams (the ram's penis is covered to prevent intromission) or vasectomized 'teaser' rams, fitted with harnesses containing marking crayons. For AI, these methods are not very useful because they are time-consuming and labour intensive. For AI using fresh semen, oestrus detection is only useful for large flocks under very special conditions and then only during the breeding season.
An alternative to oestrus detection is the control or synchronization of oestrus (see 5.3), which reduces the period during which the flock is inseminated, requires less labour and allows the more efficient management of pregnancy and parturition. It can also be used to induce oestrus and ovulation outside the normal season.

5.2.4 Mating

In natural mating conditions, the length of the oestrous cycle and the duration of oestrus mean that about 6-8% of ewes will be in oestrus each day of the breeding season. Assuming there is a ram for every 50 ewes (50:1 ratio) each will need to mate an average of 3-4 ewes per day. This is compatible with the serving capacity of the ram and allows for good fertility. The high concentration of spermatozoa per ejaculate, together with the repeated mating of the ewe throughout oestrus, ensures a good level of fertility and prolificacy. However, the reproductive performance of rams is affected by seasonal influences (Henderson and Robinson 2000) and the requirements of out-of-season breeding and the greater number of ewes coming into oestrus as a result of synchronization impose the need for a more rational use of rams.

Fertility increases as oestrus progresses, reaching a maximum towards the end of the oestrus period. Therefore, the only way to increase fertility, while at the same time optimising the use of the ram, is to practice 'hand mating'. This involves the rams being lined up in a queue in the shedding race and each ram in turn being exposed to a group of (preferably synchronized) ewes. Following an observed mating, the ewe is withdrawn from the group and the ram is taken to the back of the queue. The next ram in line is then exposed to the unmated ewes. The improvement of desirable production traits requires the selection of superior animals for breeding. Since rams are responsible for more offspring than ewes, ram selection is critical. One of the ways of managing selective breeding is batch mating; a group of ewes is mated exclusively by the same ram, using 'hand mating' after oestrus detection or synchronization, or by artificial insemination.

5.2.5 Artificial insemination

AI is the gateway to the use of top quality sires of both local and international origin. It offers progressive producers the opportunity to make previously unimaginable genetic improvements in a very short period. Considerable progress can thus be gained in respect of commercially important features such as milk production, feed conversion and growth rates of fattening lambs, as well as wool quality.

Artificial insemination (AI) brings well-known benefits for sheep production, but there are distinct differences between its use in sheep and its more common use in cattle.

Because of its different anatomy, the ovine cervix cannot be easily entered with an insemination pipette. This was the subject of extensive investigation by Kershaw et al. (2005). Essentially, the lumen of the ovine cervical canal is highly convoluted and tortuous due to the presence of 4–7 cervical rings pointing caudally. These provide a physical barrier to external contamination, but also present the major barrier to trans-cervical artificial insemination (TCAI), since they not only project into the lumen, but the second and third rings are frequently out of alignment with the first, which results in the inseminating pipette being diverted away from the lumen.
So semen must be deposited at the entrance to the cervix – intracervical/transcervical AI, or in the fundus of the vagina - intravaginal AI (Haresign 1992).
In the transcervical method, a small volume of diluted semen is inserted just inside the external os of the cervix. The ewe's hindquarters are elevated, usually by placing them over a fence rail. The inseminator uses a duck-billed speculum inserted into the vagina and a head lamp to enable him to guide the insemination pipette into the cervix. The semen is deposited no more than 10-20 mm inside the cervical canal. With the help of two catchers, a skilled operator can inseminate 100 ewes per hour using this method.
With the development of transcervical insemination skills, improved pregnancy rates are now being achieved (Anel et al., 2005; Paulenz et al., 2005).

An alternative is the use of intra-uterine AI, which is performed surgically with the aid of a laparoscope (Wulster-Radcliffe et al., 2004). In this case 0.2 ml of diluted semen containing about 15-40 x 10^6 sperm is deposited into the lumen of one or both uterine horns from a sharp-tipped glass pipette, or needle and syringe, inserted through the ventral wall of the abdomen. This technique is attractive when valuable, frozen-thawed semen is to be used, since it permits good pregnancy rates with much smaller sperm doses than those used in the intracervical and intravaginal methods.

When properly performed, depositing frozen semen into the uterine horns produces high fertility rates and lambing percentages of 60-75% (Buckrell et al., 1994; Windsor 1995;

Husein et al., 1998). These are similar to the results obtained using fresh semen, and this method is practised routinely in Australia for AI with frozen semen.
Results are good but the procedure is difficult and costs are relatively high. Nonetheless, every year, millions of sheep are inseminated laparoscopically.

Table 2 Typical results from AI in ewes

Semen type	Insemination method	Dose (in millions of sperm cells)*	Typical pregnancy rate reported	Range in pregnancy rate reported
Fresh	Intravaginal	>300	50%	40-65%
	Intracervical	150	40%	50-70%
	Laparoscopic	50	70%	60-90%
Frozen	Intravaginal	>300	10%	0-30%
	Intracervical	75-100	40-50%	30-60%
	Laparoscopic	26-60	65%	50-90%

For AI to be successful, the timing of the deposition of semen in the ewe must be accurate in relation to the time of ovulation, because the period during which fertilization can take place is limited. In most ewes, ovulation occurs at about 25 to 30 hours after the onset of oestrus.
As oestrus detection is impractical under most field conditions, AI is only used in flocks using oestrus synchronization. Artificial insemination is carried out at a fixed time, depending on the breed of ewe, the storage of the semen (chilled or frozen), the method of synchronization and the site chosen for the deposition of semen (see Table 3).

Table 3 Time of insemination in sheep according to the type of oestrus and insemination.

Type of Oestrus	Type of AI	Optimum time for AI
Natural	Cervical or vaginal	12-18 hr after onset of oestrus
Synchronised with Chrono-gest® Sponges	Cervical or vaginal	48-58 hr after sponge removal Single AI: 55 hr after sponge removal Double AI: 48-50 and 58-60 hr after sponge removal
	Intrauterine	60-66 hr after sponge removal
	Intrauterine in superovulated females	36-48 hr (preferably 44-48 hr) after sponge removal

In general, the following factors determine the success of artificial insemination in sheep:

1. *With respect to the ewe herself:*
   - age
   - general heath status and body condition
   - presence of any bacterial or viral infections affecting reproductive function
   - seasonality
   - oestrus type (spontaneous, induced/synchronized)
   - management and nutritional plane in the post AI period
2. *With respect to the insemination procedure:*
   - type of insemination method: intravaginal, transcervical, laparoscopic
   - type of semen used: fresh, frozen
   - quality of semen used
   - service timing and oestrus management in inseminated ewes (synchronization technique and PMSG/eCG dose)
   - insemination technique and handling of semen
3. *Environmental factors*
   - season
   - temperature and humidity during peri-insemination period
   - availability of water and feed during the peri-insemination period

5.3 Management of oestrus

The management of reproduction in ewes can be classified as natural (by altering the photoperiod, flushing, the ram effect) or pharmacological (using progestagens, prostaglandins and melatonin). Only adjusting the photoperiod, the use of the ram effect and the various pharmacological methods allow for actual oestrus synchronization in sheep.

The most important factors to be considered before deciding which method to use are:
- The degree of synchronization needed.
- The season.
- Economic and market factors.

The pharmacological methods are effective in the tight synchronization of oestrus in the majority of situations, ensuring good production figures following fixed time insemination, but with the disadvantage of the expense of the product and its administration.
The natural method is cheaper, but results in less tight synchronization and is only useful in certain conditions.

Flushing
Flushing involves increasing the ewes' plane of nutrition (intake of protein and energy) approximately 3-4 weeks before the planned beginning of the breeding season. Ewes in improving body condition benefit from increased ovulation and therefore lambing percentages. Flushing is an established method for boosting ovulation rate but the response to the improved quality of forage in the weeks prior to mating varies with the breed and the season. Ewes usually respond best to flushing when they are in medium body condition (2.5-3.5 Body Condition Score (BCS)). Flushing should be used as a method of improving prolificacy and fecundity, not in the hope of inducing or synchronizing oestrus.

5.3.1 Altering the photoperiod

This technique involves exposing ewes to an artificially reduced daylight length, following a period of extended daylight length. Used alone, it will hasten the onset of the breeding period, but with variable results, and an unpredictable spread in the onset of cyclicity.

Nowadays, it is widely used for ewes in intensive production systems in combination with other artificial methods, and for rams in AI centres. Sheep and goat AI centres equipped with dark housing use alternate light regimes with a month of long and a month of short days, which allows permanently high levels of semen production in rams and bucks, with no seasonal variation in sperm quality. If year-round production of semen is not required, AI centres tend to maintain their rams in open barns and expose them to a period of 2-3 extra months of long days (Dec-Feb) followed either by return to the natural photoperiod or by prolonged treatment with melatonin (subcutaneous implants). Such a treatment stimulates good quantities of high quality semen in spring, mimicking the normal season of sexual activity which itself last only around 2-3 months.

5.3.2 The Ram Effect

Social influences (e.g., chemosensory, tactile, visual) are known to have potent effects on reproductive function in a variety of species. Rams can stimulate gonadotrophin secretion and ovulation in the anoestrus ewe through chemosensory input (Henderson and Robinson 2000).
The ram effect involves the introduction of rams to ewes that have been separated from males for several weeks beforehand (at least 3-4 weeks). It has only proved to be effective at certain times of the year, usually just before the start of the natural breeding season, when the majority of ewes are not cycling. It is not effective for ewes already cycling or for those in deep anoestrus.
The majority of ewes ovulate within 6 days of the introduction of the ram, but the first oestrus is often silent, and is often followed

by one or two short cycles (of 6-7 days), or by a cycle of normal length with several peaks of oestrus activity. It is the reason for this induced oestrus not being synchronized tightly enough to allow for fixed time insemination. It has been shown that the treatment of ewes with progesterone before, or at the time of, the introduction of the rams, can improve the efficiency of this stimulatory technique, by increasing the percentage of females showing oestrus behaviour at the first ovulation, and by reducing the number of unpredictable short cycles.
It should be stressed that the efficacy of the ram effect varies with several factors, including breed, location, the time of year, nutritional status and the age of the animals. Moreover, use of the ram effect alone does not synchronize oestrus and ovulation tightly enough to allow for fixed time artificial insemination.

5.3.3 Progestagen-based methods

These methods are based on the use of progesterone or its analogues. The latter are usually more potent allowing for a smaller dose. The degree of synchronization obtained and the interval between the end of treatment and the onset of oestrus depends on the product used.
In cyclic females the treatment acts by suppressing the pre-ovulatory pituitary release of gonadotrophins, and therefore follicular development and ovulation. After the withdrawal of the progestagen, the increasing amounts of gonadotrophin released lead to oestrus and ovulation. Although some progestagens can shorten the life-span of the corpus luteum, for effective synchronization in sheep, the duration of treatment must be at least 12- 14 days, mirroring the length of the luteal phase.

Oestrus synchronization with progestagens and artificial insemination
For artificial insemination, accurate oestrus detection and precise service timing are essential. Due to poor oestrus expression in ewes this can be difficult to achieve, which is the reason for most AI in ewes taking place after pharmacologically synchronized oestrus. Among the various methods in current use, progestagens offer the most precise synchronization of

both oestrus and ovulation and, to all intents and purposes, progestagens are what make AI in sheep feasible. No other method used alone (ram effect, melatonin implants etc.) can ensure synchronization tight enough for AI.

Progestagens can be administered in a variety of ways (sponges, implants, etc.), via several routes (intravaginal, i.m., s.c.), and at different doses (Haresign 1992; Godfrey et al., 1999; Bari et al., 2000; Henderson and Robinson 2000). Intravaginal sponges are by far the most widely used as they are easy to insert and provide reliable results after natural mating or AI. Sponges are impregnated with fluorogestone acetate (Chronogest CR®) or medroxyprogesterone acetate (MAP), and are inserted into the vagina using a dedicated applicator.

As sheep are generally perceived as a more 'green' species than cows and pigs, the new Chronogest CR® sponge with a reduced cronolone load (20mg) offers an interesting option for equally efficient oestrus management and lambing rates, but using less exogenous hormone. Letelier et al. (2009) compared the ovarian follicular dynamics and plasma steroid concentrations in ewes given intravaginal Chronogest® sponges containing either 20 or 40 mg of fluorogestone acetate. None of the features monitored (including by daily ultrasonography) differed significantly between the two groups. Ovulatory follicles grew at a similar rate, with comparable initial and maximum diameters. Moreover, ten days after sponge removal, ovulation rates and plasma progesterone concentrations were similar. These authors concluded that reducing the dose of fluorogestone acetate from 40 to 20 mg in Chronogest® sponges did not significantly affect ovarian follicular dynamics or the other ovarian functions measured.

Use of PMSG/eCG in progestagen-treated ewes

In ewes in anoestrus, progestagens must be supplemented with follicle stimulating treatments (e.g. pregnant mare serum gonadotrophin, PMSG/equine chorionic gonadotrophin, eCG) to induce follicular growth, oestrus and ovulation.

When ewes are being synchronized for fixed time AI using progestagen-based programmes, PMSG/eCG should always be used, to reduce the spread in the timing of ovulation due to individual variation between ewes. A normal fertile oestrus follows the progestagen/PMSG treatment. Ali (2007) demonstrated that PMSG/eCG administration to Ossimi ewes treated with fluorogestone sponges, in the subtropics, stimulated follicular development and increased prolificacy. In this experiment, the administration of PMSG/eCG before sponge removal resulted in a shorter interval to oestrus, and ovulation linked to the earlier development of large follicles. This could be beneficial in the use of fixed-time AI. Furthermore, Luther et al. (2007) revealed that pregnancy rates following laparoscopic AI were higher in ewes treated with a combination of progestagens and PMSG/eCG (73.7%) than in those treated with progestagens alone (41.2%)

Table 4 Adjustment of PMSG dose in ewes treated with Chronogest CR® method

	Reproductive status	PMSG (Folligon®) dose
Ewes	In season	300-500 IU
	Out of season	400-600 IU
Ewe lambs	In season	250-400 IU
	Out of season	300-500 IU

For the superovulation of donor ewes in embryo transfer, eCG/PMSG may be administered at about 28 hours before sponge removal and at a higher than normal dose (Folligon®,1500 IU; Bari et al., 2000; Henderson and Robinson 2000). ECG/PMSG may also be followed by an intramuscular injection of GnRH at the onset of oestrus, for the same purpose (Türk et al., 2008).

Recently, reports have appeared suggesting a positive effect of GnRH administration prior to the standard progestagen+PMSG/eCG regime. Karaca et al. (2009) reported that the pre-treatment of ewes with 10mcg buserelin before progestagen-based synchronization (7 day progestagen program in combination with $PGF_{2\alpha}$ administration) resulted in increased multiple birth rates and litter size.

Breeding management in flocks synchronized using progestagens

One of the main advantages of this method is that it can be used to induce and/or synchronize oestrus. The high degree of synchronization obtained allows for very good reproductive performance under a variety of conditions. Ewes will begin to come into oestrus from around 24 to 48 hours after sponge removal.

The fertility of the oestrus will depend upon a number of factors related to both ewes and rams.

Ram introduction

The timing of introduction of the ram following the removal of sponges is crucial. Ewes will begin to show behavioural signs of oestrus from approximately 24 hours after sponge removal. However, most of them will not be in oestrus until 36-48 hours after removal. Consequently, rams introduced immediately after the removal of sponges will repeatedly serve the first ewes to demonstrate oestrus. This may lead to the depletion of their semen reserves, poor conception rates to the induced oestrus, extended lambing and a poor lamb crop. The ram should not therefore be introduced until 36-40 hours after the sponges have been removed from the ewes.

Ram-to-ewe ratio

In synchronized flocks, large numbers of ewes are mated over a relatively short period. This means that special attention must be paid to an appropriate ram-to-ewe ratio. During the breeding season, both ram fertility and libido should be satisfactory and one ram to 10 ewes should be adequate. However, outside the breeding season, both libido and fertility are usually reduced. Therefore, the ram-to-ewe ratio should be increased to roughly one to five. If the requirement for high numbers of rams poses a problem, then the use of AI should be considered (see 5.2.5).

Lambing period and returns to oestrus

A population of ewes conceiving to a synchronized oestrus will generally lamb over a 1-week period. None should be expected to lamb during the following week, but any repeat breeders should start lambing in the next 8-10 days. The whole of lambing should be completed in approximately 3-4 weeks if one repeat mating was allowed.

5.3.4 Prostaglandins

Prostaglandin $F_{2\alpha}$ ($PGF_{2\alpha}$) and its analogues can be used to synchronize oestrus in cyclic ewes. Their luteolytic effect leads to regression of the corpus luteum and a lowering of progesterone concentrations in the blood. The resultant increase in the amount of gonadotrophin released by the pituitary gland stimulates follicular development, and oestrus occurs within 2-3 days, and ovulation about 24 hours later. Several prostaglandin analogues are available in injectable form but only a few of the commercially available products are in fact licensed for use in sheep.

Because the corpus luteum is only responsive to prostaglandins between days 5 and 14 of the oestrous cycle, two injections 10-14 days apart are required for optimum synchronization. The wide variability of the response, and the need to inject cyclic animals twice, explains the limited used of these products in sheep, under field conditions (Henderson and Robinson 2000).

Furthermore, the fertility of the induced oestrus is generally poor, probably because the reproductive tract has been less than normally exposed to progesterone. However, this can be overcome. An abbreviated period (5 days) of progestagen priming (e.g. Chronogest CR®), followed by an injection of $PGF_{2\alpha}$ at sponge withdrawal, has been shown to be highly effective in synchronizing oestrus during the breeding season.

5.3.5 Combination of prostaglandins and GnRH

Some authors have recently reported the use of prostaglandins and GnRH in cycling ewes with reasonable results as long as the ewes are within their normal breeding season, and depending on the stage of the oestrous cycle when the treatment is begun (Cardenas et al., 2004; Deligianis et al., 2005). The results of these studies indicate that using a modified Ovsynch protocol in cycling ewes, can achieve an acceptable conception rate which could be further improved by modifying the intervals between injections.

On the other hand, Husein et al. (2005) reported that 4-day progesterone priming ahead of the treatment was essential for the effectiveness of this procedure, to maintain follicular response to GnRH. Their results showed an increased response with respect to oestrus, and improved pregnancy rates, in ewes and goats treated in this way (Husein and Kridli 2003; Husein et al. 2005). Titi et al. (2009, in press) reported encouraging results of a synchronization protocol in ewes when progestagen-loaded sponges were used between GnRH and $PGF_{2\alpha}$ injections.

5.3.6 Melatonin

Melatonin, a hormone produced by the pineal gland, mainly during the hours of darkness, is considered to be the chemical trigger which allows the photoperiod to control the secretion of hormones by the pituitary gland (Chemineau 1992). Exogenous melatonin can also be used in controlling the timing of the breeding season.

Many methods involve the continuous administration of melatonin, rather than attempting to mimic the natural daily fluctuations. In some countries, melatonin has been marketed as a slow-release implant. Apparently, elevated blood concentrations of melatonin must be maintained for at least five weeks in order to bring the breeding season forward. There is some evidence that this treatment may increase ovulation rate (Symons et al., 1988; Henderson and Robinson 2000).

Slow-release melatonin implants are often used in conjunction with other environmental techniques, such as the ram effect, especially in extensively managed flocks that are not practising artificial insemination (Zuniga et al., 2002). In the northern hemisphere, melatonin implants have been used in adult ewes, traditionally around the time of the summer solstice, in order to advance the breeding season. In commercial Mediterranean flocks implants are usually inserted at about the time of the spring equinox, as they have an earlier breeding season than genotypes kept at higher latitudes, even when subjected to the same treatment to adjust the photoperiod (Abecia et al., 2007). These workers concluded that melatonin could be a useful tool for improving lamb production in the three breeds they studied, but within each breed, the degree of success varied according to the farm and the season.

It must be stressed that treatment with melatonin alone does not synchronize oestrus and ovulation tightly enough to allow for fixed time artificial insemination. One of the possible options could be a combination of melatonin pre-treatment with precise oestrus synchronization via a progestagen-based program.
DeNicolo et al. (2008) evaluated the effect of treatment with melatonin implants followed by a progesterone-releasing device and eCG/PMSG synchronization. The results of this experiment suggest that melatonin implants, in conjunction with the administration of progesterone and eCG/PMSG, may be a suitable means of increasing the number of lambs born per ewe in an out-of-season breeding program.

5.4 Factors affecting oestrus and ovulation

Although most breeds of sheep can carry and rear at least two lambs, lambing percentages are usually lower than 200%. Manipulating the ovulation rate when breeding in or out of season, by pharmacological or natural methods, can improve lambing rates.

5.4.1 Ram effect

This is a method of inducing oestrus and ovulation in anoestrus ewes during the end of the anoestrus period season (see 5.3.1 and 5.3.2).

5.4.2 Genetics

Breeds differ considerably in terms of ovulation rate, and crossbreeding is probably the simplest method of increasing the fecundity of a flock. On the other hand, there are individual animals, or strains of animals, in several breeds world-wide, which have a considerably higher ovulation rate than the mean for their flock or breed. The best-known examples are those Merino sheep carrying the Booroola or 'F' gene. Because this characteristic lies in a single gene, it can be used, by back-crossing, to increase the ovulation rate substantially in any sheep population (Henderson and Robinson 2000).

5.4.3 Nutrition

Ewes maintained on a low plane of nutrition usually have a low ovulation rate. It has been known for many years that a rising plane of nutrition, commonly known as 'flushing', may stimulate ovulation and increase litter size. However, the response to better quality feeding in the weeks prior to mating varies with the breed. Ewes generally respond best to flushing when in medium body condition (2.5-3.5 BCS) rather than when excessively thin or fat (Henderson and Robinson 2000).

On the other hand, it has been demonstrated that low dietary intake can reduce ovulation rate in sheep and that dietary supplements containing high energy and protein can increase ovulation even in ewes in poor body condition and not being stimulated with exogenous gonadotrophins (Downing et al., 1995). O'Callaghan et al. (2000) found that non-stimulated ewes on a high quality dietary intake had a greater number of follicles compared with the ewes on a lower dietary intake. In general, in order to achieve reliable results, ewes should be allocated to groups, after weaning, depending on their condition score, and each group managed so that the majority are in the appropriate body condition prior to mating.

In Australia, supplementation of the diet with lupin seeds has been found to improve ovulation rate. This effect appears to be independent of body condition and over-stimulation seems not to occur. Animals need to be fed lupin seeds at a rate of 500-750 g/head/day for a minimum of 6 days before oestrus, when a modest increase in ovulation rate of 20-30 ovulations per 100 ewes can be expected.

5.4.4 Gonadotrophins

Gonadotrophins, such as eCG/PMSG or porcine follicle stimulating hormone (pFSH), can be used to superovulate ewes (Henderson and Robertson 2000). These treatments need to be administered to cyclic ewes during the follicular phase of the oestrous cycle, or after a period of progesterone priming when used outside the breeding season. The pituitary-derived gonadotrophins (e.g. pFSH) are short-acting and require frequent injections, so their use is restricted, in practice, to embryo transfer programmes (Haresign 1992).

PMSG/eCG (e.g. Folligon®) is longer lasting and usually used for inducing oestrus and ovulation outside the normal breeding season or for ensuring good conception rates at a synchronized oestrus in a fixed timed insemination programme during the breeding season (Husein et al., 1998; Henderson and Robertson 2000). The dose required depends largely on the conditions of use, breed and season. As a general rule, a dose of 300-500 IU should be used for females in the breeding season and 400-600 IU out of the breeding season. These doses should allow for a moderate increase in the prolificacy of the flock.

5.4.5 Immunization techniques

Immunization reduces the inhibitory effect of the ovarian steroids or ovarian inhibin on the hypothalamus and pituitary, resulting in an increase in the ovulation rate. Immunization against inhibin has been tested experimentally (Anderson et al., 1998; Dhar et al., 2001) but this technique is not yet widely used.

Androstenedione, a steroid secreted by the ovarian follicle, has a regulatory effect on ovulation rate through its feedback action on the hypothalamic-pituitary axis (Cognie 1988; Henderson and Robinson 2000). There is one vaccine (Androvax®) available commercially. The timing of vaccination is important to the success of this technique. Ewes must be sexually active when the rams are introduced. Therefore, if the technique is to be used out-of-season, the ewe flock needs to be primed with progesterone sponges and eCG/PMSG to stimulate oestrus activity. The dose of eCG/PMSG must then be carefully evaluated, as the effects of eCG/PMSG and the vaccine will be additive (Henderson and Robinson 2000).

5.5 Fertilization rate and embryonic losses in sheep

Data available in the literature suggest that, as observed in cattle, a fertilization rate of 90-95% appears to be normal in ewes, under natural mating conditions. When biotechnical methods involving artificial insemination, and especially with frozen semen, are used, much lower fertilization rates are to be expected.

Compared to cattle, there are far fewer reports and reviews defining the extent of embryonic losses in sheep. Most studies have focused either on early embryonic survival or perinatal mortality. The fact that a ewe can often ovulate more than one oocyte further complicates the interpretation of the available data.

Most embryonic mortality has been reported to occur before day 18 of pregnancy, while losses between day 18 and lambing are estimated at 9.4% and late embryonic or foetal losses from day 30 to term, as little as 1- 5%. It is now well-established that losses increase with increasing ovulation rate (Knights et al., 2003; Kleemann and Walker 2005b). It can therefore be stated that, in sheep, embryo survival rate is a function of ovulation rate.

Dixon et al. (2007) investigated patterns of late embryonic and foetal mortality in this species. Cumulatively, a greater percentage of ewes lost 1 or more, but not all, embryos or foetuses of a multiple pregnancy between day 25 and parturition (36.7%) than those that lost a single pregnancy (20.5%) or all of a multiple pregnancy (3.8%). Mean losses of embryos or foetuses averaged 3.7% of embryos from day 25 to 45, 4.3% from day 45 to 65, 3.3% from day 65 to 85, and 11.5% from day 85 to parturition; thus approximately 3 to 4% for each 20-day period of pregnancy beyond day 25. The authors found that late embryonic and foetal losses occurred at similar rates in the anoestrus and transitional seasons.

Embryonic survival and the age of the dam

There is evidence, at least in some breeds, that embryo survival is lower in ewe lambs than in adult ewes. It is believed that this impaired survival is attributable to the inherent quality of the embryo rather than to any deficiency of the uterine environment.

A study by Khan et al., (2003) demonstrated that treatment of ewe lambs with 150 IU of hCG at the time of mating improves the growth of the conceptus, placentation and the number of lambs born.

Luteal function and embryonic losses

Based on the similarities in pregnancy recognition between cattle and sheep, it is quite plausible that progesterone concentration, during the early luteal phase and placentation, does affect embryonic and foetal survival. In fact, much of the basic research on the relationship between early luteal function and embryonic development, as well as on the mechanisms of pregnancy recognition in ruminants, were carried out in sheep. Moreover, Dixon et al., (2007) found that lower concentrations of progesterone on day 25 or 45 of pregnancy were predictive of a greater chance of the complete loss of pregnancy.

Many authors postulate that the timing of breeding (i.e. in or out of season) may affect early luteal function and thus contribute to the lower pregnancy rates usually obtained with out-of-season breeding. Mitchell et al. (2002) found, however, that season did not affect the numbers of corpora lutea per ewe, nor the numbers of ova recovered, but the proportion of the recovered ova that was unfertilised/degenerate was lower in October than in April. Moreover, their results indicated that during the late, as compared with the peak breeding season, there was an increased incidence of fertilization failure as a possible consequence of seasonal shifts in LH secretion and/or the associated effects on follicular function. It is therefore more probable that the lower pregnancy rates observed in ewes bred outside the normal reproductive season are associated with low ovulation rate and poor oocyte quality, rather than a significant luteal insufficiency following induced ovulation. DeNicolo et al. (2009) evaluated plasma progesterone concentrations during early pregnancy in spring- and autumn-bred ewes, and found that early luteolysis, low progesterone secretion from corpora lutea and embryo mortality did occur, but only in a small proportion of ewes. Progesterone concentrations indicated that a majority of mated non-pregnant ewes had elevated progesterone concentrations necessary for the production of at least one viable embryo/foetus.

Nutrition and embryonic losses

Ewes carrying two or more foetuses can suffer from pregnancy toxaemia towards the end of pregnancy as a result of inadequate nutrition. A varying degree of metabolic imbalance, accompanied by hypoglycaemia and ketosis, is caused by a less than adequate feed intake for the number of lambs carried. There may also be other predisposing factors involved. The clinical signs are anorexia and a range of nervous signs, leading to abortion and/or death of the ewe. As the prognosis is poor unless ewes are treated in the very early stages of the disease, control relies heavily on prevention - identification of ewes carrying more than one foetus, and attention to their nutrition, especially in the last third of pregnancy.

Heat stress and embryonic losses

Heat stress is generally considered to have a direct negative effect on embryo survival rates in sheep. Although normal diurnal variation in temperature, and acclimatization, will moderate this effect in the field, it should not be overlooked in areas where high ambient temperatures are expected. Heat stress can also reduce foetal growth, by retarding uterine blood flow (Henderson and Robinson 2000).

5.6 Reproductive disorders

Investigation of reproductive problems in sheep must focus on the flock rather than on the individual. The most relevant losses of reproductive efficiency in sheep can be the consequence of:

- Environmental and social factors causing embryo mortality and infertility.
- Infections causing infertility, enzootic abortion and perinatal losses.
- Inadequate nutrition.

5.6.1 Infectious diseases

There are several infectious diseases that can interfere with fertility and cause pregnancy losses in sheep (Table 5). Without adequate control measures many of them carry the risk of severe financial losses due to reduced fertility, limited possibilities for replacements from within the flock, and in some cases, restrictions on the movement of animals. Moreover some infections are potential zoonoses, posing a severe threat to human health. Table 6 summarizes the most commonly encountered causative agents and the main signs relevant to each.

5.6.1.1 Toxoplasmosis

Toxoplasmosis in sheep is caused by *Toxoplasma gondii*, an intracellular protozoan parasite. Clinical toxoplasmosis occurs following a primary infection in pregnant sheep triggered by the ingestion of sporulated *T. gondii* oocysts. In the small intestine sporozoites are released from the ingested oocysts and by the fourth day the next developmental form, tachyzoites, can be found multiplying in the mesenteric lymph nodes (Buxton et al., 2007; Dubey 2009).
The main source of infection for sheep is feed and pasture contaminated with cat faeces containing infectious oocysts. Although precise data are not available, it is thought that <2% of sheep become congenitally infected with *T. gondii* and less than 4% of persistently infected sheep transmit the organism to their progeny (Buxton et al., 2007; Dubey 2009).

The pathogenesis of ovine toxoplasmosis resembles, to some extent, the mechanism found in bovine neosporosis. In sheep, due to a specific immune state which ensures the tolerance of a semi-allograft foetus, there is minimal maternal expression of cytokines, such as interleukin 2 (IL-2), tumour necrosis factor alpha (TNFα) and interferon gamma (IFNγ) (Entrican and Wheelhouse, 2006). While allowing a successful pregnancy, these mechanisms also render the placenta and foetus peculiarly susceptible to certain pathogens. That is the reason for toxoplasms, circulating in the blood of a pregnant ewe, being able to become established in the placenta. They cross the maternal caruncular septa in the placentome before invading the adjacent trophoblast cells of the foetal villi, from where they can spread to the rest of the foetus (Buxton et al., 2007).

Clinical consequences of infection during pregnancy
Toxoplasmosis has a profound effect on the reproductive health of the ewe when the animal becomes infected for the first time in mid-pregnancy. Typical signs include abortion or stillborn and/ or weakly lambs often along with a small, mummified foetus. Placental cotyledons of the accompanying placentas will show characteristic 'white spot' lesions, visible to the naked eye.
Following infection, sheep acquire an immunity through a cell-mediated immune response. They remain immune but infected

for life (with bradyzoites in tissue cysts in brain and muscle) and will not usually abort due to toxoplasmosis in future pregnancies. This represents a major difference compared with cows infected with *N.caninum* that acquire the infection transplacentally and may abort during each consecutive pregnancy throughout their life (Dubey et al., 2003; 2006). Infection of ewes with *T. gondii* earlier in gestation can result in foetal death and resorption or abortion, while infection in the latter part of gestation, when foetal immunity is relatively well-developed, may have no clinical effect, with the lambs being born normal, but infected and immune.

Control measures include good management of food and water sources to limit the contamination with cat faeces, as well as vaccination (Ovilis Toxovax®).
The diagnosis of toxoplasmosis in sheep is by the histology of samples of cotyledons and/or foetal brain, as well as by various serological tests or PCR.

Toxoplasmosis is an important zoonosis. Humans become infected post-natally by ingesting tissue cysts in undercooked meat, or consuming food or drink contaminated with oocysts. Undercooked lamb is considered an important source of infection. Most infections in humans are asymptomatic, but the parasite can produce devastating disease at times. Congenital infection occurs only when a woman becomes infected during pregnancy, and infections acquired during the first trimester are more severe than those in the second and third trimester. A wide spectrum of clinical disease occurs in congenitally infected children. Mild disease may consist of slightly diminished vision, whereas severely diseased children may have the full tetrad of signs: retinochoroiditis, hydrocephalus, convulsions, and intracerebral calcification. It should be also born in mind that Toxoplasmosis ranks high on the list of diseases which lead to the death of patients with acquired immunodeficiency syndrome (AIDS).

5.6.1.2 Enzootic abortion (EA)

Enzootic abortion is caused by a gram-negative, obligate intracellular bacterium *Chlamydophila abortus* (formerly *Chlamydia psittaci*) and represents an important production disease of sheep flocks in many countries (Kerr et al., 2005). It is the most common infectious cause of abortion in intensively managed lowland flocks near lambing time, and has a major economic impact on sheep farming worldwide.

The infection is commonly transmitted between flocks by means of infected replacement ewes. The main routes of transmission of *C. abortus* are through ingestion of the bacteria shed in vaginal fluids and placental membranes at the time of abortion or lambing, or through inhalation of aerosols from the contaminated environment. There is also some evidence of venereal transmission, but so far it has been difficult to estimate the degree to which this route contributes to the epidemiology of enzootic abortion. Another potential route of transmission is through direct infection of the foetus via the placenta, although again it is unclear what contribution this might have to the spread of the infection within the flock.

Clinical consequences of infection

Infection during pregnancy may result in abortion, stillbirth, birth of weakly, premature or clinically normal but infected lambs (Tab 5). Abortions occur typically during the last 2-3 weeks of gestation.

An initial outbreak that may be associated with only a few abortions, can lead to over 30% of the flock aborting or producing stillborn or weak offspring in the following year (Aitken 2000). In subsequent lambing seasons the incidence of abortion is likely to remain at 5–10% if affected animals are left untreated.

Table 5 Clinical picture of *C.abortus* infection during pregnancy in sheep (adapted from Kerr et al., 2005)

Timing of infection	Clinical consequences
Up to 5-6 weeks prior to parturition	Clinical disease. Abortion in the final 2–3 weeks of gestation, or birth of stillborn or weak lambs that frequently die in the first few days of life
Last 5–6 weeks of pregnancy	Commonly development of a latent infection, no clinical signs until the next lambing season. Surviving lambs born to infected mothers may be affected in their first pregnancy.

Typically, placentitis represents the major gross pathological feature of chlamydial abortion (Aitken 2000). The infection is associated with severe and extensive pathological changes in the foetal membranes. The bacterium targets the placenta, causing tissue damage and inflammation, resulting in abortion (Kerr et al. 2005).

Although there are generally no clinical signs to herald the impending abortion, a vaginal discharge can be observed up to 48 hours prior to the foetus being expelled. The foetal membranes may display varying degrees of necrosis, thickening, oedema and suppurative exudate (Williams and O'Donovan 2009). However, the aborted foetuses are usually well-developed and not autolysed, indicating that foetal death has been a fairly recent event. The discharge can persist for 2–3 weeks, adding to the environmental spread of infection. Infected ewes may also give birth to weak lambs that usually fail to survive.

Following abortion, ewes develop a protective immunity that prevents abortion from *C. abortus* infection in subsequent pregnancies.

Management of Enzootic Abortion should always include the rapid removal of aborting ewes, aborted foetuses and foetal membranes from the lambing pen, followed by cleaning and disinfection. Antimicrobial treatment of ewes with long-acting oxytetracyclines in the face of an outbreak is commonly practised, but the benefit of this treatment is difficult to evaluate. Currently available vaccines (e.g. Ovilis Enzovax®) are used to prevent Enzootic Abortion in uninfected ewes and reduce the spread of the disease within the flock.

It is important to remember that Enzootic Abortion is a zoonosis which can have particularly serious consequences for pregnant women (Longbottom and Coulter 2003).
Infection with *C. abortus* is usually due to exposure to infected foetal fluids and membranes of sheep or goats. In some countries, women who are, or may be, pregnant are advised to avoid involvement with the flock at lambing time.

The definitive method of diagnosis of *C. abortus* or *T. gondii* infection is the isolation of the pathogen from infected tissues. However, this method is labour intensive and time-consuming and relies upon the submission of fresh material to the diagnostic laboratory.
Tests such as ELISAs can detect ewes which have seroconverted after exposure to *Chlamydophila*, but it is not possible to distinguish between naturally infected and vaccinated animals. A serum agglutination test and an ELISA can be used to detect antibodies to confirm *T. gondii* infection in ewes, most infected ewes remaining seropositive for at least six months following infection. For both Enzootic Abortion and Toxoplasmosis, the PCR technique allows the identification of the antigen in aborted foetuses and foetal membranes.

5.6.1.3 Q fever

Q fever (short for 'query' fever), a zoonosis caused by the obligate intracellular micro-organism *Coxiella burnetii*, is wide spread throughout the world and affects a range of animals, including sheep. A comprehensive review of the main features of Q fever in small ruminants was published by Rodolakis (2006).

In ewes, *C. burnetii* infections are generally asymptomatic, but can have a negative effect on the reproductive performance of the flock leading to abortions, stillbirths and weak or non-viable lambs. In the majority of cases, abortion occurs at the end of gestation without any specific prior clinical signs. Aborted foetuses appear normal, but intercotyledonary fibrous thickening and discoloured exudates can be found in their placenta. Aborting ewes shed large amounts of *Coxiellae* with aborted foetuses and foetal membranes, and in vaginal discharges, urine, faeces and milk. The abortion rate is usually low.

In humans, the acute disease is associated with flu-like symptoms. However, more severe complications are possible, such as endocarditis in patients suffering from valvulopathy, as well as premature delivery or abortion in pregnant women.
Routine diagnosis of Q fever in sheep is usually established by histological examination of samples from the placenta or by serology. A recently introduced PCR allows for the accurate diagnosis of infection, and even the identification of asymptomatic animals which are shedding the microorganism.
Preventive measures include adequate management of the aborted material and adequate disinfection. Treatment with oxytetracyclines is possible in aborting flocks although this treatment does not fully suppress the abortions and the shedding of *C. burnetii* at lambing. In ruminants, the only way to prevent the disease is vaccination of the infected flocks, as well any uninfected neighbouring flocks .

Natural infection with *Neospora caninum* appears to be uncommon in sheep, and only a few cases of abortion or congenital disease have been reported (Dubey 2003). However, the role of *N. caninum* as a cause of abortion in small ruminants needs further investigation, since experimental inoculation with *N. caninum* during pregnancy produces similar effects to those observed in cattle.

Table 6 The most relevant infectious diseases causing ovine abortion and perinatal losses

Disease	Clinical signs	Lesions	Diagnostic	Control
Brucellosis 1. Brucella melitensis	Abortions in the second half of pregnancy. Stillbirth. Perinatal mortality. Systemic effects in the ewe: fever, lameness, etc.	Placentitis with oedema and necrosis of cotyledons.	Culture Direct microscopy Complement fixation test Rose Bengal test Milk-ring test	Eradication: test and slaughter Vaccination Antibiotics: usually not recommended
2. Brucella ovis	Orchitis. Infertility. Occasionally, abortions.	Ram: Epididymitis Orchitis Ewes: Placentitis	As above. Testicular palpation. Staining of semen/cotyledonsmears by acid-fast or Kösters	Eradication: test and slaughter.
Salmonellosis (paratyphoid abortion) Salmonella abortus ovis	Abortion that in endemic situations tends to affect only younger ewes. Stillbirth and perinatal mortality. Some ewes and lambs can show diarrhoea.	Non-specific lesions of the placenta. In cases of perinatal death	Culture Serum agglutination test	Vaccination Antibiotics
Enzootic Abortion (Chlamydial abortion) Chlamydia psittaci	Late abortions Premature lambing, Stillbirth Mummification Perinatal losses Usually second gestation abortion Placental retention	Placentitis with necrosis of the cotyledons and oedema and thickening of the intercotyledonary spaces. Similar to ovine brucellosis.	Placental smears and smears of vaginal discharges. Fluorescent antibody technique. Chicken embryo culture. Complement fixation test.	Hygienic measures Vaccination Antibiotics (oxytetracycline)
Toxoplasmosis (Toxoplasma gondii)	Infertility. Mummification. Abortion in late pregnancy that in endemic areas affects only younger ewes. Perinatal losses.	Gross lesions of cotyledons (grey-white foci). Mummified foetuses. Focal leucomalacia in the brain of lambs dying.	Histological examination of cotyledons and foetal brain Serological tests.	Vaccination

5.6.2 Pregnancy toxaemia

Ewes carrying two or more foetuses can suffer from pregnancy toxaemia towards the end of pregnancy as a result of inadequate nutrition. A varying degree of metabolic imbalance, accompanied by hypoglycaemia and ketosis, is caused by a less than adequate feed intake for the number of lambs carried. There may also be other predisposing factors involved. Teeth or feet problems, as well as heavy parasitic burdens may also lead to the disease, due to the associated decrease in body condition. Obese or lean ewes are more likely to develop the disorder.

Affected animals are usually in poor condition and exhibit depression, selective anorexia (initially eating only hay and straw, then only straw and finally not feeding at all) and tend to separate themselves from the rest of the flock. Soon afterwards they develop neurological signs such as tremors of the head and the neck, wandering, excessive salivation, unusual head carriage, absence of menace reflex and blindness. Finally, the affected ewe becomes recumbent and comatose.

As the prognosis is poor unless ewes are treated in the very early stages of the disease, control relies heavily on prevention - identification of ewes carrying more than one foetus, and attention to their nutrition, especially in the last third of pregnancy.

5.6.3 Clostridial infections ('post-parturient gangrene')

The condition occurs immediately post-partum when the external reproductive organs of ewes become infected with *Clostridium chauvoei*. Infection is facilitated if the vulva, vagina, or perineum has been damaged during a difficult lambing or obstetrical intervention (Lewis, 2007).

The infected animal develops high fever. The skin or the mucosa of the infected region may be discoloured, which may be accompanied by subcutaneous oedema, particularly of the perineum. Occasionally, there may be a sanguineous, malodorous vulval discharge. The infection may extend to the thigh muscles, which become dark and swollen.

Diagnosis is based on clinical and pathological examination. Vaccination of pregnant ewes is essential for the prevention of the disease. Good hygiene during lambing, especially when obstetrical assistance is provided, also helps to minimize the incidence.

5.6.4 Puerperal metritis

Factors such as dystocia followed by obstetrical assistance, prolapse of the uterus, retained placenta and post-parturient ketosis predispose ewes to infections of the uterus and puerperal metritis. The bacteria most commonly isolated are *A. pyogenes* and *E. coli*. The clinical manifestation includes swollen vulva and vagina, vaginal discharge and retention of foetal membranes, which can be accompanied by more systemic signs such as anorexia, dehydration, fever and toxaemia.
If the condition remains untreated, it can be life-threatening. Treatment should include the systemic administration of antibiotics of an adequate spectrum of activity, oxytocin and non-steroidal anti-inflammatory drugs (NSAIDs). Ewes treated at an early stage respond rapidly to treatment and there are usually no consequences for their future fertility.

5.7 Induction of parturition

Parturition may be induced if a very short lambing period is required, whether to optimize supervision for maximum lamb survival, or to simplify the management of the flock thereafter, or both. It is only practical when oestrus has already been synchronized so that mating data are available. Ewes must not be induced before day 144 of pregnancy, if the birth of premature lambs is to be avoided.
Prostaglandin $F_{2\alpha}$ cannot be used to induce parturition in sheep because pregnancy does not depend on progesterone from the corpus luteum; the placenta producing its own, and luteolysis therefore has no effect. However, both oestrogens and corticosteroids can be used successfully. Some researchers have reported higher rates of dystocia and peri-natal mortality following oestrogen treatment. Betamethasone and dexamethasone, at a dose rate of 8 to 16 mg, are the most commonly used corticosteroids. Intramuscular injection at the higher dose rate results in parturition within 26-62 hours of treatment (Henderson and Robinson 2000).

5.8 Ram

As mentioned in chapter 5.1.1, the sexual activity and breeding efficiency of rams are both subject to seasonal influences. In temperate climates, seasonal variations in the photoperiod and other environmental changes affect rams' reproductive activity, testicular size, gonadal endocrine balance, sperm quantity and quality and sexual behaviour.
In rams, sexual activity is usually stimulated 1–1.5 months earlier than in ewes, so that they are already fully sexually active when the ewes begin to cycle. In subtropical and tropical zones, it is the availability of forage and humidity that seem to have the greatest influence on the seasonality of reproductive efficiency in rams.

Evaluation of ram's suitability for breeding
It is not uncommon for poor fertility in a sheep flock to be caused by the poor quality of the rams . To avoid such situations, rams and bucks should be evaluated by a veterinary practitioner or experienced technician for breeding soundness 30 to 60 days before the breeding season, allowing time to recheck or replace those which are subfertile.

- Physical examination
  This should include careful observation of the general physical condition of the ram, body condition, alertness and especially the locomotor system. In rams used in so-called harem mating in extensive breeding systems, eyesight is also of prime importance. Signs of any general illness and parasite infestation should be noted. Also, a ram's libido can be assessed in the presence of ewe in oestrus.

- Fertility examination
  Examination of the reproductive tract consists of both an external examination of the reproductive organs and a rectal examination of internal reproductive structures and accessory glands.
  Scrotal circumference is one of the most useful measurements of a ram's testicular health and breeding ability. As in bulls, scrotal circumference is closely related to semen quality,

quantity, and reproductive success.
Careful examination should also include the penis, urethral process, and prepuce. The presence of sores, swellings, or blood clots may indicate penile or preputial injuries. Rams occasionally suffer from adhesions on the surface of the penis, which make it difficult or impossible to extrude the penis for intromission. While this problem may be corrected surgically, it is often an inherited defect, so rams exhibiting it should not be used for breeding.

- Semen evaluation
  Semen evaluation is unfortunately not a common enough practice even on well-managed sheep farms that use natural mating. Nonetheless it is an extremely important element of the management of rams, since poor quality semen may contribute substantially to a decline in the reproductive performance of the flock leading to economic losses, if undetected.
  Collection of semen can be performed in rams using an artificial vagina and spontaneous mounting. Rams quickly learn to mount a restrained ewe, and intromission and ejaculation are extremely rapid. Alternatively, electro-ejaculation can also be used and may well be required in rams not trained in the use of an artificial vagina. Electro-ejaculation is the less reliable method, as samples vary in quality and can be contaminated with urine. The volume of semen collected with the artificial vagina is 0.5-1.8 ml, while the ejaculates obtained by electro-ejaculation are of greater volume but with a lower concentration of sperm.

Good quality semen will have a milky or creamy appearance and, when examined under a stereomicroscope, will give an impression of boiling or rolling due to the intense motion of the spermatozoa.
Much as with bovine semen, evaluation consists of defining the percentage of motile spermatozoa using a simple preparation from a drop of semen on a pre-warmed microscope slide. Morphology of the spermatozoa is studied in microscopic preparations stained with eosin-nigrosin. Table 7 gives the normal parameters of sperm expected in a mature ram during the breeding season.

Table 7 Normal semen parameters in mature ram

Parameter	Normal value (during breeding season)
Volume	1 (0.8 to 1.2) ml
Sperm concentration	2.5 (1 to 6) billion/ml
Percentage of motile spermatozoa	75 (60 to 80) %
Percentage of morphologically normal spermatozoa	90 (80 to 95) %

Storage of ram semen

Ram semen may be stored for up to 24 hours by cooling the extended semen down to 2-5°C over 90-120 min. This is the approach often used by AI insemination centres during the breeding season when both the supply and the demand for semen are high. Fertility of cooled semen decreases rapidly and is usually too low after 48 hours.

The freezing and storage of ram semen in 0.25-0.3 ml, 3-dose pellets, or in 0.25 ml single-dose synthetic straws in liquid nitrogen at -196°C is successful in maintaining sperm viability, but there may be high variability in post-thaw motility and fertility between rams or batches of semen from the same ram. Semen stored this way is widely used in countries where intensive sheep production and breeding are practised (e.g. France, Australia, Spain).

Management of rams prior to breeding

Properly planned management is necessary to optimize reproductive efficiency in rams, and thus improve the chances of achieving better lambing percentages. Rams should be in good health and condition, well in advance of the breeding season, in order to correct any possible deficiencies, as well as to allow the evaluation of soundness and semen quality. Infertile rams can also be identified and removed at this stage.

Table 8 Suggested evaluation of rams before the breeding season:

Time-to-mating	Procedures
12 weeks before mating	Correction of possible selenium deficiency
6 weeks before mating	Flushing aimed at achieving 3.5 BCS at the start of mating Treatment to remove endo-and ectoparasites Foot care Separation from ewes at least 3 weeks before mating Clinical examination
2 weeks before mating	Detailed clinical examination Semen evaluation

The general health and performance of breeding rams should be also monitored closely throughout the breeding season. Adjustments can be made to feeding to ensure optimum breeding condition, and replacements can be arranged for any problem animals.

5.9 Embryo technology

Embryo transfer and embryo production in vitro are well established in sheep although their wide scale commercial use is very limited. This results directly from the adverse cost:benefit ratio of embryo transfer in sheep, when the value of a single animal, even one of high genetic merit, is usually relatively low. Nonetheless, the production of embryos in vitro provides a rich source of relatively low-cost embryos for basic research, as well in the development of the commercial use of emerging techniques such as nuclear transfer and transgenetics.

5.10 References

Abecia JA., Valares JA., Forcada F., Palacin I., Martin S., Martino A. The effect of melatonin on the reproductive performance of three sheep breeds in Spain. Small Rum Res 2007;69:10–16

Aitken ID. Chlamydial abortion. In: Martin, W.B., Aitken, I.D. (Eds.), Diseases of Sheep, third ed. Blackwell Science, Oxford 2000, pp. 81–86

Ali A. Effect of time of eCG administration on follicular response and reproductive performance of FGA-treated Ossimi ewes. Small Rum Res 2007;72:33–37

Anel L., Kaabi M., Abroug B., Alvarez M., Anel L., Boixo JC., de la Fuente LF., de Paz P. Factors influencing the success of vaginal and laparoscopic artificial insemination in Churra ewes: a field assay. Theriogenology 2005;63:1235–1247

Anderson ST., Bindon BM., Hillard MA., O'SheaT. Increased ovulation rate in Merino ewes immunized against small synthetic peptide fragments of the inhibin alpha unit. Reprod Fertil Dev 1998;10: 421-431

Bari F., Khalid M., Olf B., Haresign W., Murray A., Merrel B. The repeatability of superovulatory response and embryo recovery in sheep. Theriogenology 2001;56:147-155

Buckrell BC., Buschbeck C., Gartley CJ., Kroetsch T., McCutcheon W., Martin J., Penner WK., Walton JS. Further development of a transcervical technique for artificial insemination in sheep using previously frozen semen. Theriogenology 1994;42:601-611

Buxton D., Maley SW., Wright SE., Rodger S., Bartley P., Innes EA. Toxoplasma gondii and ovine toxoplasmosis: New aspects of an old story. Vet Parasitol 2007;149: 25–28

Cardenas H., Wiley TM., Pope WF. Prostaglandin $F_{2\alpha}$-induced estrus in ewes exhibiting estrous cycles of different duration. Theriogenology 2004;62:123–129

Chemineau P. Medio ambiente y reproducción animal. 6as jornadas Int. Reprod. Anim. e I.A., Salamanca, 2-5 Junio, libro de ponenecias y mesas redondas, 1992:292-306.

Cognie Y. Nouvelles méthodes utlisées pour améliorer les performances de reproduction chez les ovins. INRA Prod Anim, 1988;1:83-92.

Deligiannis C., Valasi I., Rekkas CA., Goulas P., Theodosiadou E., Lainas T., Amiridis GS. Synchronization of ovulation and fixed time intrauterine insemination in ewes. Reprod Domest Anim 2005;40:6-10.

DeNicolo G., Parkinson TJ., Kenyon PR., Morel PCH., Morris ST. Plasma progesterone concentrations during early pregnancy in spring- and autumn-bred ewes. Anim Reprod Sci 2009;111:279–288

Dhar A., Doughton BW., Pruysers E., Brown RW., Findlay JK. Effect of immunization against the alpha N (alphaN) and alpha C (alphaC) peptides of the alpha 43 subunit of inhibin on antral follicular growth and atresia and the patterns of gonadotrophin secretion in ewes. Reprod 2001;121:707-718

Dixon AB., Knights M., Winkler JL., Marsh DJ., Pate JL., Wilson ME., Dailey RA., Seidel G., Inskeep EK. Patterns of late embryonic and fetal mortality and association with several factors in sheep. J Anim Sci 2007;85:1274-1284.

Downing JA., Joss J., Connell P., Scaramuzzi RJ. Ovulation rate and the concentrations of gonadotrophic and metabolic hormones in ewes fed lupin grain. J Reprod Fertil 1995;103:137-145

Dubey JP. Review of Neospora caninum and neosporosis in animals. Korean J Parasitol 2003; 41:1-16

Dubey JP. Toxoplasmosis in sheep – the last 20 years. Vet Parasitol 2009;163:1-14

Entrican G., Wheelhouse NM. Immunity in the female sheep reproductive tract. Vet Res 2006;37:295–309.

Evans ACO. Ovarian follicle growth and consequences for fertility in sheep. Anim Reprod Sci 2003;78:289–306

Godfrey RW., Collins JR., Hansley EL., Wheaton JE. Estrus synchronization and artificial insemination of hair ewes in the tropics.
Theriogenology 1999; 51:985-997

Haresign W. The influence of nutrition on reproduction in the ewe. I . Effects on ovulation rate, follicle development and luteinizing hormone release. Anim Prod 1981;32:197-202

Haresign W. Manipulation of reproduction in sheep. J Reprod Fertil 1992; Suppl. 45:127-139.

Henderson DC and Robinson JJ. The reproductive cycle and its manipulation. In: Martin WB, Aitken ID. Diseases of Sheep. 3rd ed. Oxford: Blackwell Scientific Publications, 2000.

Husein MQ., Bailey MT., Ababneh MM., Romano JE., Crabo BG., Wheaton JE. Effect of eCG on the pregnancy rate of ewes transcervically inseminated with frozen-thawed semen outside the breeding season.
Theriogenology 1998;49:997-1005

Husein MQ., Kridli RT. Effect of progesterone prior to GnRH–PGF$_{2\alpha}$ treatment on induction of oestrus and pregnancy in anoestrous Awassi ewes. Reprod Dom Anim 2003;38:228–232.

Husein MQ., Ababneh MM., Haddad SG. The effects of progesterone priming on reproductive performance of GnRH–PGF$_{2\alpha}$-treated anestrous goats. Reprod Nutr Dev 2005;45:689–698.

Karaca F., Ataman MB., Coyan K. Synchronization of estrus with short- and long-term progestagen treatments and the use of GnRH prior to short-term progestagen treatment in ewes. Small Rum Res 2009;81:185-188

Kerr K., Entrican G., McKeever D., Longbottom D. Immunopathology of Chlamydophila abortus infection in sheep and mice. Res Vet Sci 2005;78:1–7

Kershaw CM., Khalid M., McGowan MR., Ingram K., Leethongdee S., G Wax., Scaramuzzi RJ. The anatomy of the sheep cervix and its influence on the transcervical passage of an inseminating pipette into the uterine lumen. Theriogenology 2005;64:1225–1235

Khan TH., Hastie PM., Beck NFG., Khalid M. hCG treatment on day of mating improves embryo viability and fertility in ewe lambs.
Anim Reprod Sci 2003;76:81–89

Kleemann, D. O., S. K. Walker, and R. F. Seamark. 1994. Enhanced fetal growth in sheep administered progesterone during the first three days of pregnancy. J Reprod Fertil 102:411–417.

Knights, M., Q. S. Baptiste, A. B. Dixon, J. L. Pate, D. J. Marsh, E. K. Inskeep, and P. E. Lewis. Effects of dosage of FSH, vehicle and time of treatment on ovulation rate and prolificacy in ewes during the anestrous season. Small Rum Res 2003;50:1–9.

Letelier CA., Contreras-Solis I., Garcia-Fernandez RA., Ariznavarreta C., Tresguerres JAF., Flores JM., Gonzalez-Bulnes A. Ovarian follicular dynamics and plasma steroid concentrations are not significantly different in ewes given intravaginal sponges containing either 20 or 40 mg of fluorogestone acetate. Theriogenology 2009;71:676–682

Lewis CJ . Clostridial diseases. In: Aitken, I.A. (Ed.), Diseases of Sheep, 4th edn. Blackwell, Oxford 2007, pp. 156–167.

Longbottom D., Coulter L.J. Animal chlamydioses and zoonotic implications. J Com Pathol 2003;128:217–244.

Luther JS., Grazul-Bilska AT., Kirsch JD., Weigl RM., Kraft KC., Navanukraw C., Pant D., Reynolds LP., Redmer DA. The effect of GnRH, eCG and progestin type on estrus synchronization following laparoscopic AI in ewes. Small Rum Res 2007;72:227–231

Mann GE., Lamming GE., Fray MD. Plasma oestradiol and progesterone during early pregnancy in the cow and the effects of treatment with buserelin. Anim Reprod Sci 1995; 37: 121-131

Marai IFM., El-Darawany AA., Fadiel A., Abdel-Hafez MAM. Physiological traits as affected by heat stress in sheep—A review. Small Rum Res 2007;71:1–12

Mitchell LM., Dingwall WS., Mylne MJA., Hunton J., Matthews K., Gebbie FE., McCallum GJ., McEvoy TG. Season affects characteristics of the pre-ovulatory LH surge and embryo viability in superovulated ewes.
Anim Reprod Sci 2002;74:163–174

O'Callaghan D. Physiology of seasonality in sheep: role of photoperiod and melatonin. Proceedings of the First European Conference on Progress in embryo technology and genetic engineering in cattle and sheep breeding, Krakow 1994, 35-43

O'Callaghan D., Yaakub H., Hyttel P., Spicer LJ., Boland M. Effect of nutrition and superovulation on oocyte morphology, follicular fluid composition and systemic hormone concentration in ewes. J Reprod Fertil 2000;118:303-313.

Paulenz H., Söderquist L., Ådnøy T., Nordstoga AB., Andersen Berg K. Effect of vaginal and cervical deposition of semen on the fertility of sheep inseminated with frozen-thawed semen. Vet Rec 2005;156:372-375

Rodolakis A. Q fever, state of art: Epidemiology, diagnosis and prophylaxis. Small Rum Res 2006;62:121–12

Rosa HJD., Bryant MJ. Seasonality of reproduction in sheep: Review. Small Rum Res 2003;48:155–171

Sammin D., Markey B., Bassett H., Buxton D. The ovine placenta and placentitis-A review. Vet Microbiol 2009;135:90–97

Symons AM., Arendt J., Poulton AL., English J. The induction of ovulation with melatonin. Proceedings of the 11th International Congress on Animal Reproduction; Dublin, June 26-30,1988:155-9.

Titi HH., Kridli RT., Alnimer MA. Estrus Synchronization in Sheep and Goats Using Combinations of GnRH, Progestagen and Prostaglandin $F_{2\alpha}$. Reprod Domest Anim 2009;in press)

Türk G., Gür S., Sönmez M., Bozkurt T., Aksu EH., Aksoy H. Effect of exogenous GnRH at the time of artificial insemination on reproductive performance of Awassi ewes synchronized with progestegen-PMSG-$PGF_{2\alpha}$ combination. Reprod Dom Anim 2008;43:308-313

Williams EJ and O'Donovan J. Ovine abortion: an overview. Irish Veterinary Journal 2009;62: 342-346

Windsor DP. Factors influencing the success of transcervical insemination in merino ewes. Theriogenology 1995;43:1009-1018

Wulster-Radcliffe MC., Wang S., and Lewis GS. Transcervical artificial insemination in sheep: effects of a new transcervical artificial insemination instrument and traversing the cervix on pregnancy and lambing rates. Theriogenology 2004;62:990–1002

Zúñiga O., Forcada F., Abecia JA. The effect of melatonin implants on the response to the male effect and on the subsequent cyclicity of Rasa Aragonesa ewes implanted in April. Anim Reprod Sci 2002;72:165-74.

6 Caprine Reproduction

6.1 Physiology

6.1.1 Seasonality of sexual and ovarian activity

The female goat is seasonally polyoestrous. The length of the breeding season is governed mainly by a combination of genetic and environmental factors. Various climatic elements, such as temperature and photoperiod, regulate the physiological response. In temperate zones, the goat behaves as a seasonal breeder, with a definite anoestrus period dependent on changing daylight length.

The goat is a so-called 'short day breeder' (see Ovine Reproduction chapter). In tropical goats, the photoperiod is less important than temperature, rainfall, vegetation and availability of pasture. The oestrus season of most of the dairy breeds in the Northern Hemisphere is usually restricted to the period between September and December. Meat-producing goats have a short anoestrus period in spring. Anglo-Nubian and Pygmy goats have extremely long breeding seasons. Seasonal influence should always be considered when designing breeding programmes for imported goats, as those recently transferred from another region may take some time to adjust to the difference in the seasons.

The onset of puberty is related to body weight, which, in turn, depends on the level of nutrition, age, type of birth and the season in which it takes place. Most breeds reach puberty between 5 and 10 months of age, but the more seasonally dependent breeds may approach 15-18 months before being developed enough to exhibit signs of oestrus. The climate, nutrition and the presence of a buck can modify the age at puberty. It is not advisable to breed young does before they have reached at least 60-75% of their adult body weight, for the sake of their own development, as well as for the viability of any offspring. Most of the European breeds are usually put in kid for the first time when they reach 7-8 months of age and a body weight of at least 30-35 kg.

Decreasing daylight length also stimulates reproductive activity in the buck. Although most bucks will mate at any time of the year, reductions in libido and semen quality have been observed when they have been worked out of season (Ahmad and Noakes 1996).
Bucks are at peak reproductive activity in late summer and autumn, in response to declining daylight length.
This period, known as the rut, is associated with:
- peak testosterone production
- high sebaceous gland activity (characteristic odour)
- agonistic behaviour (fighting)
- courting behaviour in the presence of females

Testicular weight, in the breeds with a strong seasonality, is usually minimal in spring and maximal in late summer, associated with marked changes in sperm production. Alpine bucks display dramatic variations in sexual behaviour between the spring-summer and autumn-winter periods (0–1.5 matings in 10 min), individual sperm motility (2.5–3.5 to over 5) and fertilizing ability (20%–70% of kiddings after AI) (Delgadillo et al., 1991).

6.1.2 The oestrous cycle.

The duration of the oestrous cycle varies widely, from as short as 3 days, to as long as 62 days. The majority of oestrous cycles are 19-21 days in length, but a proportion of them are shorter (<12 days), and others longer (>26 days). The occurrence of short cycles is influenced by the season of the year, the onset of the oestrus season or a transitional period, a 'buck effect' and the early post partum period. Short cycles are frequently observed, in particular, in does in tropical regions, when they are housed. The longer cycles are commonly encountered at the end of the breeding season before the does enter anoestrus. They can also be associated with embryonic death or persistence of the corpus luteum.
The follicular phase of the oestrous cycle is relatively short, 3-4 days, while the luteal phase occupies the rest of the cycle (i.e. about 17 days in a 'normal' cycle). Daily ultrasonographic studies have indicated that between ovulations there is a wave-like pattern of follicular development, as occurs in other ruminant species (Rubianes et al., 2003; Medan et al., 2005).

Different authors report the number of follicular waves ranging between two and five waves per cycle, but the pattern in a 'normal' cycle usually consists of four waves (de Castro et al., 1999; Schwarz and Wierzchos 2000; Menchaca et al., 2002). Evidence of follicular dominance in goats remains equivocal. Some authors have even postulated that, in goats, more than one follicle may 'cooperate' in exerting a functional dominance over the growth of others (Medan et al., 2005).

Oestrus appears to be variable in length, generally reported as 36 hours, ranging from 22 to 60 hours. Ovulation takes place a few hours after the end of visible oestrus.
The average number of ovulations varies from 1-4 per cycle, with reduced kidding rates due either to fertilization failure or early embryonic mortality.

6.1.3. Pregnancy

Pregnancy in the doe is dependent on progesterone from the corpus luteum, throughout the whole period, and any interference with the function of the corpus luteum will result in abortion.
The caprine placenta produces a considerable quantity of prostaglandin throughout pregnancy which, together with luteinising hormone (LH) and placental lactogen, forms a luteotrophic complex that ensures the continuous production of progesterone by the ovaries and thus the maintenance of pregnancy (Ford et al., 1995).
Gestation length varies from 144 to 151 days, with a typical mean of 149 days.
The length of post partum anoestrus (between parturition and first oestrus) can vary from 5 weeks (or even less) to 27 weeks, and is influenced by breed, lactation length and nutrition.

6.2 Herd reproduction management

6.2.1 Introduction

Goats are usually classified into four types according to their production: milk, meat and pelt, fibre, and dual-purpose (milk and meat). For small farmers and rural dwellers who are not land-owners, goats are unique among the domestic ruminants because of their ability to survive and reproduce under unfavourable conditions.

There is a great diversity in production systems, which makes it difficult to characterize the industry, but, regardless of the type of goat being produced, their reproductive performance is a major determinant of productivity and therefore the economic viability of commercial goat farms.

The control of reproduction may be necessary to avoid undesirable cross-breeding, in-breeding or inappropriate timing, as well as to produce animals better adapted to various environmental conditions.

The more sophisticated methods for controlling reproduction are restricted to use in intensive and highly profitable systems. Extensive and low income flocks must rely on more simple measures, such as modifications to the environment, e.g. the male effect, altering the photoperiod, dietary modifications (e.g. flushing), and modifying the breeding pattern (e.g. exogenous hormones, weaning). Both management and pharmaceutical methods can be combined, of course.

The seasonality of reproduction in goats results in lower reproductive efficiency (delayed puberty, prolonged kidding interval, etc.) while the seasonality of production leads to variations in market prices. So any improvements in reproductive performance will contribute to improvements in the efficiency of meat or milk production, and therefore profitability.

The 'kidding interval', which can range from 240 to 350 days, is defined as the period between two consecutive parturitions, comprising the very variable period from kidding to conception, and the gestation period. The kidding interval is affected by breed, age and parity of the doe, level of milk production, kidding rate, season of the year and level of nutrition. These influences can be grouped into husbandry (i.e. interval between kidding and introduction of the bucks), physiological (seasonal and post partum anoestrus, conception rate) and pathological (embryonic death, abortion).

Differences in litter size are mainly associated with breed, season, parity and body condition. The kidding rate (number of kids born/does giving birth) varies by breed from 1.01 to 2.05. In seasonal breeders, the prolificacy following the autumn mating is generally greater than that for the rest of the year. Kidding rate usually increases from the first to the fifth parity, and declines thereafter.

6.2.2 Pregnancy diagnosis

The main indications for pregnancy diagnosis in the goat are better management (feeding strategy, labour, vaccination, etc.) and to reduce the number of barren females. Most animals which are not successfully mated will return to oestrus 17-23 days after mating. Towards the end of the breeding season, longer cycles are likely to occur and, in some cases, non-pregnant animals remain in anoestrus. Goats frequently show signs of oestrus during pregnancy. Care must therefore be taken to distinguish between pregnancy, normal cyclical activity, and pseudopregnancy.

Several methods have been devised for pregnancy diagnosis in goats, because the signals which are commonly relied upon in other ruminants, do not apply in goats. For instance, non-return to oestrus is not reliable. Many does do not exhibit signs of oestrus throughout their breeding season, which may be associated with seasonal anoestrus or pseudopregnancy. Mammary gland development in primiparous goats should not be relied upon either, as 'maiden milkers' are common.

Hormone levels in blood, milk and urine do provide a means by which to confirm the presence or absence of pregnancy.
Oestrone sulphate concentrations in milk and plasma increase steadily during pregnancy and can be used to diagnose pregnancy approximately 50 days post service. Progesterone secreted by the corpus luteum of a pregnant goat can be detected with RIA or ELISA assays in milk or plasma. Random sampling can produce misleading results, however, because the corpus luteum of cyclic goats, and those with a false pregnancy, also produces progesterone. Nevertheless, a low progesterone level will always indicate non-pregnancy and can be considered to be 100% accurate.

Recently, so-called Pregnancy Associated Glycoproteins (PAGs) have received increasing attention in ruminants, including goats, as potential markers of pregnancy, and therefore useful candidates for the development of tools for early pregnancy diagnosis. Three different PAG molecules have been isolated, and partially characterised, from goat placenta. During gestation, PAG concentrations reach maximal levels during week 8, reduce between weeks 12 and 14 and then remain relatively constant until parturition (Sousa et al., 2006). After parturition, concentrations decrease rapidly to very low levels by the 4th week post partum.
Although using RIA or ELISA, these molecules can be detected in goats after day 26 and 32 in plasma and milk, respectively, no test is currently commercially available for routine use in the field.

With the advent of ultrasound, efficient and safe methods of pregnancy detection have become available.
A-mode *ultrasonography* is based on the detection of the fluid-filled uterus and is thus not specific for pregnancy. A-mode units emit ultrasonic waves from a hand held transducer placed externally against the skin of the abdomen and directed towards the uterus. The examination is carried out in a standing doe with the transducer placed against the lower part of the right flank near the udder. Clipping a small area of hair in this region is recommended to allow for optimal contact. Examination between 60 and 120 days post breeding should allow an accuracy of 80-85%.
Techniques based on the *Doppler effect* can detect blood flow in the middle uterine artery, umbilical arteries and foetal heart as well as foetal movement. Thus the foetal pulse can be detected after approximately two months of gestation, either via a transrectal or external/transabdominal probe. The accuracy of pregnancy detection approaches 100% during the last half of gestation but the technique is less effective between 50 and 75 days or earlier. The transrectal technique may be attempted as early as 25 to 30 days post breeding but false negative results are common, so it is advisable to wait until day 35 to 40 of gestation.
Real-time (B-mode) ultrasound devices produce a 2-dimensional picture on the screen, including a moving image of the uterus, foetus, foetal fluids, foetal heart and placentomes. With the

aid of real-time ultrasound, pregnancy can be detected from 40 days of gestation onwards, but is best done between 50 and 100 days. Ultrasound scanning is estimated to be virtually 100% accurate in determining pregnancy and 96-97% accurate in diagnosing twins and triplets. The ability to identify multiple foetuses with real-time ultrasonography has a clear advantage over other ultrasound techniques. Feeding management can be adjusted for does carrying multiple foetuses and appropriate care can be planned in advance of the expected kidding. The optimal time for estimating foetal numbers is probably between 40-70 days, because after 70 days, additional foetuses may lie beyond the depth range of a 5 MHz linear-array transducer. Experienced operators can distinguish pseudopregnancy and resorbed foetuses, as well as identify live kids.

Trans-abdominal scanning is usually carried out with the goat standing.

6.2.3 Oestrus detection and mating

Oestrus is preceded by pro-oestrus, which usually lasts about a day during which the doe is followed around closely by the buck, but will not stand to be mounted. The only sure sign of oestrus is the female standing and allowing the male to mount (the 'standing reflex'). Does actively seek the presence of the male when in oestrus, and the odour of the buck has a stimulating effect on the expression of oestrus signs. The buck may exhibit the flehmen reaction, flick his tongue and strike the doe with a forelimb (Ott 1980). Signs of oestrus in does also include tail-wagging, bleating and urination when near the buck. There may also be swelling of the vulva and a mucous discharge. Some does show no signs other than limited tail-wagging and standing to be mounted by the buck. By contrast with cows, however, most does will not stand to be mounted by other females, even when in oestrus.

As oestrus progresses, a variable amount of transparent mucus is visible in the cervix and on the floor of the vagina. This mucus later turns cloudy and finally, cheesy-white, at the end of oestrus. Conception is most likely to take place if the doe is bred when her cervical mucus is cloudy and the cervix is relaxed.

Silent heat is not as common in goats post partum, as it is in

sheep. Under field conditions, oestrus detection is of little importance. Several matings will usually occur within the flock, so timing will not necessarily be of any great interest. However, if artificial insemination (AI) is to be practised, it should be carried out near the end of oestrus. Therefore with the use of AI in dairy goats, for example, oestrus detection may well be important.
Ovulation is spontaneous and takes place about 30-36 hours after the onset of oestrus. Although it generally occurs late in oestrus, when the cycle is short it may be after the end of oestrus.

6.2.4 Artificial insemination

In countries such as France, where the genetic improvement of dairy goats is pursued systematically, AI has become part of the management routine. It is important in genetic improvement programmes in allowing the use of semen from males of high genetic merit, even those in distant locations, which are likely to have been bred from planned matings between the very best females and males in the population. Moreover, AI is helpful in reducing the spread of infectious diseases by reducing the need to transport animals for natural breeding and the opportunity for venereal transmission.

Semen collection and storage

Collection of semen from males requires a teaser and an artificial vagina, and is a well-established technique. Undiluted fresh semen can be used where donors and recipients are reared in close proximity. The main advantage is that it requires only simple equipment, but has the disadvantage in that it is difficult to assess semen quality.

Diluted chilled semen allows more time between collection and AI (12 hours) in which to assess sperm motility. Chilled goat semen is usually maintained at 4°C (Leboeuf et al., 2008). However, it requires the use of special diluents and rather more equipment. Because the motility and fertilising capacity of some bucks' sperm is reduced during the non-breeding season, their stored semen should not be used to inseminate does which have been induced to ovulate out of season.

Goat semen is stored, long term, in 0.2 ml straws containing 1×10^8 sperm cells and frozen in liquid nitrogen down to -196°C in three progressive steps.

The use of frozen-thawed semen is unfortunately limited in countries with less advanced levels of technology (Corteel 1981).

When properly carried out, insemination of does with fresh semen yields fertilization rates comparable to natural mating. As a rule, the use of frozen semen leads to poorer conception rates. Nonetheless, fertility rates after cervical AI with frozen semen are higher in goats than in sheep. This is mainly due to structural differences in the cervix at oestrus. In a substantial number of does (50-60%), semen can be deposited deep into the cervical canal or even into the uterus.

With laparoscopic AI, even better, and more consistent, pregnancy rates can usually be achieved. However, the use of this technique is limited by the requirement for elaborate equipment and skilled operators.

Kidding rates of 71% have been reported with another technique, recently described by Sohnrey and Holtz (2005), in which semen is deposited deep in the uterine horns by the trans-cervical route. The kidding rate in the laparoscopically inseminated controls in this trial, was 53%.

The timing of AI varies according to the method of AI used, the kind of oestrus (spontaneous or induced), the age and breed of the animal, and whether single or double AI is to be performed (see Table 1). Insemination not coordinated with ovulation can be detrimental to fertility. When stored or frozen semen is used, the timing of AI is even more critical. Fixed-time insemination in goats (hormone induced oestrus) has to be gauged specifically for different breeds and physiological conditions.

Table 1 Timing of insemination in goats.

Type of oestrus	Insemination time
Natural*	12-18 hours after onset of oestrus
Induced by Chrono-gest® sponges**	Long or short progestagen treatment: two AI about 30 and 50 hours after removal of the sponges Short progestagen treatment: one single AI 43 to 46 hours after removal of the sponges, depending on the breed Kid does about 45 ± 1 hours after removal of the sponges

* According to Evans and Maxwell (1987)
** According to Corteel et al. (1988)

6.3 Control of oestrus

The control of oestrus and out-of-season breeding are of increasing interest, as they enable milk producers to maintain regular and consistent levels of production, as well as allowing three kid crops in 2 years, from fibre-producing goats. Methods of oestrus control in goats are analogous to those described for sheep, but there are some peculiarities worthy of note. Moreover, it should be highlighted that the best results are obtained when oestrus induction and synchronization are undertaken in order to extend the breeding season, rather than to breed does out of season, when they are in profound anoestrus.

6.3.1 Buck effect

Introducing bucks to anovulatory females, after a period of complete segregation (which must be at least 4-6 weeks), induces synchronous ovulations in the ensuing days (Pellicer-Rubio et al. 2007). Although an olfactory stimulus plays a predominant part, all the senses are probably involved in the does' response. The contact with males induces the appearance of a pre-ovulatory surge of LH that triggers ovulation. The first induced ovulations are silent in 40% of the does and are followed by a short luteal phase in 75% of them. Oestrous and ovarian cycles return to normal later. The quality of the response depends on the intensity of stimulation and on the depth of anoestrus at the time the males are introduced. Similarly, the fertility of the females is also variable. Generally, the closer to the breeding season, the better the oestrus response and as well as fertility. In more seasonal breeders (Alpine and Saanen), subjecting females to artificial photoperiods may be necessary to improve the response to the male effect. Under these conditions, most does exposed to males were reported to ovulate (99%), and to deliver kids (81%) (Pellicer-Rubio et al. 2007).
The buck effect is more effective in breeds with a low seasonality. However, even in breeds responding well to this stimulus, a progestagen is often needed to obtain good fertility at the first buck-induced ovulation. Artificial insemination can be used, with one or two inseminations over a 24-hour period determined by the occurrence of oestrus or by the introduction of a buck.

Relatively high rates of fertility can be achieved in this way, but the required oestrus detection and careful timing of AI are very labour intensive.

6.3.2 Photoperiod regimes

Since the seasonality of reproduction is under the control of day length, reproduction during seasonal anoestrus can be successfully achieved using artificial light, which advances the breeding season, but also induces a reproductive state in the middle of the anoestrus period (Chemineau et al., 1986, 1988, 1999; Delgadillo et al., 2002). While it induces ovulation, it does not synchronize ovulation.

Goat AI centres, equipped with dark housing, use alternating light regimes with a month of long days and a month of short days, which allows for consistently high semen production with no seasonal variation in sperm quality. Currently, in the French national genetic improvement scheme, all bucks (approximately 70 per year) are permanently treated by rapidly alternating long and short days, which increases semen production per buck by 40% per year and reduces the duration of the breeding period of males (Cheminault et al., 2008).

On goat farms (always in open barns), males and females are subjected to the other system used in AI centres (long days followed by short days). This more natural treatment needs to be used in conjunction with the buck effect (introducing treated bucks for 45 days after 35–75 of the short day phase) in order to induce oestrous behaviour and ovulation, and to achieve high fertility rates. Under such conditions, out-of-season fertility and prolificacy can be maintained at high levels (>75% kidding rate with approximately two kids per kidding). For local breeds in subtropical conditions, where seasonality is less marked than those in temperate latitudes, the treatment of females is not necessary.

6.3.3 Melatonin

It has been shown experimentally that treatment with melatonin can stimulate oestrus and ovulatory activity in anovulatory, out-of-season, dairy goats. For maximum stimulation, the melatonin has to be preceded by a 2-month period of 'long days' (using artificial light), and followed by the male effect. When used soon after kidding, however, melatonin slightly decreased milk production (Evans et al., 1987).

6.3.4 Progestagen-based methods

The use of progestagens for oestrus management in goats allows for:
- oestrus synchronization during the breeding season
- tight oestrus and ovulation synchronization for fixed time AI
- extension of the breeding season
- out-of-season breeding

There are some differences in the physiology of goat reproduction that require alterations to the schedule used in sheep.
The same progestagens are used as in sheep, but when they are used without complementary luteolytic treatment, the duration of treatment must equal or exceed the lifespan of the corpus luteum (i.e. 16-18 days) in order to achieve effective synchronization.
Because progestagens do not hasten luteolysis in the goat as they do in the ewe, a long-lasting treatment is needed. At present, the progestagens available for oestrus management in goats include: intravaginal sponges impregnated with fluorogestone (e.g. Chronogest CR®) or medroxyprogesterone and intravaginal devices impregnated with progesterone. There have been some reports of the use of norgestomet implants for oestrus and ovulation synchronization in these species.
The protocol varies according to season, method of breeding and factors specifically related to the females to be treated (see Tables 2 and 3). When natural mating is to be used, sponges may be withdrawn from 17 to 22 days after insertion. With AI, sponges must not be withdrawn before 21 days (a longer treatment).
In both cases, it is advisable to inject from 400 IU to 700 IU of pregnant mare serum gonadotrophin/equine serum gonadotrophin (PMSG/eCG; Folligon®) at the time of sponge removal (Table 3). During the pre-breeding season or shallow anoestrus periods, and even in deep anoestrus, the same progestagen regimen may be used, but it is necessary to inject even higher doses of PMSG 24-48 hours before the end of

progestagen treatment. The fertility obtained after oestrus induced by these treatments ranges from 50 to 70%; the closer to the breeding season, the better the fertility (Corteel et al., 1982).

The interval from parturition to the beginning of treatment greatly influences fertility at the induced oestrus. A minimum of four months is required in the European dairy goat to obtain good results A shorter treatment regime has been adopted, involving the intravaginal administration of 20 mg FGA sponges for 11-12 days and PMSG/eCG and a $PGF_{2\alpha}$ 48 hours before the end of progestagen treatment (see Table 2). This treatment has advantages over the long treatment: less variable ovulation rate, better synchronized oestrus and higher fertility. It produces good results with a single cervical AI, and can be used in maiden does with satisfactory results, providing the dose of PMSG/eCG (e.g. Folligon®) is reduced (250-300 IU).

Goats treated with progestagen-impregnated sponges usually show very strong behavioural signs of oestrus. Oestrus usually occurs approximately 24-72 hours after the removal of sponges, with the optimal time for fixed-time AI at 36-40 hours after sponge removal. Treated goats are usually inseminated once with a thawed dose of frozen semen containing $1x10^8$ spermatozoa.

Table 2 Treatment schedules for Chrono-gest® sponges in goats.

Treatment	Insertion of sponges	Injection of prostaglandin	Removal of sponges
Short	Day 0	Day 10	Day 12

Table 3 Adjustment of PMSG dose in does treated with Chronogest CR® method

	Milk production	PMSG (Folligon®) dose
In season	< 3.5L/day	400 IU
	< 3.5L/day	500 IU
Transitional period	< 3.5L/day	500 IU
	< 3.5L/day	600 IU
Out-of-season	< 3.5L/day	600 IU
	< 3.5L/day	700 IU

6.3.5 Prostaglandins

Prostaglandins or analogues can be used to synchronize oestrus in cyclic goats. Because luteolysis is provoked only in the presence of a functional corpus luteum (from day 5 to day 19 of the cycle), animals have to be pre-synchronized either by progestagen treatment or by a previous injection of $PGF_{2\alpha}$.
Two intramuscular injections of 8 mg $PGF_{2\alpha}$ administered 11 days apart rendered a high degree of synchronization (94% of animals in oestrus 53 ± 3 hours after the second injection) and a conception rate similar to non-treated controls after natural service (Ott et al., 1980). The most common use of $PGF_{2\alpha}$ in synchronizing oestrus is in combination with a short duration progestagen treatment, in which case a single standard dose of prostaglandin indicated by the producer for goats is used. The wider use of prostaglandins in goat breeding is often complicated by the fact that few $PGF_{2\alpha}$-based products are licensed for use in goats or supplied with detailed information about the dose in this species.

6.3.6 Prostaglandins combined with GnRH

While oestrus synchronization with progestagens generally results in good fertility, irrespective of seasonal effects (breeding or anoestrus season), some breeders are interested in alternative synchronization strategies, especially those not involving the use of steroid hormones. Systems based on the so-called Ovsynch protocol developed for cattle (Pursley et al., 1995), involving the sequential administration of GnRH and $PGF_{2\alpha}$ could therefore become an interesting possibility. Holtz et al. (2009) compared results of oestrus synchronization using the Ovsynch protocol and fluorogestone impregnated intravaginal sponges (combined with $PGF_{2\alpha}$ and PMSG/eCG treatment) in Boer does during the breeding season. Does were inseminated at pre-determined times (16 hours after the second GnRH injection and 43 hours after sponge removal). Oestrus was identified in 96% of the Ovsynch-treated goats and in 100% of the goats synchronized with progestagen sponges. Kidding rates (58% and 46% in the Ovsynch and sponge groups, respectively) and prolificacy (1.86 and 1.83 in the Ovsynch- and sponge-treated goats, respectively) were similar for both groups, as were the number of ovulations (2.9 and 3.3) and the proportion of does with premature regression of the corpus luteum (29 and 17%). The authors therefore postulated that, during the breeding season, the Ovsynch protocol may be a useful alternative to progestagen treatment. It is important to bear in mind that, just as in anoestrus in cattle, the treatment of goats outside the breeding season will produce much poorer results in terms of oestrus induction and pregnancy rates. Additionally, although very attractive, such systems have an important limitation in that only a few GnRH and $PGF_{2\alpha}$ products are actually licensed for use in this species.

6.4 Superovulation and embryo transfer

The same methods used to induce ovulation in sheep are also applicable to the goat, but the programme and the doses need to be adapted accordingly. The main purpose of this treatment is to induce superovulation for embryo transfer programmes.

Although both PMSG/eCG and porcine follicle-stimulating hormone have been used, with or without progestagen treatment, the FSHp seems to be superior with respect to ovulation rate and number of offspring born to recipients. Since the half-life of pFSH in goats is only 5 hours, FSH is administered twice daily for 3-4 days, usually in decreasing doses, beginning between 1 and 3 days before the end of the progestagen treatment (Baril et al., 1990). On average 8–16 ovulations are generated, although this is very variable between individuals. Baril et al. (1996) reported very good superovulation results with progestagen pre-treatment followed 12 hours later by administration of a GnRH antagonist.

Two papers published by Medan et al. (2003a,b) indicated the suitability of active inhibin immunization for eliciting multiple ovulations in goats. However, before this method can be used on a larger scale, even in research, there are issues to be resolved, such as the high rate of premature luteal regression occurring in treated animals and an unusually large number of non-ovulated follicles.

Whereas embryo transfer is an effective method of achieving genetic improvement in cattle, it is not widely used in goats, the main reasons being the lesser value of goats, and the considerably greater technical difficulties involved in collecting and transferring their embryos. Surgical and laparoscopic embryo transfer techniques have been developed, but they still require general anaesthesia, as well as the use of sophisticated equipment and considerable technical skill. Moreover, post-operative adhesions are a frequent complication, limiting the number of possible collections.
A novel, non-surgical method was described by Pereira et al. (1998), Holtz et al. (2000), Suyadi et al. (2000) and Holtz (2005) and has since become standard with various embryo transfer groups.

The various steps involved with the *in vitro* production of caprine embryos are quite similar to those employed in the bovine. Both the standard *in vitro* fertilization (IVF) and 'intracytoplasmic sperm injection' (ICSI) have been reported in goats, resulting in the birth of live offspring (Baldassarre et al., 2003; Wang et al., 2003).
Methods for the cryopreservation of caprine embryos are also similar to those used successfully in bovines. In favourable conditions, pregnancy rates between 45 and >80% may be expected after the transfer of cryopreserved blastocysts, depending, in part, on the number of embryos transferred per animal (Holtz et al., 2000).

Other techniques, such as embryo splitting and nuclear transfer, have been reported in goats, but are a long way from being used on a large scale, even in research. Nonetheless, there is growing interest in these technologies mainly driven by the desire to breed transgenic animals to provide substances suitable for the pharmaceutical industry.

6.5 Reproductive disorders

6.5.1 Intersexuality (polled gene)

The intersex condition, or hermaphroditism, is a common cause of infertility in does of polled breeds (Smith 1980). It is an anatomical and functional abnormality which usually involves masculinisation of females, and cryptorchid-related abnormalities in the male. The condition is associated genetically with the absence of horns in several breeds of dairy goats (Riera 1984). The polled trait is dominant while the associated hermaphroditic trait is recessive and sex-linked. If one parent is horned, the offspring will almost never be one of the intersexes. The use of a horned buck is the standard method of avoiding the condition (Smith 1980).

6.5.2 Pseudopregnancy

This condition, also known as hydrometra, mucometra or 'cloudburst', consists of an accumulation of varying amounts of sterile fluid within the uterus (Pieterse et al., 1986). It is a significant cause of infertility in the goat (Smith, 1980), that causes permanent anoestrus due to a spontaneous persistence of corpus luteum function (Taverne et al., 1988).
An outward sign of hydrometra is abdominal distension caused by the fluid accumulating in the uterus. This, together with a false-positive pregnancy test, may prolong the non-productive period in affected goats because they appear to be pregnant.
The aetiology of the condition remains obscure. The term 'cloudburst' refers to those cases in which cloudy (uterine) fluid occurs around the expected time of parturition in non-mated animals (Pieterse et al., 1986). It is relatively easy to diagnose with the aid of real-time ultrasound, and can be treated with prostaglandins, after which pregnancy is once again possible.

6.5.3 Infectious abortion

Abortion is a relatively common cause of loss of reproductive efficiency in goats, as it is in sheep. The most frequent causes of infectious abortion in goats are *Brucella spp* and Chlamydia (see in Chapter 5). Brucella abortion is caused mainly by *B. melitensis* and occasionally by *B. abortus*. The main feature is abortion, usually in the 4th month of pregnancy, but it can also be associated with other clinical signs such as lameness, mastitis and orchitis. Chlamydia causes enzootic abortion, also known as viral abortion. It usually takes place after the 3rd month of pregnancy, and most frequently during the last two weeks of pregnancy (Smith 1980). Other infectious diseases associated with reproductive failure and abortion in goats include Q fever (*Coxiella burnetii*) Listeriosis (*Listeria monocytogenes*), Leptospirosis (*Leptospira spp*) and Toxoplasmosis (*Toxoplasma gondii*).

6.5.4 Delayed ovulation/follicular atresia

There is only limited evidence in the literature for these disorders in goats, in comparison with cattle. However, in practice, a treatment to induce ovulation using human chorionic gonadotrophin (hCG; e.g. Chorulon®, 500 IU) or GnRH (e.g. Receptal®, 2.5 ml) at the time of AI is often used to improve fertility, especially in high-yielding milking goats.

6.6 Induction of parturition

$PGF_{2\alpha}$ and its synthetic analogues have been shown to be effective in inducing parturition in does treated on day 144 of gestation (Bretzlaff et al., 1983). However, care should be taken to avoid premature treatment, as high doses of oestrogens or $PGF_{2\alpha}$ analogues will provoke abortion at any stage of pregnancy. Therefore, if the date of mating and the duration of pregnancy are not known for sure, it is more advisable to use corticosteroids which will induce parturition only if the foetuses are ready to signal the initiation of labour (Corteel et al., 1982). In practice, however, they are hardly ever used.

6.7 References

Ahmad N., Noakes DE. Seasonal variation in the semen quality of young British goats. Br Vet J 1996;152:225-236.

Baldassarre H., Wang B., Kafidi N., Gauthier M., Neveu N., Lapointe J., Sneek L., Leduc M., Duguay F., Zhou JF., Lazaris A., Karatzas CN. Production of transgenic goats by pronuclear microinjection of in vitro produced zygotes derived from oocytes recovered by laparoscopy. Theriogenology 2003;59:831–839.

Baril G., Vallet J. Time of ovulations in Dairy goats induced to superovulate with porcine follicle simulating hormone during and out of the breeding season. Theriogenology 1990;34:303-309.

Baril G., Pougnard JL., Freitas VJF., Leboeuf B., Saumande J. A new method for controlling the precise time of occurrence of the preovulatory surge in superovulated goats. Theriogenology 1996;45:697-706.

Bretzlaff KN., Ott RS. Doses of prostaglandin $F_{2\alpha}$ effective for induction of parturition in goats. Theriogenology 1983;19:849-853.

de Castro T., Rubianes E., Menchaca A., Rivero A. Ovarian dynamics, serum estradiol and progesterone concentrations during the interovulatory interval in goats. Theriogenology 1999;52:399–411.

Chemineau P. Possibilities for using bucks to stimulate ovarian and oestrous cycles in anovulatory goats - a review. Livest Prod Sci 1987;17:135-147.

Chemineau P., Pelletier J., Guerin Y., Colas G., Ravault JP., Tour G., Almeida G., Thimonier J., Ortavant R. Photoperiodic and melatonin treatments for the control of seasonal reproduction in sheep and goats. Reprod Nutr Develop 1988;28:409-422.

Chemineau P., Baril G., Leboeuf B., Maurel MC., Roy F., Pellicer-Rubio M., Malpaux B., Cognie Y. Implications of recent advances in reproductive physiology for reproductive management of goats. J Reprod Fertil Suppl 1999;54:129–142.

Corteel JM. Collection, Processing and Artificial Insemination of goat semen. In: C. Gall (ed), Goat Production. London: Academic Press Inc, 1981; pg 171-191.

Corteel JM., Gonzalez C., Nunes JF. Research and development in the control of reproduction. Proc 3rd Inter Conf Goat Prod Disease; Tucson, Arizona, 1982.

Delgadillo JA., Leboeuf B., Chemineau P. Decrease in the seasonality of sexual behaviour and sperm production in bucks by exposure to short photoperiod cycles. Theriogenology 1991;36:755-770.

Delgadillo JA., Flores JA., V´eliz FG., Hernandez HF., Duarte G., Vielma J., Poindron P., Chemineau P., Malpaux B. Induction of sexual activity in lactating anovulatory female goats using male goats treated only with artificially long days. J Anim Sci 2002;80:2780–2786.

Ford MM., Young IR., Thoburn GD. Prostaglandins and the maintenance of pregnancy in goats. J Reprod Fertil 1995;Suppl 49:555-559.

Evans G., Maxwell WMC. Salamon's artificial Insemination of sheep and goats. Sydney: Butterworths, 1987.

Holtz W., Pereira RJTA., Suyadi Wang XL., Padilla G., Sohnrey B. Collection of goat embryos via transcervical route. In: Proceedings of the 7th International Conference on Goats, Tours, France, 2000;15–21 May, pp. 490–491.

Holtz W. Recent developments in assisted reproduction in goats. Small Rum Res 2005;60:95–110

Holtz W., Sohnrey B., Gerland M., Driancourt MA. Ovsynch synchronization and fixed-time insemination in goats. Theriogenology 2009 (in press).

Leboeuf B., Delgadillo JA., Manfredi E., Piacere A., Clement V., Martin P., Pellicer M., Boue B., de Cremoux R. Management of Goat Reproduction and Insemination for Genetic Improvement in France. Reprod Dom Anim 2008;43 (Suppl. 2):379–385

Matthews J. Diseases of the goat. Blackwell Science 1992; pg 17.
Medan MS., Watanabe G., Sasaki K., Groome NP., Sharavy S., Taya K. Follicular and hormonal dynamics during the estrous cycle in goats. J Reprod Dev 2005;51:455-463
Medan MS., Watanabe G., Sasaki K., Nagura Y., Sakaime H., Fujita M., Sharawy S., Taya K. Effects of passive immunization of goats against inhibin on follicular evelopment, hormone profile and ovulation rate. Reproduction 2003a;125:751–757.
Medan MS., Watanabe G., Sasaki K., Nagura Y., Sakaime H., Fujita M., Sharawy S., Taya K. Ovarian and hormonal response of female goats to active immunization against inhibin. J Endocr 2003b;177;287–294.
Menchaca A., Pinczak A., Rubianes E. Follicular recruitment and ovulatory response to FSH treatment initiated on Day 0 or Day 3 post-ovulation in goats. Theriogenology 2002;58:1713–1721.
Ott RS. Breeding techniques for dairy goats. Inter Goat and Sheep Res 1980;1:1-5.
Ott RS., Nelson DR., Hixon JE. Fertility of goats following synchronization of oestrus with prostaglandin $F_{2\alpha}$. Theriogenology 1980;13:341-345.
Pellicer-Rubio MT., Leboeuf B., Bernelas D., Forgerit Y., Pougnard JL., Bonne JL., Senty E., Chemineau P. Highly synchronous and fertile reproductive activity induced by the male effect during deep anoestrus in lactating goats subjected to treatment with artificially long days followed by a natural photoperiod. Anim Reprod Sci 2007;98:241–258.
Pereira RJTA., Sohnrey B., Holtz W. Nonsurgical embryo collection in goats treated with prostaglandin F_{2a} and oxytocin. J. Anim. Sci.1998;76:360–363.
Pieterse MC., Taverne MAM. Hydrometra in goats: diagnosis with real-time ultrasound and treatment with prostaglandins or oxytocin. Theriogenology 1986;26:813-821.
Pursley JR., Mee MO., and Wiltbank MC. Synchronization of ovulation in dairy cows using $PGF_{2\alpha}$ and GnRH. Theriogenology 1995;44:915–923.
Riera GS. Some similarities and differences in female sheep and goat reproduction. Proc 10th Inter Cong Anim Reprod; Urbana-Champaign, Illinois, 1984.
Rubianes E., Menchaca A. The pattern and manipulation of ovarian follicular growth in goats. Anim Reprod Sci 2003;78:271–287
Schwarz T., Wierzchos E. Relationship between FSH and ovarian follicular dynamics in goats during the estrous cycle. Theriogenology 2000;53:381 (abstract).
Smith MC. Caprine Production. In: Morrow DA (ed). Current Therapy in Theriogenology: diagnosis, treatment and prevention of reproductive diseases in animals. Philadelphia: WB Saunders, 1980;pg 969-1004.
Sohnrey B., Holtz W. Transcervical deep cornual insemination of goats. J Anim Sci 2005;83:1543–1548.
Sousa NM., Ayad A., Beckers JF., Gajewski Z. Pregnancy-associated glycoproteins (PAG) as pregnancy markers in the ruminants. J Physiol Pharmacol 2006;57:153-171
Suyadi Sohnrey B., Holtz W. Transcervical embryo collection in Boer goats. Small Ruminant Res. 2000;36:195–200.
Wang B., Baldassarre H., Pierson J., Cote F., Rao KM., Karatzas CN. The in vitro and in vivo development of goat embryos produced by intracytoplasmic sperm injection using tail-cut spermatozoa. Zygote 2003;11:219–227.

7 Canine Reproduction

7.1 Physiology

7.1.1 The oestrous cycle of the bitch

Bitches are monooestrous since they have only one oestrous cycle during each breeding season. The oestrous cycle of the bitch can be divided into four phases (Figure 1). A period of sexual inactivity (anoestrus) is followed by pro-oestrus, which is characterized by vulval swelling and bleeding. Oestrus, the time during which the bitch will accept the male, immediately follows pro-oestrus, and ovulation occurs spontaneously at the beginning of this phase of the cycle. If pregnancy does not ensue, oestrus is followed by metoestrus (also known as dioestrus), which blends imperceptibly into anoestrus. The term 'heat' is used by dog owners to describe the period of pro-oestrus and oestrus together. There is no specific lay terminology for the rest of the oestrous cycle of the bitch.

Figure 1 The oestrous cycle of the bitch

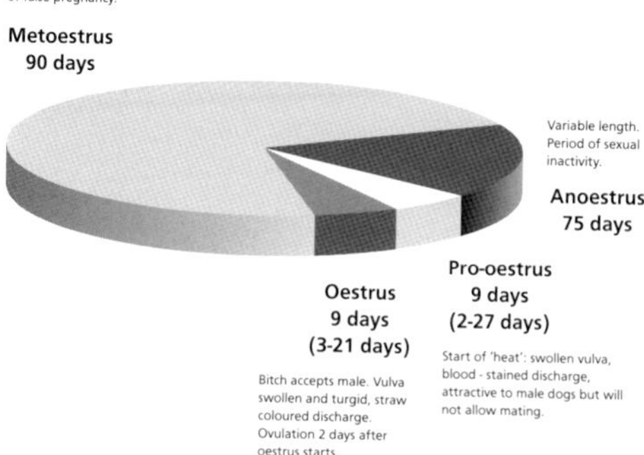

The duration of the various phases of the oestrous cycle can vary considerably between individuals. The situation is also complicated because the duration and intensity of the external changes and behavioural signs - swelling of the vulva, vaginal bleeding and acceptance of the male - by which pro-estrus and oestrus are recognized in the bitch are by no means consistent between animals. Furthermore, the beginning, end and duration of metoestrus cannot be determined by observation since this phase of the cycle is not characterized by the presence of specific external signs. All these factors, together with the fact that the external signs may not mirror the underlying hormonal status, are of great importance when considering breeding or manipulation of the cycle. Relatively simple techniques, including vaginal exfoliate cytology, the measurement of hormone concentrations (particularly progesterone) and vaginal endoscopy can reduce these difficulties substantially (Jeffcoate and Lindsay 1989) (Figure 2).

Figure 2 Hormone concentrations and vaginal cytology in pro-oestrus and oestrus

	Early pro-oestrus	Late pro-oestrus	Early oestrus	Late oestrus
Red blood cells	+++	++	+	
Keratinized cells		+	++	+++
Leucocytes	+			+
Debris	+++	++	+	

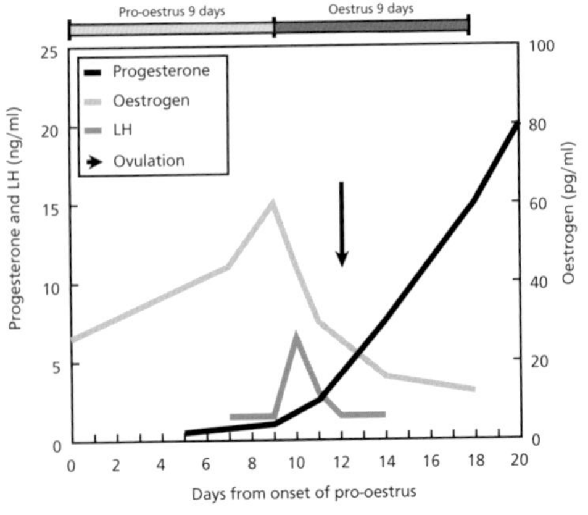

Metoestrus can be divided into progressive (phase 1) and regressive (phase 2) stages (Figure 3). Originally this division was based on the histological appearance of the uterus but the two stages can be related directly to luteal function. Phase 1 refers to the phase of post-oestrus luteal development (approximately 20 days) and Phase 2 to the time from the onset of luteal regression until the uterus returns to the anoestrus state, a further 70 days. Thus, metoestrus normally lasts for approximately 3 months with luteal function declining after the first 20 days of this phase. Endometrial desquamation starts at about day 90 of the oestrous cycle (day 0 = first day of oestrus) and continues for about 21 days, the discarded tissue being resorbed or expelled via the cervix. The endometrium has regenerated completely by day 150, on average.

Figure 3 Hormone concentrations and vaginal cytology in 'heat' and metoestrus

	'Heat'	Metoestrus
Red blood cells	+++ to +	
Keratinized cells	- to +++	++
Leucocytes	+ to 0 to +	+++
Debris	+++ to +	

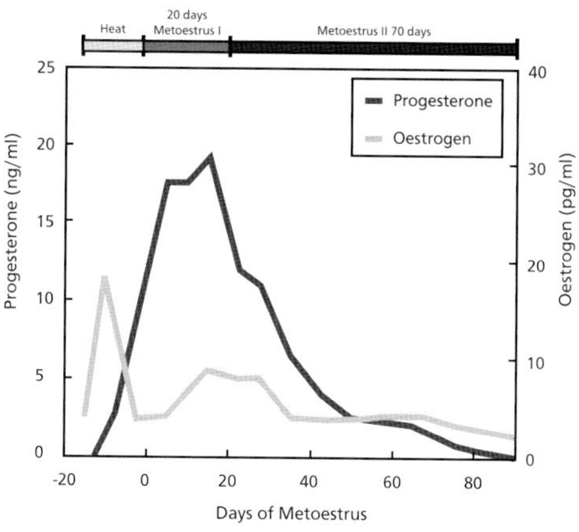

Seasonal activity may be slightly increased during the period February to May (Christie and Bell 1971), but essentially bitches commence cycling, and breed and whelp at any time throughout the year. There may appear to be some seasonality since the majority of the bitches housed together often show signs of heat within a limited period. The same is also seen in places where the population density of dogs is high, e.g. dog shelters, boarding kennels, and some urban areas. This is not true seasonality but 'natural' oestrus induction, presumably due to pheromones, and it may influence the efficacy of pharmacological intervention.

7.1.2 Hormonal changes in bitches

Hormones from a variety of origins (pituitary gland, placenta and ovary) are involved in the control of the ovarian cycle in dogs (Onclin et al., 2002). Innate cyclical activity and reproductive function are controlled by the hypothalamus, which is sensitive to both external (environmental) and internal stimuli. The oestrous cycle is therefore controlled by the complex interplay between the hypothalamus and the reproductive tract, with the anterior pituitary acting as the 'central relay station'. A summary of the hormonal changes is given below.

During the 2-3 weeks prior to the onset of pro-oestrus, the anterior pituitary secretes follicle stimulating hormone (FSH) in pulses of increasing frequency. FSH controls the development of the ovarian follicles which, in turn, principally secrete oestrogen, but also, as they reach maturity, progesterone. Low concentrations of oestrogen exert positive feedback on the anterior pituitary stimulating more FSH to be released, resulting in further follicle growth and increased oestrogen concentrations.

This process continues until the follicles are mature and about to rupture. At this stage, the higher concentrations of oestrogen have a negative feedback effect that inhibits FSH secretion and triggers the release of luteinizing hormone (LH) from the anterior pituitary in a large pulse, which causes ovulation (Figure 2).

The ruptured follicle is rapidly converted into a corpus luteum. The development of corpora lutea is initiated in response to LH and is maintained by luteotrophic factor(s)-prolactin (Okkens et al., 1990). Corpora lutea secrete progesterone, which, at high concentrations, has a negative feedback effect on the production of LH, which maintains these secretory bodies until day 35. Falling levels of progesterone have a positive feedback effect on the release of prolactin, the gonadotrophin that maintains luteal function after day 35.

The bitch is unusual in a few respects:

- Low progesterone concentrations produced by pre-ovulatory follicles are present prior to ovulation and these, in conjunction with falling levels of oestrogen, are probably responsible for the initiation of standing oestrus (Figure 2). The signal that marks the end of pro-oestrus and the beginning of oestrus are progesterone concentrations above the critical plateau of 0.5 ng/ml, in conjunction with declining oestrogen concentrations (Figure 2).
- There is a long period of progesterone dominance, probably because the canine uterus produces no luteolytic factor (Figure 3).

The unique hormonal changes involved in the oestrous cycle in bitches, lead to two distinct phenomena, false pregnancy and the cystic endometrial hyperplasia (CEH)-pyometra complex. In addition, long exposure to high progesterone concentrations during each oestrous cycle may result in a syndrome of excessive growth hormone production from the mammary gland resulting in acromegaly in some dogs (Kooistra and Okkens 2002).

7.1.3 Oestrus induction

Oestrus induction is used clinically in conjunction with routine breeding management (e.g. when breeding opportunities are missed or following conception failure) or as a treatment for primary or secondary anoestrus (oestrus interval >12 months). The different schedules that have been used (more than 40) were reviewed recently (Kutzler 2005). Not all of them are suitable for use in clinical practice. A short summary of some of the different approaches is given below.

Whatever procedure is adopted, proper timing of treatment is crucial for success, particularly if this is regarded not only as oestrus induction but also as ovulation and subsequent pregnancy. Generally dog owners should be discouraged from trying to induce oestrus in bitches in metoestrus and early anoestrus, as the results are usually poor, regardless of the treatment used. It is also not unusual for bitches, in which oestrus induction is commenced in early anoestrus, to have an anovulatory oestrus or corpus luteum insufficiency, resulting in a very low pregnancy rate (Chaffaux et al., 1984; Jeukenne and Verstegen 1997; Verstegen et al., 1999). Generally the later the induction of oestrus is performed in anoestrus the better the results, with the optimal time being 3-4 weeks before the next spontaneous heat is expected.

Gonadotrophins

The termination of anoestrus in bitches is associated with increased serum concentration or pulse frequency of LH (Concannon 1993). PMSG/eCG (Folligon®) has potent effects and signs of pro-oestrus usually occur within one week of starting daily treatment in late anoestrus (Chaffaux et al., 1984). However, the response to treatment varies and the duration of induced oestrus is often shorter than that of spontaneous oestrus (Chaffaux et al., 1984). Since PMSG/eCG alone does not appear to be sufficient to restore complete ovarian activity, this is often followed with hCG (Chorulon®).

In fact, many of the published studies were carried out using PMSG/eCG at a dose rate of 500 IU/bitch, or 20 IU/kg for 10 consecutive days, followed by a single injection of 500 IU of hCG on day 10. Arnold et al. (1989) and Weilenmann et al. (1993) reported good results with oestrus induced in anoestrus bitches using 20 IU/kg PMSG/eCG given for 5 consecutive days with a single injection of 500 IU of hCG on day 5. Pregnancy rates after mating at the induced oestrus range between 30-50%.

Gonadotrophin-releasing hormone

Potent, synthetic GnRH-agonists can be used to induce oestrus in bitches (Cain et al., 1989; Concannon et al., 2006) but require daily administration of sufficient doses for more than 7 days. Pulsatile intravenous injections, although effective when treatment is initiated in anoestrus (Concannon et al., 1997;

Vanderlip et al., 1987), are not practical in general practice. Inaba et al. (1998) obtained encouraging results using a sustained-release formulation of a GnRH agonist. GnRH agonists formulated as a subcutaneous implant induce oestrus in the first weeks following administration to bitches unless treatment is administered before puberty (Gobello 2007, Trigg et al., 2006).

Dopamine agonists

Prolactin appears to have a role in the interoestrus interval in dogs (Kutzler 2005). Dopamine D2 agonists decrease plasma prolactin concentration and shorten the duration of anoestrus (Beijerink et al., 2004; Kutzler 2005) but likely also have other dopamine agonistic effects, probably an increase in FSH secretion (Beijerink et al., 2004). Prolactin-lowering doses of dopamine agonists administered on days 90 to 135 of the cycle can result in premature pro-oestrus and fertile oestrus. Pro-oestrus takes place between a few and several days after treatment, depending on how late in anoestrus the treatment is started. Both bromocriptine (Okkens et al., 1985; Zoldag et al., 2001) and cabergoline (Jeukenne and Verstegen 1997; Verstegen et al., 1994) have been used successfully. Cabergoline treatment produces less intensive side effects making it a more suitable choice for oestrus induction in bitches (Verstegen et al., 1999).

7.1.4 Prolonged or persistent oestrus

GnRH can be administered intramuscularly at a dose rate of 0.05 to 0.10 mg per bitch every 24 to 48 hours for a total of three doses (Davidson and Feldman 2000). Alternatively, hCG can be given at a dose rate of 22 IU/kg every 24 to 48 hours (Davidson and Feldman 2000). The success rates of medical treatment are reportedly poor.

7.1.5 Infertility in female dogs

Infertility in bitches, the failure to conceive and produce viable offspring, is most commonly associated with inappropriate breeding management (Davidson and Feldman 2000; Grundy et al., 2002). Thus most bitches that are presented for reproductive evaluation are in fact healthy. Before any treatment for infertility is undertaken, a full history and physical examination should be carried out and, where necessary, laboratory evaluations undertaken.

Specific treatment for the most common causes of infertility is centred around appropriate breeding management (Davidson and Feldman 2000; Grundy et al., 2002).

7.1.5.1 Failure to cycle

There are a number of reasons why a bitch may fail to cycle. These include previous spaying (ovariohysterectomy) and silent or missed heat.

7.1.5.2 Prolonged or primary anoestrus

A bitch that has not experienced its first oestrus by 23 months of age is generally considered to have primary anoestrus. Primary anoestrus can be associated with hermaphroditism or pseudo-hermaphroditism, thyroid insufficiency or infantilism.

Before oestrus induction is undertaken, a detailed history of the bitch should be collected and a thorough physical examination carried out. If any specific causes of prolonged/primary anoestrus are diagnosed, targeted therapeutic measures can be adopted. If no specific primary cause is found, oestrus induction can be attempted (see section 7.1.3).

7.1.5.3 Delayed puberty

Puberty is usually reached by 6-7 months of age (range 4-22 months) however there is wide individual and breed variability. Small breeds tend to have a first heat between 6 and 10 months of age, but larger breeds may not begin to cycle until 18-20 months old, and in Greyhounds this may be as late as 20-24 months of age. Absence of oestrus cycling by 24 months of age may be indicative of hypothalamic-pituitary-ovarian axis malfunction and warrants detailed reproductive evaluation (Kutzler 2005).

7.1.6 Short or prolonged interoestrus intervals and split heats

The frequency of heat in the bitch is primarily determined by the length of anoestrus, which varies from bitch to bitch. The average interoestrus interval in the dog is 7 months (Christie and Bell 1971) but varies from 4-12 months. Breed variability can be striking, e.g. German Shepherds commonly have an interoestrus interval of 4-4.5 months and African breeds, such as the Basenji (Fuller 1956), cycle only once per annum. Pregnancy increases the interval to the next heat by 28 days, on average.

In the mature, sexually active bitch an interval of more than 12 months (excluding the Basenji) is considered as a prolonged interoestrus interval. Reasons for prolonged anoestrus include hypothyroidism, progestagen administration, long-term glucocorticoid treatment and starvation/malnutrition. Failure to recognize signs of heat and poor heat manifestation should also be considered.

When the signs of heat are interrupted shortly before ovulation and recommence between 1 and 10 weeks later, this is referred to as 'split heat' (Davidson and Feldman 2000; Grundy et al., 2002). The second heat is usually associated with ovulation. Split heat is common in bitches experiencing heat for the first or second time and is less common in dogs over 2 years of age. Treatment is usually unnecessary and insemination timing can be determined using serial serum progesterone concentrations.

7.1.7 Prolonged/persistent oestrus

If ovulation has not occurred within 25 days of oestrus and external signs of heat continue, the bitch is considered to have a persistent/prolonged oestrus. The most usual cause of this condition is persistence of ovarian follicles that have failed to ovulate. Young bitches frequently have prolonged oestrus during their first or second cycles. Individual variability in the duration of heat should always be considered.

7.1.8 Failure to conceive/early resorption

One of the most common causes of failure to conceive is inappropriate breeding management. Differential diagnoses for failure to conceive include inappropriate breeding management (including male-related problems), uterine infection, uterine pathology and systemic illness.

7.2 Mating

Mating in bitches has been reviewed in depth by a number of authors (Christiansen 1984; Feldman and Nelson 2004). This is summarized below.

7.2.1 Mating behaviour

Bitches are attractive to male dogs for approximately 9 days whilst they are in pro-oestrus. Mating occurs when the bitch is in standing heat. Before mounting a bitch, the male dog may go through a relatively prolonged courtship procedure, but often will simply briefly lick the vulva before mounting the bitch. As a result of this attention, the bitch will usually stand firmly with its tail held to one side, exposing the vulva. Penetration in the dog is achieved without erection because of the presence of the os penis. However, once inside the vagina, the bulbus glandis becomes engorged and is accompanied by strong thrusting movements. This results in the ejaculation of prostatic fluid. Once pelvic thrusting ends, the dog will dismount and, by lifting one hind leg over the bitch, end up 'tied' to it, tail to tail, locked by the engorged bulbus that make separation difficult. The 'tie' can last anything from 5-60 minutes (average 20 minutes) and during this time the bitch and dog may drag each other around. During the tie ejaculation of seminal fluid continues. This second part is sperm rich. The tie finally breaks quite spontaneously and some seminal fluid may be seen draining from the bitch's vulva. The tie is not essential for conception.

7.2.2 Timing of mating

Although the majority of dogs will breed at an appropriate time to result in conception, the most common cause of mating failure is inappropriate timing (Goodman 2001). Traditionally, bitch owners have their bitches mated twice, 11 and 13 days after the onset of pro-oestrus, to try and ensure that spermatozoa are present in the female reproductive tract at or around the time of ovulation. This is generally very successful, due to the unusual longevity of dog spermatozoa (6-11 days) in the female genital tract (Concannon et al., 1989; Goodman 2001).

There is no doubt that many fertility problems result from mating being arranged at a convenient time rather than on the most appropriate day. If the timing of ovulation is more precisely determined, fertility rates are likely to increase and the expected whelping date can be predicted more accurately. In addition, conception failures are less likely and the management of the bitch can be simplified.

7.2.3 Detection of ovulation

Essentially, three methods of detecting ovulation are available to veterinary practitioners: vaginal cytology, vaginoscopy and the measurement of hormone concentrations (Feldman and Nelson 2004; Jeffcoate and Lindsay 1989; Schaeffers-Okkens 2000).

Vaginal (exfoliate) cytology

Cytological evaluation of vaginal smears can be used to monitor the progress of the so-called vaginal cycle. This is a series of consecutive changes in the number and morphological features of the vaginal epithelial cells that mirror the changes in the endocrine environment and the related changes in ovarian activity during the oestrous cycle.

During pro-oestrus the number of parabasal and small intermediate cells with easily visible nuclei decreases, whilst the number of superficial cells increases (Figure 3). As pro-oestrus develops, the number of keratinized superficial cells with pyknotic or indistinguishable nuclei increases and this reaches

60-80% at the transition into oestrus (Figure 3). Red blood cells are usually observed throughout pro-oestrus and slowly disappear as oestrus commences. However, this feature should not be relied upon since red blood cells can persist in vaginal smears. There is no reliable change in the smear indicative of the LH surge or ovulation (Concannon et al., 1989). In fact, cytology can only be used to detect the time of ovulation retrospectively because the first day of metoestrus is the only stage of the cycle that can be pinpointed precisely using this technique.

The first day of metoestrus is characterized by a dramatic fall in the percentage of superficial cells and the reappearance of white blood cells (Figure 2 and 3). In most bitches this takes place 8-10 days after the LH surge and gives a rough indication that ovulation occurred approximately 6 days earlier. This is of no practical value for breeding management. Thus, vaginal cytology is not a very reliable method for determining the appropriate time for mating bitches. In addition, vaginal cytology is a rather crude index for predicting the first day of standing heat, however it can be very useful when close monitoring of the consecutive phases of the oestrous cycle is required.

Whenever vaginal cytology is used to time mating it should never be based on a single sample, even if that was taken at the time of standing oestrus. In fact, vaginal cytology should be carried out at least three times, starting at day 5 after a bloody discharge was first detected, and subsequently on days 7 and 9. If the percentage of cornified cells has not reached 60% on day 9 the next sample should be taken within 2 days. Experienced practitioners suggest that mating should be first attempted when the amount of cornification exceeds 80%, and then repeated every second day for as long as the bitch accepts the dog.

Vaginoscopy

The changes in the lining of the vagina, as seen through a vaginoscope, parallel those seen in vaginal cytology. However, at the time of ovulation, a skilled observer will note the onset of 'wrinkling'. The wrinkles become very obvious about 4 days after ovulation, the most critical time for mating (Jeffcoate and Lindsay 1989). It is necessary, however, to become familiar with the technique and to examine bitches at least every other day, from 4-5 days after the onset of pro-oestrus, if the method is to be used effectively.

Measurement of hormone concentrations
The hormonal changes that occur during pro-oestrus and oestrus are shown in relation to the time of ovulation in Figure 2. The pre-ovulatory LH surge is commonly regarded as the central event in the cycle (Concannon et al., 1989). Most of the important events that occur in the cycle are closely synchronized with this event (Table 4).

Figure 4 Timing of major reproductive events in relation to the LH peak

Ovulation	48 hours
Oocyte maturation	4-5 days (i.e. 2-3 days post-ovulation)
Peak fertility	0-5 days
Implantation	18 days
Parturition	64-66 days

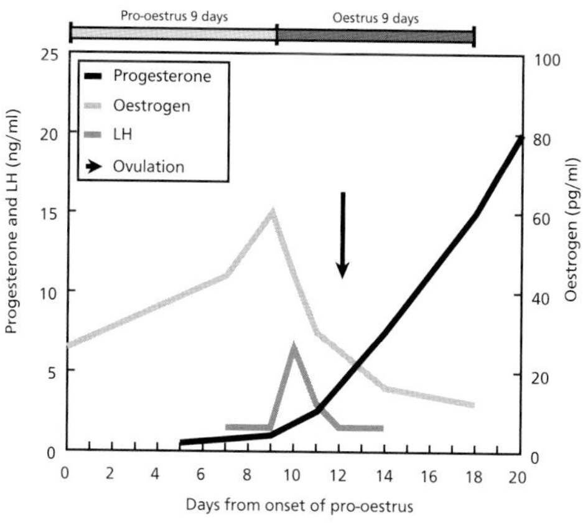

It would be ideal if the LH surge could be detected conveniently and easily. However, this is not practical, since LH concentrations are raised only transiently over a period of 1-3 days, thus frequent blood sampling would be required in order to ensure detection of this surge.

Progesterone concentrations increase during the LH surge and reach concentrations of 2-5 ng/ml around day 2 after the LH peak. Concentrations continue to rise throughout oestrus and reach peak levels 13-28 days later (Concannon et al., 1989). It is possible to measure progesterone concentrations in just a drop of blood or plasma. Based on sampling every two to three days, the optimal time for mating is around 12±3 days (6-21 days) after the onset of vulval bleeding (van Haaften et al., 1989).

7.3 Pregnancy

7.3.1 Duration

The duration of pregnancy in the bitch has always been regarded as being 63 days post-mating. However, a range of 56-72 days from the first mating to the potential whelping date is more likely to be correct (Linde-Forsberg and Eneroth 2000). This large variation is due, at least in part, to the longevity of canine spermatozoa (Concannon et al., 1989). There is also some interbreed variation and variation associated with litter size: bitches carrying four or fewer pups have a significantly longer gestation than those carrying five or more (Eilts et al., 2005). Despite this, gestation length is in fact remarkably constant at 65±1 days after the LH peak, with implantation occurring 18 days after the LH peak (Figure 4).

7.3.2 Hormonal changes during pregnancy

The endocrine changes that occur during pregnancy in bitches have been described in detail by a number of authors (Concannon et al., 1975; Concannon et al., 1989; Feldman and Nelson 2004). It is well established that circulating concentrations of progesterone, oestrogen and prolactin in pregnant bitches, unmated bitches in metoestrus, and bitches that have failed to become pregnant are very similar (Figure 3). The luteal phase in pregnant and non-pregnant bitches is remarkably similar with high levels of progesterone maintained for 50–60 days after the LH peak. However, in the pregnant bitch there are often secondary increases in circulating progesterone concentrations between days 25 and 40 that may reflect pregnancy-specific mechanisms that result in additional stimulation of progesterone production. Functional corpora lutea are essential for pregnancy: after day 30 of gestation, abortion occurs within 24-72 hours of ovariectomy. During the last third of pregnancy elevated oestrogen concentrations can be detected. Luteal function in pregnant bitches is terminated abruptly by luteolysis 62-65 days after the LH surge (Concannon 1986).

Prolactin concentrations rise post oestrus in both pregnant and non-pregnant bitches, although the concentrations are somewhat higher in pregnant bitches and show a transient surge during the rapid decline in progesterone concentrations that occur 1-2 days before whelping. Prolactin concentrations remain elevated post-whelping until the puppies are weaned. The pregnancy-specific hormone relaxin can be detected in the blood of a pregnant bitch 26-30 days after the LH peak but is not present in non-pregnant dogs (Concannon et al., 1996).

7.3.3 Pregnancy diagnosis

The average bodyweight gain of a pregnant bitch from oestrus to parturition is 36% (range 20-55%), with the increase being most marked in the last third of pregnancy. A change in body shape is usually visible by about day 56 of pregnancy and foetal movements may also be noted around this time. The nipples enlarge and mammary development occurs during the second half of pregnancy and serous secretion may be present shortly before parturition (Christiansen 1984).

Bitch owners frequently want to know whether their bitch is pregnant following a planned mating, principally out of curiosity, but also so that adequate plans can be made in advance of the anticipated whelping date.

Abdominal palpation

Abdominal palpation, usually 3-4 weeks post-mating, is used commonly for the diagnosis of pregnancy in the bitch. Although false positive results are rare in the hands of experienced veterinarians, it is difficult to be certain that a bitch is not pregnant.

Problems can be encountered in certain breeds, fat animals and in bitches that guard their abdomens.

Radiography

Radiography can be used to confirm canine pregnancy but foetal skeletons do not become radio-opaque until day 45.

Ultrasonography

Ultrasonography can be used to visualize foetal vesicles from day 16-20 of pregnancy. Foetal heart beats can be seen, using real time ultrasound, from day 24-28 of pregnancy.

Hormone measurements

Levels of conventional hormones (e.g. progesterone) cannot be used to diagnose pregnancy. Acute phase protein levels are significantly elevated from day 21-50 post-mating in pregnant bitches, compared to non-pregnant animals (Concannon et al., 1996; Evans and Anderton 1992). Not all acute phase proteins are useful for early pregnancy diagnosis and bitches must be healthy and mating dates known in order to avoid false positive or false negative results (Vannucchi et al., 2002).

7.4 Parturition

Several authors have described the events, which take place immediately before and during parturition (Christiansen 1984; Concannon et al., 1989; Feldman and Nelson 2004; Linde-Forsberg and Eneroth 2000; von Heimendahl and Cariou 2009).

7.4.1 Initiating events

The precise hormonal mechanisms that precipitate parturition have not been clearly elucidated in bitches. It is thought that whelping is brought about by a series of hormonal changes, starting with rising oestrogen and falling progesterone concentrations and the production of luteolytic amounts of prostaglandin $F_{2\alpha}$ by the foeto-placental unit. This prostaglandin induces the production of relaxin, which results in the relaxation of the pelvis and reproductive tract, and causes uterine contractions and abdominal straining, both directly and via the release of oxytocin from the pituitary. Rising cortisol concentrations, which result from the maturation of the foetal hypophyseal-pituitary-adrenal axis, trigger this whole cascade of events.

7.4.2 Pre-partum signs

During the last 2-3 days before parturition bitches usually exhibit characteristic behaviour, such as seeking solitude, restlessness and nest making. The presence or absence of milk is too variable to be a reliable sign of impending parturition. Just prior to whelping it is not uncommon for the vagina to become oedematous and a slight vaginal discharge may be visible. Bitches frequently refuse food for 1-2 days prior to parturition.

Body temperature decrease, frequently taken by breeders as an indication that whelping will occur within the next 24 hours, is not a reliable indicator of impending parturition in the bitch (Veronesi et al., 2002). There is a significant decrease in progesterone concentrations from 24 h prior to whelping onwards (Veronesi et al., 2002).

7.4.3 Labour

Classically, labour is divided into three stages, with the stage altering as each individual foetus is produced:

First stage of labour: cervical relaxation and dilation
During this stage, which lasts between 4 and 36 hours, the cervix relaxes and dilates. The bitch becomes more restless and nervous, shivers, pants, may vomit and/or tear up bedding material. Weak uterine contractions may be apparent.

Second stage of labour: the production of young
This stage is characterized by strong uterine contractions and visible straining. Between contractions the bitch will lick its vulva, especially once the foetal sac ruptures and placental fluid is released. Once the foetal head or pelvis is engaged, strong abdominal straining is stimulated. The duration of the second stage of labour is extremely variable between individuals and between puppies within a litter. As a rule of thumb, however, no more than 6 hours should be allowed to elapse after the delivery of the first puppy before an investigation is carried out, since a long delay may result in placental separation and the death of any remaining viable puppies. The interval between births is also variable. Second and subsequent puppies are usually produced after no more than 30 minutes of straining. Rest periods of more than 3-4 hours should be regarded as abnormal. It is not uncommon for a large litter to take up to 24 hours to be produced. Bitches that are good mothers will clean and suckle the puppies between successive births.

Third stage of labour: the expulsion of the placenta
This is the stage during which the foetal membranes are expelled. Puppies may be born with the membranes intact or they may be born simply attached by the umbilical cord with the placenta remaining in the genital tract. In the latter case the placenta will be expelled separately before, with or after subsequent births. The bitch may eat the placenta; it has been suggested that placental hormones promote uterine involution and milk production. It is probably unwise to let a bitch eat every placenta if the litter is large.
The end of whelping is signaled by a bitch relaxing and nursing its pups contentedly.

7.4.3.1 Induction of parturition

Treatment with the progesterone-receptor antagonist aglepristone on two occasions at a 9 hour interval on day 58 of pregnancy has been reported to be suitable the for induction of parturition in the bitch (Baan et al., 2005).

7.4.3.2 Delayed parturition (Uterine inertia)

Uterine inertia or the failure of uterine contractions is probably the most common and worrying cause of dystocia in bitches. The cause is not entirely clear but mechanical, physical, genetic and hormonal factors are involved, possibly in concert. Two types of uterine inertia are recognized.

Primary inertia
When there is total uterine inertia, the bitch fails to show any signs of impending parturition or fails to progress from the first to the second stage of labour. Injections of oxytocin have very little or no effect in such cases. Caesarean section is indicated if live puppies are to be produced. The production of copious amounts of dark green/black fluid by bitches not showing any signs of first stage of labour also indicates the need for Caesarean section. In cases of partial primary uterine inertia it is important to be sure that no maternal or foetal obstructions are present. If no obstructions are present, medical management is usually successful. Oxytocin, by intramuscular or intravenous injection, is best given in small (1-12 IU intravenously or 2.5-10 IU intramuscularly), repeated doses 30 minutes apart (Linde-Forsberg and Eneroth 2000). If the response is insufficient, each oxytocin injection can be preceded by slow intravenous infusion (1 ml/min) of 2-20 ml calcium gluconate (Linde-Forsberg and Eneroth 2000).

Secondary inertia
This is most frequently due to exhaustion of the uterine musculature and follows protracted straining in cases of obstructive dystocia, or the delivery of large litters. Unless large numbers of foetuses remain, an injection of oxytocin will often successfully restart uterine contractions. If this is not effective or if large numbers of foetuses remain, Caesarean section is indicated.

7.4.3.3 Retained placentas

Expulsion of retained placentas can be stimulated using oxytocin at a dose of 1-5 IU oxytocin per dog administered subcutaneously or intramuscularly two to four times daily for up to 3 days (Linde-Forsberg and Eneroth 2000).

7.5 Unwanted pregnancy (Misalliance)

It is important that a full history is taken for cases in which mismating (also known as misalliance or mésalliance) is suspected. Where mating has not been observed, the presence of spermatozoa or sperm heads in a vaginal smear is evidence that mating did occur. However, negative vaginal cytology should be interpreted with extreme caution, since the lack of spermatozoa in a sample is not evidence that mating did not occur.

7.5.1 Bitches not intended for breeding

Ovariohysterectomy (spaying) is the treatment of choice in bitches which have been mated but are not intended for breeding and should be advised especially when the management indicates that there is a real risk that the bitch will escape and be mated again. Surgery can be carried out 3-4 weeks post mating. This time schedule offers the additional possibility for pregnancy diagnosis prior to surgery. Ovariohysterectomy is relatively safe and removes the future risk of other reproductive problems, such as CEH-pyometra complex.

Despite the indisputable advantages of spaying a mismated bitch, many owners will not accept this option due to fear of the risks connected with any surgical procedure (Burrow et al., 2005) or concerns about future complications, such as urinary incontinence or behavioural changes. The high cost of the procedure can also deter the owners from having their bitch spayed, in which case pharmacological termination of unwanted pregnancy can be considered.

7.5.2 Bitches intended for breeding

A number of different pharmaceutical treatments can be used to terminate pregnancy (Verstegen 2000). The owner of the bitch should always be informed about the predicted efficacy and possible side-effects of the treatment chosen.

Oestrogens

In the bitch, egg cells are fertilized in the Fallopian tube and take 6-10 days to migrate into the uterine horns. Large doses of oestrogen prolong the oviductal transport time and tighten the utero-tubular junction. This results in failure of implantation in the uterus and death of the embryo (Feldman and Nelson 2004). In this respect treatment with oestrogens should be perceived as a means to prevent implantation rather than an abortifacient.

Several oestrogens, including oestradiol benzoate, have been used successfully for many years to prevent pregnancy in bitches.

Traditionally, a single, relatively large dose of oestradiol benzoate (0.3 mg/kg up to a maximum of 10 mg per bitch) was administered by intramuscular or subcutaneous injection between 24 and 96 hours (1-4 days) post-mating. This dosing regime was associated with a relatively high risk of side-effects such as iatrogenic pyometra, bone marrow suppression, infertility and prolonged oestrus behaviour.

In order to reduce these possible drawbacks, an alternative low dose regime was developed. A field study involving 358 bitches showed that this new dosage regime is associated with a reduced risk of side-effects (Sutton et al., 1997).

In order to avoid further complications and possible complaints, owners of treated bitches should be clearly instructed that the bitch has to be supervised so as to avoid another unwanted mating. Supervision should be maintained throughout treatment and continued until vaginal discharge is no longer observed and the bitch is no longer attractive to male dogs. In some bitches oestrus signs can be prolonged following oestradiol administration.

Progesterone antagonists

Progesterone antagonists or anti-progestins are synthetic steroids that bind with strong affinity to progesterone receptors, thus preventing progesterone from exerting its biological effects (Hoffmann et al., 2000). Pregnancy termination is possible from the time of mating until day 45 of gestation. Aglepristone is indicated for pregnancy termination and seems to be safe and effective (Galac et al., 2000; Gobello 2006). This treatment has few side-effects.

Dopamine agonists

Prolactin secretion provides essential luteotrophic support and is required to maintain pregnancy in dogs. Ergot alkaloids such as bromocriptine, cabergoline and metergoline are effective abortifacient agents when used after day 30-35 of pregnancy (Feldman and Nelson 2004).

- Bromocriptine can be given orally at a dose of 0.1 mg/kg once daily for 6 consecutive days from day 35, or at a dose of 0.03 mg/kg twice daily for 4 consecutive days from day 30 (Feldman and Nelson 2004). Side-effects such as anorexia, vomiting and depression are quite common.
- Cabergoline can be given orally at a dose of 0.005 mg/kg once daily from day 40. Cabergoline causes fewer side-effects than bromocriptine (Feldman and Nelson 2004).
- Metergoline administered orally at a dose rate of 0.6 mg/kg twice daily from day 28 resulted in pregnancy termination in eight out of nine bitches, although the treatment interval showed considerable variation between individuals (3-23 days) (Nöthling et al., 2003).

Prostaglandins

Prostaglandins work via the induction of luteolysis, stimulation of uterine contractions and dilation of the cervix. Prostaglandins have significant limitations as abortifacients in dogs (Feldman and Nelson 2004; Verstegen 2000). High doses of prostaglandins are required to induce luteolysis in early metoestrus and terminate pregnancy. Such high doses produce intense side-effects (which usually last for around 20-30 minutes), including vomiting, salivation, diarrhoea, and respiratory distress.

Low doses of prostaglandin analogues (0.03 mg/kg twice daily) have been reported to be efficient in terminating pregnancy from day 35 onwards (Concannon and Hansel 1977; Wichtel et al., 1990). In spite of some encouraging results, the success of pregnancy termination using prostaglandins is variable, so the use of prostaglandins alone for pregnancy termination in bitches is not recommended.

Bitches treated during the second half of pregnancy should be hospitalized due both to the possible side-effects and the variable time to foetal expulsion post-treatment. Entirely formed foetuses are aborted; thus this procedure is even more unacceptable to many owners and veterinary practitioners. Radiography or ultrasonography should be used to confirm the complete expulsion of all the foetuses.

Dopamine agonists plus prostaglandins
A combination of a dopamine agonist and a prostaglandin can be used to interrupt pregnancy successfully from day 25 after the LH peak (Gobello et al., 2002; Onclin and Verstegen 1990). These agents reduce circulating progesterone concentrations.

Using the agents in combination reduces the risk of side-effects (associated with the prostaglandin). Low doses of either cabergoline or bromocriptine combined with cloprostenol have been shown to be relatively safe and effective (Onclin and Verstegen 1990;1996) and result in foetal resorption if treatment is started on day 25. Bromocriptine mesylate (oral, 0.015-0.030 mg/kg, twice daily) combined with either dinoprost tromethamine (subcutaneous injection, 0.1-0.2 mg/kg, once daily) or cloprostenol (subcutaneous injection, 0.001 mg/kg, every second day) until pregnancy termination, has been reported to be effective and to produce minimal side-effects (Gobello et al., 2002).

Glucocorticoids
Glucocorticoids are not as consistently effective in terminating pregnancy in bitches as they are in ruminants (Wanke et al., 1997).

7.6 Oestrus control

The over-production of puppies necessitates the destruction of large numbers of unwanted dogs. Thus, control of oestrus in bitches is of great socio-economic importance. Furthermore, if carried out properly it provides a health advantage for bitches. There are two methods of oestrus control: surgical (ovariectomy or ovariohysterectomy) and medical.

7.6.1 Surgical control of oestrus

There is a trend towards early spaying in a number of countries (Root Kustritz and Olson 2000). Surgical removal of the ovaries and/or uterus (ovariectomy or ovariohysterectomy; spaying) is usually very effective and safe, and offers many benefits. However, although it is cost-effective in the long-term, spaying may not be suitable for all bitches, and obviously not for those intended for future breeding. Ovariohysterectomy is not entirely without hazard and some owners are unhappy about letting their pet undergo major surgery (Burrow et al., 2005). Side-effects can be encountered, such as urinary incontinence (especially in large, docked breeds), obesity, infantile vulva, hair loss and changes in coat colour and texture.

7.6.2 Medical control of oestrus

The majority of agents used for the chemical control of oestrus are natural or synthetic steroid hormones: primarily progestagens or androgens. More recently, non-steroidal approaches (e.g. vaccines, GnRH agonists, GnRH antagonists) have been researched (Gobello 2006; Verstegen 2000) but, as yet, none of these agents is approved for use in bitches.

Progestagens
Studies in a number of animal species have shown that progestagens have a number of actions:
- Anti-gonadotrophic: suppress follicular development and thus the production of oestrogen, and prevent ovulation and the formation of corpora lutea
- Anti-oestrogenic: control vaginal bleeding

- Anti-androgenic: reduce sex drive in male dogs
- Contraceptive: interfere with sperm transport and desynchronize the events that need to be critically timed if pregnancy is to result
- Progestagenic: maintain pregnancy and produce a secretory endometrium

The relative potency of the different progestagens varies and thus findings related to one compound do not apply to others. A number of synthetic steroids including progestagens (e.g. proligestone (Covinan®, also known as Delvosteron®), medroxyprogesterone acetate, megestrol acetate (Burke and Reynolds 1975), chlormadinone acetate and androgens (e.g. mibolerone acetate) are used to control ovarian cyclicity in dogs (Verstegen 2000).

The oestrous cycle in bitches can be controlled in three ways:

- Suppression of oestrus (heat) and prevention of conception can be achieved by treatment at the onset of pro-oestrus.
- Temporary postponement of oestrus to a more convenient time can be achieved by treatment just before an anticipated heat.
- Permanent postponement of oestrus can be achieved by repeated treatment, starting in anoestrus or pro-oestrus.

Proligestone is a second-generation synthetic progestagen (Van Os 1982). It can be used for suppression, temporary postponement or permanent postponement of heat in bitches. The incidence of false pregnancy in bitches with permanent postponement of oestrus induced by injections of proligestone is only 3.9%, lower than in bitches left to cycle normally (van Os and Evans 1980).

Large individual differences have been reported in the time from the last proligestone administration to the commencement of cyclic activity. In the majority of bitches heat will be evident within 3-6 months after the last dose of proligestone. In individual cases however, the blockade of reproductive activity may last for up to 2 years. This means that not all bitches will show heat 3-6 months after a single administration of proligestone. This is an important consideration if only the temporary postponement of heat is intended. The fertility at the first heat following the withdrawal of proligestone treatment is not adversely affected.

Whenever long-acting progestagens are used the following factors, which might affect the efficacy of the treatment, should be considered:

Individual/breed variability
There is individual variation in the duration of the blocking effect of progestagens on the reproductive activity in bitches. After the initial dosing regime, continuation with one injection every 5-6 months is efficient for the prevention of oestrus in the majority of bitches. However, in some individuals the duration of action of long-acting progestagens is less than 5-6 months. In such bitches, shortening the time interval between consecutive injections is advisable (e.g. to every 4 months). The progestagen should be administered at the manufacturer's recommended dose rate.

Environmental factors
In general, environmental and/or seasonal influences do not affect the efficacy of progestagen treatment in bitches. However, bitches housed together (i.e. with other cycling bitches) may require a shorter interval between consecutive injections.

Phase of oestrous cycle
Anoestrus is the most appropriate time for the initiation of progestagen treatment in bitches. Long-acting progestagens are the most effective when administered during anoestrus. The efficacy of these preparations may be decreased if administered during pro-oestrus. Suppression of heat during pro-oestrus is better achieved using short-acting, oral progestagens.

Progestagens have a number of well-known side-effects and contraindications. Side-effects of exogenous progestagens may manifest themselves as a transient increase in appetite, weight gain, and rarely lethargy. Bitches treated with progestagens during pregnancy may have delayed parturition, with the subsequent death of the foetuses, if effective progestagens concentrations persist for longer than the normal duration of pregnancy (van Os 1982).

- Due to the potential diabetogenic effect of long-term therapy with progestagens, diabetic bitches should not be treated with these preparations. Spaying is the treatment of choice in such animals. This should be carried out as soon as possible, even before initiating insulin treatment.
- Medroxyprogesterone acetate has stimulated the development of hyperplastic and neoplastic nodules in the mammary glands of treated bitches (van Os et al., 1981). Bitches with any neoplastic or hyperplastic changes in the mammary glands should be spayed rather than treated with progestagens.
- If any pathological endometrial changes have been diagnosed, treatment with long-acting progestagens is contraindicated. Finally, the injectable compounds may cause local reactions at the injection site, such as hair loss, hair discoloration and possibly atrophy of the skin and surrounding tissues, often referred to as 'pitting'. These effects can be minimized if the injection is given strictly subcutaneously (Evans and Sutton 1989; van Os 1982).

Androgens

Testosterone and mibolerone have been used to suppress oestrus, but have several disadvantages. Although very efficient, androgens are known to produce severe side-effects in bitches, which are directly associated with their androgenic activity including masculinisation (characterized by clitoral hypertrophy), recurrent colpitis and behavioural changes. Bitches treated long-term with androgens become attracted to other female dogs and exhibit typical male behaviour (e.g. mounting, territorial urination). Androgen therapy in female dogs has been also associated with iatrogenic hypertrophic changes in the endometrium and with pyometra and liver disease.

Androgen therapy should not be used in pregnant bitches because this produces masculinisation and severe abnormalities of the reproductive and urinary tracts in female foetuses. Administration of androgens in pro-oestrus should also be avoided, as there is always a risk that the bitch may escape and mate.

7.7 Other conditions of the female urogenital tract

7.7.1 False pregnancy

False pregnancy (pseudopregnancy or pseudocyesis) occurs in intact bitches within 6 to 8 weeks after oestrus. The signs may vary in intensity from abdominal distension with mammary hyperplasia and milk production, to an almost complete replication of parturition (including nervousness, excitability and panting) and nursing (including the production of variable amounts of milk) (Harvey et al., 1999). The bitch may also show mothering behaviour towards inanimate objects.

The incidence of false pregnancy is difficult to assess since the signs may be very mild in some cases. However, it is generally considered that the majority of bitches (50-75%) will show some signs of this normal physiological condition.

Prolactin is recognized as being the most important luteotrophic factor from day 35 of the cycle, its release from the anterior pituitary being stimulated by falling progesterone concentrations. Prolactin is the key hormone for lactogenesis and the initiation and maintenance of lactation. False pregnancy is thought to result from the rising prolactin concentrations that are stimulated by falling progesterone concentrations as metoestrus progresses. This is supported by the fact that very prolonged lactation occurs if the ovaries are removed from bitches that have signs of false pregnancy. Moreover, bitches with false pregnancy have significantly lower progesterone and significantly higher prolactin concentrations than unaffected bitches at a comparable stage of the oestrous cycle (between 50 and 95 days after the onset of pro-oestrus) (Tsutsui et al., 2007).

There is no evidence that bitches that show significant signs of false pregnancy are any more likely to suffer from CEH-pyometra complex or infertility.

The requirement for treatment of false pregnancy depends on the type and severity of the signs shown. The condition is usually mild and most cases recover spontaneously within a few weeks. In more severe cases, medical treatment (with a dopamine agonist) is indicated (Harvey et al., 1997).

Dopamine agonists effectively inhibit prolactin via a direct action (bromocriptine, cabergoline) on D2-dopamine receptors of the lactotrophic cells of the anterior pituitary gland (Gobello 2006). Treatment with bromocriptine is, however, frequently associated with side-effects such as vomiting. Cabergoline, a newer dopamine agonist, seems to be associated with far fewer side-effects (Harvey et al., 1997; Feldman and Nelson, 2004). Progestagens inhibit milk production via negative feedback on the anterior pituitary, which inhibits prolactin production. Progestagens may also help reduce the behavioural signs of false pregnancy due to their calming effect on the hypothalamus.

In bitches that suffer from severe bouts of false pregnancy after each oestrus, surgery (ovariectomy/ovariohysterectomy) is the treatment of choice since this will prevent recurrence of the condition. The surgery should not be carried out whilst signs of false pregnancy are present (Harvey et al., 1999) or whilst being suppressed medically. Failure to observe this rule may result in untreatable persistent lactation.

7.7.2 CEH-pyometra complex

The CEH-pyometra complex is a severe condition in which the uterus becomes filled with fluid, and may also be contaminated by bacteria (Feldman 2000). The toxaemia that results gives rise to characteristic clinical signs particularly excessive thirst (due to (initially reversible) glomerulonephritis), vomiting, inappetance, shock and death. Typically the condition occurs 4-6 weeks after oestrus, but it has been diagnosed in some bitches as early as the end of oestrus and as late as 12-14 weeks after standing heat. Pyometra occurs primarily in older bitches (>5 years) that have not been used for breeding. However, the condition can occur in young bitches and has even been recorded in bitches after their first heat.

Two main types of pyometra occur, open and closed. In open pyometra, the contents of the uterus are lost, at least in part, through the vagina via the open cervix. In closed pyometra, there is no vaginal discharge (closed cervix) and the bitch is usually much more acutely ill.

The cause of CEH-pyometra complex is not entirely clear but it is thought to be associated with progressive hormonal imbalance linked to the progesterone-sensitivity of the canine uterus. It is thought that sequential periods of oestrogen dominance, which enhance the stimulatory effects of progesterone on the uterus, followed by prolonged progesterone dominance, either natural (metoestrus) or following progestagen administration, lead to the development of CEH, which in turn may be followed by mucometra or pyometra.

Surgical removal of the uterus and ovaries, following adequate rehydration (intravenous fluid therapy), is the treatment of choice (Nelson & Feldman, 1986). Medical treatment of CEH-pyometra can be used in bitches intended for breeding (Nelson and Feldman 1986). A combination of prostaglandin and the progesterone antagonist aglepristone has proved the most successful medical approach to date (Gobello et al., 2003).

Prostaglandins increase myometrial contractions and are luteolytic, decreasing serum progesterone concentrations, but produce variable cervical relaxation in bitches. The use of prostaglandins in the treatment of closed pyometra (i.e. the cervix is closed) is associated with a very high risk of uterine rupture, a life-threatening complication. Prostaglandin administration can also be associated with both circulatory and respiratory depression, serious complications that may easily lead to a fatal outcome and should therefore be administered with great care.

Aglepristone is a progesterone antagonist (or anti-progestin) that binds with great affinity to uterine progesterone receptors, thus preventing progesterone from exerting its biological effects (Hoffmann et al., 2000). The combination of the synthetic prostaglandin analogue cloprostenol (0.001 mg/kg subcutaneously) and agelpristone (10 mg/kg subcutaneously) on a number of occasions over a 15 day period has been shown to be quite effective (Gobello et al., 2003).

7.7.3 Urinary incontinence

Urinary incontinence is a lack of control of voluntary urination, and results in the uncontrolled loss of urine. In females the *M. sphincter urethrae* contains oestrogen-receptors through which oestrogens influence muscle tone and the closure of the urethral sphincter. Thus, (relative) oestrogen deficiency can cause urinary incontinence. Oestrogen deficiency can be a result of spaying and/or increased age.

Factors predisposing to urinary incontinence include:
- early spaying
- breed (large size, heavy breed, tail docking)
- obesity

There are also differences in plasma gonadotrophin levels between continent and incontinent spayed bitches (Reichler et al., 2006).Oestrogens are used to treat urinary incontinence to try to restore the normal tonus of the urethral sphincter. Although there are no major differences in oestrogen concentrations between spayed and anoestrus intact bitches, the majority of spayed bitches with urinary incontinence respond to oestrogen therapy.

Oestrogens, such as ethinyl oestradiol and diethylstilboestrol, have been used for this indication, but cause so-called long-term oestrogenic effects, such as bone marrow suppression. More recently, one of the natural oestrogens, oestriol (Incurin® tablets) has been registered for the treatment of urinary incontinence in spayed bitches.

Oestriol is a short-acting oestrogen, due to its short receptor occupancy time. Oestriol is safe for the treatment of urinary incontinence and is not associated with long-term oestrogenic side-effects. In a field study of 133 bitches with urinary incontinence, 83% had a positive response to treatment (Mandigers and Nell 2001). Short term oestrogenic effects (e.g. vulval swelling) were seen in approximately 5-9% of spayed bitches treated with oestriol. GnRH-agonists have also been used successfully to treat urinary incontinence in bitches, although it is not absolutely clear why bladder function is improved after GnRH administration (Reichler et al., 2006).

7.8 Male dogs

In male dogs, secondary sexual characteristics and behaviour occur as a result of the interplay between hormones produced by the anterior pituitary (the gonadotrophins), gonads and hypothalamus. In response to gonadotrophin releasing hormone (GnRH), secreted from the hypothalamus, two gonadotrophic hormones, FSH and LH are released from the anterior pituitary. FSH is responsible for spermatogenesis, while LH, also known as interstitial cell stimulating hormone (ICSH), maintains androgen (testosterone and dihydrotestosterone) production. LH is released continually in an episodic fashion; concentrations vary throughout the day.

The main androgen, testosterone, acts on target organs to maintain the male secondary sexual characteristics and function, including libido, and helps to maintain spermatogenesis. This hormone also exerts a negative feedback effect on the anterior pituitary and/or hypothalamus. Thus it can be seen that androgens not only control reproductive processes but also associated behaviour - mounting, aggression and territory marking. Parts of the cerebral cortex in the hypothalamic region are also involved in determining sexual behaviour.

7.8.1 Hypersexuality

As already noted, there are two different mechanisms controlling sexual behaviour - the male sex hormones and parts of the cerebral cortex. These systems are related because steroids, including the sex hormones, are thought to bind to the hypothalamic region and control both positive and negative feedback mechanisms for hormonal activity and sexual behaviour.

It is important to note that there are large differences in the relative dependence of sexual behaviour upon androgens and the cerebral cortex, both between species and between individuals within a species (Dunbar 1975).

Hypersexuality is essentially excessive or aberrant sexual behaviour, although it is sometimes also taken to encompass normal sexual behaviour that is misplaced within modern society, and manifests as:

- Aggression
- Mounting other dogs, people, inanimate objects
- Territory marking, especially urination in the house
- Roaming
- Destructive behaviour
- Excitability, including excessive barking

Most owners are not concerned about this type of behaviour in their dogs and do not seek treatment. This is probably because this type of behaviour is accepted as part and parcel of owning an entire male dog. In fact, some of these traits are normal in male dogs and it is merely a question of severity, frequency and place that makes the behaviour unacceptable.

Surgical or medical castration and behavioural training are used to treat hypersexuality in dogs (Andersson and Linde-Forsberg 2001). However the success of treatment depends on the main clinical sign: intermale aggression has often a poorer response to treatment than other manifestations of hypersexuality.

- Surgical castration removes the main source of androgens but has no effect on the cerebral cortex and will have no effect on the actions of androgens from alternative sources, such as the adrenal glands.
- Progestagens, such as medroxyprogesterone acetate, delmadinone acetate and proligestone, have been used to control hypersexuality in male dogs. These agents can be effective. Side-effects include lethargy and increased appetite.
- Behavioural training is often effective but the efficacy varies depending on the behavioural signs exhibited. The hormonal status of the dog remains unaffected. Behavioural training requires considerable owner time and commitment.

7.8.2 Cryptorchidism

The testes of the dog are intra-abdominal at birth and normally descend into the scrotum during the first 7-10 days of life. At 2 weeks of age, the testes can often be palpated in either the scrotum or inguinal canal, although descent may be delayed in some individuals.

Unilateral cryptorchid dogs are often fertile since the descended testicle usually functions normally. Dogs that have bilaterally retained testicles are infertile but usually have normal libido and male secondary sexual characteristics. The main significance of cryptorchidism in pet dogs is that there is a significant risk that the retained testicle(s) will undergo neoplastic change and/or torsion of the spermatic cord.

About 6-12% of dogs are cryptorchid (one or both testicles have not descended normally by puberty). The exact cause is unknown but it is likely that there is an underlying, inherited hormonal abnormality since the incidence is noticeably higher in some breeds (e.g. Boxers). For this reason cryptorchid dogs should not be used for breeding. In view of the probable hereditary nature of the condition, medical treatment is considered unethical. If a testicular tumour is already present, surgical removal of both testes is advocated.
GnRH can be administered at 0.002 mg/kg intravenously or 0.050 mg/kg intramuscularly with blood samples taken for testosterone prior to GnRH administration, and 60 minutes later, to test if a dog has an abdominal testicle (Purswell and Wilcke 1993). In dogs more than 12 months of age (i.e. post-puberty), retained testicles should be removed surgically, ideally before the dog is middle aged (4-6 years old) to avoid neoplasia.

7.9 References

Anderson A and Linde-Forsberg C. Castration and progestagen treatment of male dogs, part 2. Svensk Veterinar tidning 2001;53:391-397

Arnold S., Arnold P., Concannon P., Weilenmansn R., Hubler M., Casal M., Fairburn A., Eggenberger E., Rusch P. Effect of duration of PMSG treatment on induction of oestrus, pregnancy rates and complications of hyperoestrogenism in dogs. J Reprod Fertil Suppl 1989;39:115-122

Baan M., Taverne MAM., Kooistra HS., De Gier J., Dieleman SJ., Okkens AC. Induction of parturition in the bitch with the progesterone receptor blocker aglepristone. Theriogenology 2005;63:1958-1972.

Beijerink NJ., Kooistra HS., Dieleman SJ., Okkens AC. Serotonin antagonistinduced lowering of prolactin secretion does not affect the pattern of pulsatile secretion of follicle-stimulating hormone and luteinizing hormone in the bitch. Reproduction 2004;128:181-188.

Burke TJ., Reynolds HA Jr. Megestrol acetate for estrus postponement in the bitch. J Am vet Med Assoc 1975;167:285-287.

Burrow R., Batchelor D., Cripps P. Complications observed during and after ovariohysterectomy of 142 bitches at a veterinary teaching hospital. Vet Rec 2005;157:829-33.

Cain JL., Lasley BL., Cain GR., Feldman EC., Stabenfeldt GH. Induction of ovulation in bitches with pulsatile or continuous infusion of GnRH. J Reprod Fertil Suppl 1989;39:143-147

Chaffaux S., Locci D., Pontois M., Deletang F., Thibier, M. Induction of ovarian activity in anoestrus beagle bitches, Br Vet J 1984;140:191-195.

Christiansen IB J. Reproduction in the dog and cat. Eastbourne, England: Balliere Tindall 1984:80-109.

Christie DW., Bell ET. Some observations on the seasonal incidence and frequency of oestrus in breeding bitches in Britain. J Small Anim Pract 1971;12:159-167.

Concannon PW. Canine pregnancy and parturition. Vet Clin North Am Small Anim Pract 1986;16: 453-475.

Concannon PW. Biology of gonadotropin secretion in adult and prepubertal female dogs. J Reprod Fertil Suppl 1993;47:3-27.

Concannon PW., Gimpel P., Newton L., Castracane VD. Postimplantation increase in plasma fibrinogen concentration with increase in relaxin concentration in pregnant dogs. Am J Vet Res 1996;57:1382-1385.

Concannon PW., Hansel W. Prostaglandin $F_{2\alpha}$ induced luteolysis, hypothermia and abortions in Beagle bitches. Prostaglandins 1977;13:533-542.

Concannon PW., Hansel W., Visek WJ. The ovarian cycle of the bitch: plasma estrogen, LH and progesterone. Biol Reprod 1975;13:112-121.

Concannon PW., McCann JP., Temple M. Biology and endocrinology of ovulation, pregnancy and parturition in the dog. J Reprod Fertil Suppl 1989;39:3-25.

Concannon PW., Lasley B., Vanderlip S. LH release, induction of oestrus and fertile ovulations in response to pulsatile administration of GnRH to anoestrus dogs. J Reprod Fertil Suppl 1997;51:41-54.

Concannon P., Temple M., Montanez A., Newton L. Effects of dose and duration of continuous GnRH-agonist treatment on inductionof estrus in beagle dogs: Competing and concurrent up-regulation and down-regulation of LH release. Theriogenology 2006;66:1488-1496.

Eilts BE., Davidson AP., Hosgood G., Paccamonti DL., Baker DG. Factors affecting gestation duration in the bitch. Theriogenology 2005;64:242-251.

Evans JM., Sutton DJ. The use of hormones, especially progestagens, to control oestrus in bitches. J Reprod Fertil Suppl1989;39:163-173.
Evans JM., Anderton DJ. Pregnancy diagnosis in the bitch: the development of a test based on the measurement of acute phase protein in the blood. Ann Zootech 1992;41:397-405.
Feldman EC. Cystic Endometrial Hyperplasia, Pyometra, and fertility. In: Textbook of Veterinary Internal Medicine, 5th edn. Eds. SJ. Ettinger and EC. Feldman. Saunders 2000; XIII: 1549-1565
Feldman EC., Nelson RW. Canine & Feline Endocrinology and Reproduction. Philadelphia: WB Saunders, 2004;7:751-1014.
Fuller JL. Photoperiodic control of estrus in the Basenji. J Hered 1956;47:179-180.
Galac S., Kooistra HS., Butinar J., Bevers MM., Dieleman SJ., Voorhout G, et al. Termination of mid gestation pregnancy in bitches with aglepristone, a progesterone receptor antagonist. Theriogenology 2000;53:941-950.
Gobello C. Dopamine agonists, anti-progestins, anti-androgens, long-term release GnRH agonists and anti-estrogens in canine reproduction: A review. Theriogenology 2006;66:1560-1567
Gobello C., Castex G., Corrada Y., Klima L., de la Sota RL., Rodriguez, R. Use of prostaglandins and bromocriptine mesylate for pregnancy termination in bitches. J Am Vet Med Assoc 2002;220:1017-1019.
Gobello C., Castex G., Klima L., Rodriguez R., Corrada Y. A study of two protocols combining aglepristone and cloprostenol to treat open cervix pyometra in the bitch. Theriogenology 2003;60:901-908.
Gobello C. New GnRH analogs in canine reproduction. Anim Reprod Sci 2007;100:1-13.
Goodman M. Ovulation timing. Concepts and controversies. Vet Clin North Am Small Anim Pract 2001;31:219-234.
Grundy SA., Feldman E., Davidson A. Evaluation of infertility in the bitch. Clin Tech SA Pract 2002;17:108-115.
Harvey MJA., Cauvin A., Dale M., Lindley S., Ballabio, R. Effect and mechanisms of the anti-prolactin drug cabergoline on pseudopregnancy in the bitch. J Small Anim Pract 1997;38:336-339.
Harvey MJA., Dale MJ., Lindley S., Waterston MM. A study of the aetiology of pseudopregnancy in the bitch and the effect of cabergoline therapy. Vet Rec **1999;144:433-436.**
Hoffmann B and Schuler G. Receptor blockers – general aspects with respect to their use in domestic animal reproduction. Anim Reprod Sci 2000;60-61:295-312
Inaba T., Tani H., Gonda M., Nakagawa A., Ohmura M., Mori J., Torii R., Tamada H., Sawada T. Induction of fertile estrus in bitches using a sustainedrelease formulation of a GnRH agonist (leuprolide acetate). Theriogenology 1998;49(5):975-982
Jeffcoate IA., Lindsay FEF. Ovulation detection and timing of insemination based on hormonal concentrations, vaginal cytology and the endoscopic appearance of the vagina in domestic bitches. J Reprod Fertil Suppl 1989;39:277-287.
Jeukenne P., Verstegen J. Termination of dioestrus and induction of oestrus in dioestrus nonpregnant bitches by the prolactin antagonist cabergoline. J Reprod Fert Suppl 1997;51:59-66.
Kooistra HS., Okkens AC. Secretion of growth hormone and prolactin during progression of the luteal phase in healthy dogs: a review. Mol Cell Endocrinol 2002;197:167-172.
Kutzler MA. Induction and synchronization of estrus in dogs. Theriogenology 2005;64:766-75.
Linde-Forsberg C and Eneroth A. Abnormalities in Pregnancy, Parturition, and the Periparturient Period. In: Textbook of Veterinary Internal Medicine, 5th edn. Eds. SJ. Ettinger and EC. Feldman. Saunders 2000; XIII:1527-1238

Mandigers PJ., Nell T. Treatment of bitches with acquired urinary incontinence with oestriol. Vet Rec 2001;149:764-7.

Nelson RW., Feldman EC. Pyometra. Vet Clin North Am Small Anim Pract 1986;16:561-576.

Nöthling JO., Gerber D., Gerstenberg C., Kaiser C., Döbeli M. Abortifacient and endocrine effects of metergoline in beagle bitches during the second half of gestation. Theriogenology 2003;59:1929-40.

Okkens AC., Bevers MM., Dieleman SJ., Willems AH. Shortening of the interoestrous interval and the lifespan of the corpus luteum of the cyclic dog by bromocryptine treatment. Vet Q 1985;7:173-176.

Okkens AC., Bevers MM., Dieleman SJ., Willemse AH. Evidence for prolactin as the main luteotrophic factor in the cyclic dog. Vet Q 1990;12:193-201.

Onclin K., Murphy B., Verstegen JP. Comparisons of estradiol, LH and FSH patterns in pregnant and nonpregnant beagle bitches. Theriogenology 2002;57:1957-1972.

Onclin K., Verstegen JP. Comparison of different combinations of analogues of $PGF_{2\alpha}$ and dopamine agonists for termination of pregnancy in dogs. Vet Rec 1990;144:416-19

Onclin K., Verstegen JP. Practical use of a combination of a dopamine agonist and a synthetic prostaglandin analogue to terminate unwanted pregnancy in dogs. Journal of Small Animal Practice, 1996; 37:211-216.

Purswell BJ., Wilcke JR. Response to gonadotrophin-releasing hormone by the intact male dog: serum testosterone, luteinizing hormone and follicle-stimulating hormone. J Reprod Fertil Suppl 1993;47:335-341.

Reichler IM, Barth A, Piché CA, Jöchle W, Roos M, Hubler M, Arnold S. Urodynamic parameters and plasma LH/FSH in spayed Beagle bitches before and 8 weeks after GnRH depot analogue treatment. Theriogenology 2006;66:2127-2136.

Root Kustritz MV and Olson PN. Early Spy and Neuter. In: Textbook of Veterinary Internal Medicine, 5th edn. Eds. SJ. Ettinger and EC. Feldman. Saunders 2000; XIII:1539-1541

Schaefers-Okkens AC. Estrous Cycle and Breeding Management of the Healthy Bitch. In: Textbook of Veterinary Internal Medicine, 5th edn. Eds. SJ. Ettinger and EC. Feldman. Saunders 2000; XIII:1510-1519

Sutton DJ., Geary MR., Bergman JGHE. The prevention of pregnancy in bitches following unwanted mating: a clinical trial using low dose oestradiol benzoate. J Reprod Fert Suppl 1997;51: 239

Tsutsui T, Kirihara N, Hori T, Concannon PW. Plasma progesterone and prolactin concentrations in overtly pseudopregnant bitches: a clinical study. Theriogenology 2007;67(5):1032-1038.

Trigg TE., Doyle AG., Walsh JD., Swangchan-Uthai T. A review of advances in the use of the GnRH agonist deslorelin in control of reproduction. Theriogenology 2006;66:1507-1512.

Vanderlip SL., Wing AE., Felt P., Linkie D., Rivier J., Concannon PW., Lasley BL. Ovulation induction in anoestrus bitches by pulsatile administration of gonadotrophin-releasing hormone. Lab Anim Sci 1987;37:459-64

Van Haaften B., Dieleman SJ., Okkens A.C, Wirllemse AH. Timing the mating of dogs on the basis of blood progesterone concentration. Vet Rec 1989;125:524-26.

Van Os JL. Oestrus control in the bitch with proligestone. A clinical study [Thesis]. Utrecht University: 1982.

Van Os JL., Evans JM. False pregnancy and proligestone. Vet Rec 1980;106:36.

Van Os JL., van Laar PH., Oldenkamp EP., Verschoor JSC. Oestrus control and the incidence of mammary nodules in bitches, a clinical study with two progestagens. Vet Quar 1981;3:46-56.

Vannucchi CI., Mirandola RM., Oliveira CM. Acute-phase protein profile during gestation and diestrous: proposal for an early pregnancy test in bitches. Anim Reprod Sci 2002;74:87-99.

Veronesi MC., Battocchio M., Marinelli L., Faustini M., Kindahl H., Cairoli F. Correlations among body temperature, plasma progesterone, cortisol and prostaglandin $F_{2\alpha}$ of the periparturient bitch. J Vet Med A 2002;49:264-268.

Vestergen J. Contraception and Pregnancy termination. In: Textbook of Veterinary Internal Medicine, 5th edn. Eds. SJ. Ettinger and EC. Feldman. Saunders 2000; XIII:1542-1548

Verstegen J., Onclin K., Silva L., Concannon PW. Early termination of anestrus and induction of fertile estrus in dogs by the dopamine superagonist cabergoline. Biol Reprod 1994; Suppl 1:157

Verstegen JP., Onclin K., Silva LDM., Concannon PW. Effect of stage of anestrus on the induction of estrus by the dopamine agonist cabergoline in dogs. Theriogenology 1999;51:597-611

von Heimendahl A., Cariou M. Normal parturition and management of dystocia in dogs and cats. In Practice 2009;31:254-261.

Wanke M., Loza ME., Monachesi N., Concannon P. Clinical use of dexamethasone for termination of unwanted pregnancy in dogs. J Reprod Fertil Suppl 1997;51:233-238.

Wichtel JJ., Whitacre MD., Yates DJ and Van Camp SD. Comparison of the effects of $PGF_{2\alpha}$ and bromocriptine in pregnant beagle bitches. Theriogenology 1990;33:829-836

Weilenmann R., Arnold S., Dobeli M., Rusch P., Zerobin K. Estrus induction in bitches by the administration of PMSG and HCG. Schweiz Arch Tierheilkd 1993;135: 236-241

Zoldag L., Fekete S., Csaky I., Bersenyi A. Fertile estrus induced in bitches by bromocrytpine, a dopamine agonist: a clinical trial. Theriogenology 2001;55:1657–66.

8 Feline Reproduction

8.1 Physiology

8.1.1 The oestrous cycle

Female domestic cats usually reach puberty by 6-9 months of age or 2.3 to 2.5 kg bodyweight (Verstegen 2000). Sexual activity of free-ranging cats is photoperiod-dependent, thus the onset of puberty can be influenced by the time of year the queen is born (Goodrowe et al., 1989).

The queen is seasonally polyoestrous with prolonged anoestrus resulting from decreasing or short day length (Johnston et al., 1996). The onset and duration of ovarian activity is also linked closely to day length. In the northern hemisphere, queens cycle between January and September with peaks of sexual activity in February, May and June, and occasionally in September.

In terms of behaviour, the oestrous cycle of the queen can be divided into the heat and non-heat periods (Verstegen 2000). Heat periods are observed every 4-30 days (mode 14-19 days) throughout the breeding season (Lawler et al., 1993; Root et al., 1995; Verstegen 2000). The duration of, and signs evident in, each phase are indicated in Table 1.
The average duration of the oestrous cycle is around 6 days (range 2-19 days) (Root et al., 1995). The heat period can be divided into pro-oestrus and oestrus. Pro-oestrus (1 to 4 days) is followed by oestrus (3-10 days). This is followed by a short period of sexual inactivity (interoestrus) when plasma oestrogen concentrations usually decline to basal values. In the absence of mating or spontaneous ovulation (Gudermuth et al., 1997), this cycle of events is repeated until the end of the breeding season. The last interoestrus of the breeding season is followed by a longer non-breeding season (anoestrus), which lasts until the first pro-oestrus of the next period of sexual activity. This usually occurs when natural day length is short (September to late January in the Northern hemisphere) and can be absent in cats submitted to artificial constant day length (e.g. indoors).

Pseudopregnancy, lasting about 36 days (range 25-45 days), can occur following any non-fertile mating or if ovulation is stimulated artificially. Pseudopregnancy in the cat is not usually associated with behavioural changes or lactation (Christiansen 1984). The subsequent oestrus is delayed by 45 days on average (range 35-70 days), i.e. about half the normal duration of a feline pregnancy. The delay will be longer if anoestrus follows pseudopregnancy.

Table 1 The phases of the oestrous cycle in the cat

Stage of cycle	Duration	Comments
Proestrus	1-4 days	The period when males are attracted to non-receptive females. Proestrus is characterized by behavioural changes, such as rubbing the head and neck against convenient objects, constant vocalising, posturing and rolling. This stage often goes unnoticed. Affectionate behaviour may be the only obvious sign.
Oestrus	3-10 days	The stage when the queen will accept a male. In the presence of a male oestrus lasts 4 days (range 3-6 days), but it is extended to up to 10 days if the queen is not mated. Ovulation occurs 27 hours (range 24-30 hours) after mating. The signs of oestrus are similar to those described under proestus but are much more exaggerated. Oestrous queens may urinate more frequently, be more restless and show an increased desire to roam. Some queens become more affectionate towards their owners whereas others become aggressive.
Interoestrus	6-16 days	Characterized by sexual inactivity
Anoestrus	3-4 months	Prolonged sexual inactivity

Hormonal changes

Behavioural oestrus occurs during peak follicular growth. Pro-oestrus is associated with an abrupt rise in circulating oestrogen (oestradiol-17β) concentrations, heralding the onset of the follicular phase. During this phase, oestrogen concentrations rise rapidly from basal concentrations (15-20 pg/ml) to more than 40-80 pg/ml, remain elevated for 3-4 days and then decline over the next 2-3 days to basal levels.

Coital stimulation of the vagina is followed immediately by an increase in neural activity in the hypothalamus, which is followed by the release of luteinizing hormone (LH). The LH response varies considerably between individuals and does not correlate with plasma concentrations of oestradiol or progesterone (Johnson and Gay 1981). Multiple matings may be required to stimulate the release of gonadotrophin-releasing hormone (GnRH), which is thought to cause the LH surge that initiates ovulation (Concannon et al., 1980). The coitus-to-ovulation interval is not a reliable indicator of the time of ovulation in the cat since neither LH response nor ovulation are ensured by single or multiple copulations (Wildt et al., 1981).

Ovulation is followed by the formation of a corpus luteum or corpora lutea. Progesterone concentrations rise 2-3 days after a successful mating and peak at around 30-60 ng/ml around day 20-25 after mating. Thereafter concentrations decrease and then remain stable around 15-30 ng/ml until just before parturition (around day 60 when they decrease to below 1-1.5 ng/ml) (Figure 1) (Verstegen et al., 1993). The corpora lutea of pregnancy are functional throughout gestation (Goodrowe et al., 1989; Schmidt et al., 1983; Verhage et al., 1976).

In the pseudopregnant cat, progesterone concentrations mimic those seen in pregnant animals and peak at around day 20-25 but return to basal values around days 30-40 (Figure 1). The decline in progesterone in these animals is slow and progressive, probably due to the lack of a luteolytic factor (Verstegen 2000).

Figure 1 Average concentrations of progesterone and oestradiol in pregnant and pseudopregnant queens (after Verhage et al., 1976)

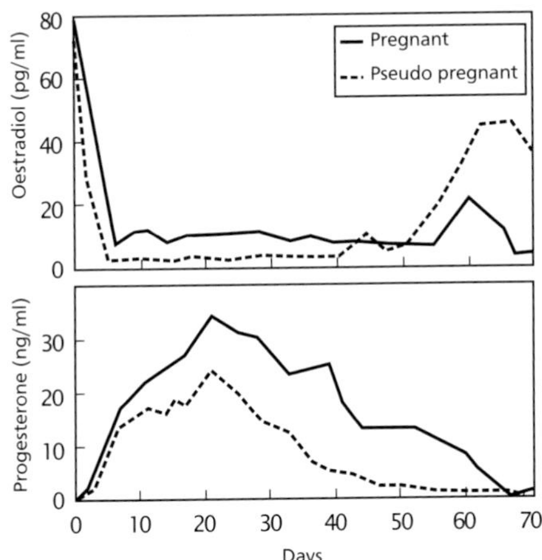

Relaxin is a pregnancy specific hormone. It is secreted mainly by the placenta. Relaxin concentrations are basal during oestrus and pseudopregnancy but rise from day 25-30 after mating. This is coincident with, or slightly before, the increase in prolactin. Prolactin appears to play a major luteotrophic role: its suppression, by the administration of a dopamine agonist such as cabergoline, results in a rapid fall in progesterone concentrations and abortion. Prolactin concentrations are basal during oestrus and increase around day 30-35 of gestation, reaching a maximum a few days before parturition. Prolactin plays a major role in mammary gland secretion and the maintenance of lactation. Thus prolactin concentrations remain high during lactation but decline during the last 2 weeks of milk production.

During anoestrus, plasma oestrogen and progesterone concentrations remain at basal levels and gonadotrophin concentrations undergo only minor fluctuations.

8.1.2 Hormonal changes in tom cats

Tom cats reach sexual maturity at 9 months of age (range 7-12 months) (Christiansen 1984). Spermatogenesis is seen around 20 weeks and the first spermatazoa appear in the spermatic cord at 30-36 weeks of age (Verstegen 2000).

The release of LH is controlled by feedback effects of testosterone on the anterior pituitary. There is considerable variation between individuals in LH and testosterone concentrations (Goodrowe et al., 1989). Basal levels of LH in adult tom cats are similar to those seen in anoestrus queens. Basal concentrations of testosterone are high (around 4-8 ng/ml) in both intact and castrated male (and female) cats (Verstegen 2000). Administration of an exogenous GnRH agonist or human chorionic gonadotrophin (hCG) causes the release of LH and a consequent rise in circulating testosterone concentrations (Verstegen 2000). Maximal testosterone concentrations of 12-16 ng/ml are reached 20-24 hours after administration.

8.2 Mating

During oestrus the queen will, as in pro-oestrus, rub its neck against various objects and people's legs. Typically, queens crouch, hold their tails to one side and show frequent rolling and treading when 'calling'. Vocalization, often involving the production of a low moaning sound, occurs more frequently than in pro-oestrus. Such signs often go unrecognized in normally affectionate cats, but may be interpreted by cat owners as a sign of illness or pain (Christiansen 1984; Feldman and Nelson 2004; Verstegen 2000).

During mating the tom cat bites the neck of the queen firmly and mounts, grasping the queen's chest with its forelegs. Usually at this stage, both cats tread actively and the queen adopts a posture, which makes the vulva more accessible. The penis of the tom cat normally points posteriorly but as it becomes erect it is directed forwards. Intromission is followed rapidly by ejaculation. This whole sequence of events can occur in as little as 30 seconds and rarely lasts for more than 5 minutes.

As the tom cat withdraws, the queen typically gives a loud, piercing 'copulatory call' and the tom cat retires to a safe distance.
Mating is usually repeated 6-7 times at varying, but often quite frequent, intervals until the queen no longer allows the tom cat to mount. Mating may be repeated over 2-4 days (Christiansen 1984; Feldman and Nelson 2004; Verstegen 2000).

8.3 Pregnancy

Fertilization in the queen is presumed to occur in the oviducts and the blastocysts migrate into the uterus 4-5 days post mating. Implantation is thought to occur at around 15 days post-mating. The duration of pregnancy is 63 days (range 61-69 days) under controlled conditions, but can range from 56-72 days (Feldman and Nelson 2004; Verstegen 2000). Variation in the coitus-to-parturition interval is probably best explained by the fact that coitus does not always produce an ovulatory surge and ovulation, rather than by breed differences.
Pregnancy is most commonly confirmed by abdominal palpation: a series of discrete, firm, spherical uterine enlargements can be readily felt by 17-25 days of gestation (Feldman and Nelson 2004, Verstegen 2000). Ultrasound can be used to detect pregnancy as early as days 11-15 and foetal heartbeats can be seen from days 22-24. Foetal skeletons can be visualized radiographically from days 38-43 onwards. Radiography after day 45 is least likely to yield inconclusive results.

8.4 Parturition

8.4.1 Normal parturition

Parturition in queens can be split into three stages (von Heimendahl and Cariou 2009).
The first stage of labour, which usually lasts for about 24 hours, is characterized by restlessness, vocalization and nesting behaviour. Some normally affectionate queens may show signs of aggression as the time of parturition approaches.
Once second stage labour commences, the kittens are usually produced quite quickly with relatively little abdominal straining.

The birth of the first kitten usually takes 30-60 minutes and the interval between the delivery of subsequent kittens varies from 5-60 minutes.
Third stage labour, the expulsion of the placenta, usually occurs after each kitten is delivered. Most queens will sever the umbilical cords, eat the placenta and clean the kittens, without requiring any assistance.

There are a few key differences between parturition in the dog and cat (Feldman and Nelson 2004; Verstegen 2000):
- The placenta is red-brown in the cat (it is dark green in dogs)
- Kittening can be as short as 1 hour but can also last 1-2 days
- Delayed parturition may occur in a stressful environment
- Second stage labour may be divided, with the queen resting for as long as 12-24 hours between the production of two batches of kittens (Christiansen 1984).

The breed and condition of the queen and the number of litters produced affect litter size. Litter size increases up to the fourth parturition and then declines. The number of kittens born alive per litter is 4 (range 1-8) (Christiansen 1984; Root et al., 1995). Mortality by 8 weeks of age is around 30% (range 15-45%; Root et al., 1995).
Pro-oestrus may follow soon after parturition or may be preceded by a period of anoestrus. On average, queens will call 4-8 weeks (range 1-21 weeks) after having a litter. The interval is dependent on the age at which kittens are weaned and, in cats with a non-breeding season, upon the time of the year when kittens are born.

8.4.2 Dystocia

Dystocia is rare in queens. This can result from maternal factors, such as a congenitally narrow pelvis, poorly healed pelvic fractures, uterine torsion or uterine inertia, which may be linked with obesity, or foetal factors, such as relative foetal oversize and malpresentation. Some breeds, notably Siamese and Persians, have been reported to have a higher prevalence of dystocia (von Heimendahl and Cariou 2009). Remedial action should be considered if unproductive straining occurs for more

than an hour or if a large quantity of blood-stained vaginal discharge is seen (Feldman and Nelson 2004). If a kitten is present in the vagina, manual removal may be possible, but this must been done carefully.
If uterine inertia is suspected in queens with small litters, oxytocin (e.g. Oxytocin-S®, Intertocin-S®), at a dose rate of 2-4 IU/ queen by intravenous or intramuscular injection, may help (Feldman and Nelson 2004). If this has no effect, treatment can be repeated 20 minutes later after administering 1-2 ml 10% calcium gluconate, which can be followed after 20 minutes by 2 ml 50% dextrose intravenously and a further oxytocin treatment (Feldman and Nelson 2004). If there is still no effect then Caesarean section should be performed.

8.5 Mismating and prevention of implantation

Veterinary surgeons in practice are not commonly asked to treat mismating or terminate an unwanted pregnancy in cats, since pregnancy often goes unsuspected. A number of options are available after attempting to determine whether mating actually occurred. These methods, with the exception of a single oral dose (2 mg) of the progestagen, megestrol acetate during oestrus (Feldman and Nelson 2004), are usually carried out after pregnancy has been confirmed. Surgical removal of the uterus after confirmation of pregnancy is possible but is obviously not suitable for queens intended for breeding.

Dopamine agonists and/or prostaglandins
The dopamine agonist cabergoline, may be administered on food at a dose rate of 0.005-0.015 mg/kg once daily, from day 36 until pregnancy termination (usually a few days) (Jöchle and Jöchle 1993). Cabergoline alone may not be effective when treatment is started later in gestation (after day 45) (Erünal-Maral et al., 2004) with 9 days or more treatment being required, and resulting in premature parturition of live rather than dead kittens and insufficient lactation (Jöchle and Jöchle 1993). The efficacy can be increased by combining cabergoline (0.005 mg/kg orally once daily) with a synthetic prostaglandin $F_{2\alpha}$ ($PGF_{2\alpha}$) analogue, such as cloprostenol (0.005 mg/kg every 2 days by subcutaneous injection) (Onclin and Verstegen 1997).

Progesterone receptor antagonists

The progesterone receptor antagonist aglepristone administered subcutaneously, at a dose rate of 10 mg/kg, on days 25 and 26 after mating was effective in terminating pregnancy around 5 days (range 4-7 days) after the start of treatment in 87% of the cats (n=23) tested (Georgiev and Wehrend 2006). In a second study in 61 queens in mid-pregnancy, the efficacy of two injections of aglepristone (15 mg/kg) 24 hours apart was 88.5% (Fieni et al., 2006). Irritation at the injection site immediately after injection was observed infrequently and was the only side-effect reported (Georgiev and Wehrend 2006).

8.6 Control of reproduction

Although surgical methods (neutering: ovariohysterectomy (spaying) and castration) are widely used to control reproduction in cats, this approach is obviously not suitable for breeding animals. In addition, pet owners may be reluctant to consider surgery (Kutzler and Wood 2006).

8.6.1 Surgical methods

Ovariohysterectomy (spaying), complete removal of the ovaries with the uterus is the method of choice for queens not intended for breeding. Castration, complete removal of both testes is the method of choice for tom cats not intended for breeding. The surgical procedures are relatively inexpensive and generally very safe and free from side-effects, especially when performed around puberty.

Neutering prior to puberty, also known as prepubertal gonadectomy, has increased in popularity in a some countries, particularly the United States. It does not appear to stunt growth but may alter the metabolic rate in cats (Olson et al., 2001; Root Kustritz and Olson 2000). To date, adverse side-effects are apparently no greater in animals neutered early (7 weeks) than in those neutered at the conventional age (>4 months old, around puberty) (Olson et al., 2001; Root Kustritz and Olson 2000).

8.6.2 Non-surgical methods

Non-surgical control of reproduction in queens is possible by inducing ovulation or by suppressing or postponing oestrus, using hormones. Currently there is no suitable alternative to the surgical neutering in male cats.

8.6.2.1 Induction of ovulation without copulation

Human chorionic gonadotrophin

There is a linear response between hCG dose and the ovulatory response in queens in the dose range 0-500 IU (Wildt and Seager 1978). Usually, a dose of 50-250 IU of hCG given by intravenous or intramuscular injection will induce ovulation and also delay subsequent calling (Verstegen 2000). This is a safe and relatively efficient means of terminating calling in queens with seasonal oestrus. Using this regime, the behavioural signs of heat cease within 1-2 days of the injection and the next period of calling does not take place until the subsequent season starts.

In queens with less marked seasonality, the results are not as long-lasting. However once calling has been temporarily interrupted, the queen can be spayed or progestagen therapy can be initiated.

Vaginal stimulation

Mechanical vaginal stimulation using a glass rod or similar object, introduced at least 4-8 times at 5-20 minute intervals for 2.5 seconds per time has been suggested (Feldman and Nelson 2004). This action will not shorten the oestrus period but, if successful, will delay the onset of the next oestrus.

8.6.2.2 Postponement or suppression of oestrus using progestagens

Progestagens are synthetic exogenous steroid hormones that have been used widely for many years in queens, however much of the data available is based on extrapolation from their use in bitches (Kutzler and Wood 2006).

Proligestone (Covinan®, Delvosteron®) is a unique (second generation) progestagen that has weaker progestational activity than other synthetic progestagens. In queens, proligestone acts principally as an antigonadotrophin.

There are three ways in which progestagen treatment can be used to control oestrus in queens which should ideally be given during anoestrus (Feldman and Nelson 2004) to minimize the risk of inducing untoward side-effects.

- *Permanent postponement:* Doses repeated at regular intervals during the lifetime of the cat starting either in anoestrus or interoestrus
- *Temporary postponement:* A single dose given during anoestrus or interoestrus to postpone the subsequent oestrus
- *Suppression:* A single dose given as soon as signs of calling are seen. Progestagens suppress the call and may prevent conception during that call should mating occur.

Administration of any progestagen, particularly for a prolonged period, can result in cystic endometrial hyperplasia (CEH), pyometra or mammary hyperplasia and/or neoplasia, diabetes mellitus and other side-effects, such as depression and increased appetite (Feldman and Nelson 2004; Kutzler and Wood 2006).

Postponement of oestrus

The first generation progestagens, e.g. depot injections of medroxyprogesterone acetate (MPA) or by tablets containing MPA or megestrol acetate (MA), can be used to postpone calling. Depot injections, usually given at 6 monthly intervals, have the advantage of convenience but the occurrence of the next call is unpredictable as their duration of action can vary widely from queen to queen. Tablets containing MPA or MA (e.g. 5 mg per cat) can be given orally either daily or once weekly to postpone calling (Kutzler and Wood 2006).

The second generation progestagen, proligestone, can be used for the permanent postponement of oestrus in cats using a dosage regime similar to that advised for bitches, namely injections (1 ml per cat) at 3, 4 and 5 monthly intervals. If the timing of the next dose and the breeding season are expected to coincide, it is advisable to shorten the time between injections to 4 months. In fact, it might be necessary to administer treatment every 4 months to avoid any breakthrough during the period when there is an intense seasonal influence, particularly in queens that exhibit strictly seasonal reproductive activity. Similarly, queens housed together with other intact female cats might require a tighter treatment regime. An increase in dose rate is inadvisable.

Suppression of oestrus

Orally administered (first generation) progestagens are suitable for the prevention of oestrus once signs of calling have been observed. This is achieved by giving a fairly high dose of an orally active progestagen for a short time (1-3 days), beginning as soon as the signs of calling are seen. Often the queen will have stopped showing signs of sexual behaviour after only one dose, but the signs may persist for longer.

Oestrus postponement, rather than oestrus suppression, is often the method of choice for a planned breeding. Following an injection of proligestone (1 ml per cat) at the onset of calling, the signs of oestrus will usually abate within 1-4 days, but may persist for as long as 7 days. Queens may conceive during the few days after proligestone has been administered for the suppression of calling, even although the signs of oestrus may have already disappeared. Contact with males should therefore be prevented for the first five days following injection at this stage of the oestrous cycle.

Return to oestrus

The recurrence of calling after treatment is very variable. It is not possible to say precisely when a cat will call again following postponement of oestrus with progestagens.

Following the oral administration of an MA or MPA to postpone oestrus, queens may call soon after dosing ceases, but a delay of 2-3 months is more usual. Generally cats call sooner after the suppression than after the postponement of oestrus; 4 weeks after treatment ceases is usual. This means that there is only a slight extension of the normal interval between cycles.

For injectable preparations, it is even more difficult to predict when a queen will return to oestrus. Following treatment with proligestone, the majority of queens will call 6-7 months after administration. It is important to remember that following suppression or postponement of oestrus the subsequent onset of calling will depend on the time of year. If the queen is treated at the end of the breeding season, the next period of calling may not occur until the beginning of the next breeding cycle, so calling could be delayed by as much as six months.

Safety

First generation progestagens are associated with quite a high incidence of side-effects (Kutzler and Wood 2006), such as CEH, pyometra or mammary hyperplasia and/or neoplasia, diabetes mellitus and others such as depression and increased appetite. The second generation progestagen proligestone did not promote the development of uterine disease or mammary neoplasia during extensive clinical trials in dogs (Van Os et al., 1981). Progestagens are contraindicated in cats with genital tract infection.

8.6.3 Alternatives for the control of reproduction in cats

A number of alternatives for non-surgical control of reproduction in cats have been examined. Some of them approaches have been reviewed recently (Kutzler and Wood 2006) and a few of these are summarized below. The search for a suitable non-surgical alternative for controlling cat populations continues.

Chemical vasectomy

Intra-epididymal injection of 4.5% chlorhexidine digluconate has been tested in cats (Poineda and Doohey 1984). Although this successfully neutered the cats, administration was associated with pain and swelling for up to 2 weeks post-injection and with intra-epididymal granuloma formation. This approach has not found widespread acceptance.

GnRH agonists

Sustained exposure to GnRH reduces the GnRH-stimulated secretion of gonadotrophins through the down-regulation and internalization of GnRH receptors and signal uncoupling. This can be used to produce reversible contraception (Kutzler and Wood 2006).

Immunocontraception

A number of components of the reproductive system (including LH and its receptors, oocyte zona pellucida and GnRH) have been identified as suitable targets for an immunocontraceptive vaccine. Immunocontraception appears to offer some promise for the control of reproduction in cats, and further developments are expected in this field. A summary of some of the immunological targets and their use in cats is presented below.

Oocyte zona pellucida vaccines have been used successfully in many species but to date have proved problematic in queens (Kutzler and Wood 2006; Levy et al., 2005). Vaccination of queens with an LH-receptor vaccine has been shown to suppress oestrus for more than 11 months in queens via suppression of corpus luteum function (Saxena et al., 2003).

Development of GnRH vaccines has been problematic, primarily due to the poor immunogenicity of GnRH. In male cats, a single injection of synthetic GnRH coupled to keyhole limpet haemocyanin and combined with a mycobacterial adjuvant to enhance immunogenicity, was effective (basal testosterone concentrations and testicular atrophy) for between 3 and 6 months in two-thirds of the nine cats tested (Levy et al., 2004). A recombinant GnRH antigen has been shown to produce biologically relevant anti-GnRH antibody titres for 20 months in cats following administration on two occasions to 8- and 12-week old cats (Robbins et al., 2004). Booster vaccination after 20 months resulted in a significant anamnestic response.

8.7 Disorders of the reproductive tract

8.7.1 Queens

8.7.1.1 Cystic endometrial hyperplasia-pyometra complex

This condition is less common in cats than in dogs (Verstegen 2000). It is more usually seen in queens aged 5 years or older (Potter et al., 1991) presumably due to the elevated progesterone concentrations that occur during pseudopregnancy in non-pregnant cats (Christiansen 1984; Verstegen 2000). CEH-pyometra complex may also be brought about iatrogenically by the administration of exogenous hormones, particularly the first generation progestagens.

Queens with CEH-pyometra complex do not always show clinical signs; these can be an incidental finding during routine ovariohysterectomy in queens (Potter et al., 1991). If clinical signs are present, they are less prominent than in dogs (Kenney et al., 1987) and usually include vaginal discharge, abdominal distention, dehydration, a palpable uterus, and pyrexia (Kenney et al., 1987).

Surgical treatment
Surgery (ovariohysterectomy) is the treatment of choice, particularly in severe cases.

Medical treatment
Medical treatment (e.g. using natural prostaglandins (dinoprost) or progesterone-receptor antagonists) can be attempted (Davidson et al., 1992) but is rarely the treatment of choice. Side-effects of prostaglandin treatment have been seen (Christiansen 1984; Feldman and Nelson 2004) and repeated low doses of $PGF_{2\alpha}$ are reportedly better tolerated (Verstegen 2000). A small, preliminary study on the progesterone-receptor antagonist aglepristone (two doses at 10 mg/kg, 24 hours apart) suggests that this agent is both effective and free from side-effects in cats (Hecker et al., 2000).

8.7.1.2 Failure to cycle

Apparently prolonged anoestrus may result from poor oestrus detection and poor management, or be secondary to progestagen administration (Verstegen 2000). Queens with strictly seasonal reproductive behaviour might give a poorer response when oestrus induction is attempted during anoestrus. The closer the time of treatment to the beginning of the reproductive season, the better the results. Stress, poor nutrition, systemic disease, temperature extremes, inadequate lighting (lack of exposure to daylight), iatrogenic (progestagen or glucocorticoid administration) or cystic follicles all cause oestrus failure in queens. Silent oestrus may result from overcrowding, especially in the case of very subordinate queens (Feldman and Nelson 2004).

Treatment

The treatment chosen will depend on the underlying cause. It is important to eliminate functional, anatomical and infectious causes before instigating treatment with exogenous hormones. Adjusting the lighting pattern (exposure to 14 hours daylight/day or 12 hours/day after a period of shorter day length), and/or housing with other cycling queens may be successful (Christiansen 1984).

Stimulation of ovarian activity by oestrus induction using 150 IU of pregnant mare serum gonadotrophin/equine chorionic gonadotrophin (PMSG/eCG) followed 3-4 days later by 100 IU hCG, both by intramuscular injection, may be successful (Donoghue et al., 1993; Swanson et al., 1997). Higher doses of PMSG can cause ovarian hyperstimulation and the development of cystic follicles and abnormal endocrine profiles (Wildt et al., 1978; Cline et al., 1980).

8.7.1.3 Ovarian remnant syndrome

This condition is defined as the presence of functional ovarian tissue despite previous ovariohysterectomy (spaying). In most cases, it is clear that the surgery has been incomplete. Ovarian remnant syndrome manifests as oestrous behaviour of variable intensity with or without a seasonal pattern. In affected queens, the onset of oestrus behaviour may be days to years after spaying (Johnston et al., 1996).

Exploratory laparotomy can be performed when the cat is in behavioural oestrus, however this is associated with an increased risk of bleeding. It is more advantageous to perform the surgery 2-3 weeks later and especially after induction of ovulation with hCG (250 IU/queen) or a GnRH agonist (0.025 mg/queen) (Johnston et al., 1996). The increased risk of bleeding is then removed by the onset of pseudopregnancy and the corpora lutea formed make the search for the ovarian remnant far easier. A recent study showed that administration of the a GnRH agonist buserelin resulted in an increase in oestradiol (based on blood samples for oestradiol taken before and two hours after treatment) that could help the reliable diagnosis of the presence of ovarian tissue in queens (Axnér et al., 2008).

8.7.1.4 Mammary hypertrophy

Mammary hypertrophy (also known as fibroadenomatosis or fibroadenomatous hyperplasia) is a non-neoplastic hyperplasia of the mammary glands. Falling progesterone (endogenous or exogenous) concentrations are thought to stimulate prolactin production, which in turn stimulates the growth of mammary tissue (Feldman and Nelson 2004). The condition is progesterone-dependent and develops in post-ovulatory (including pregnant) and progestagen-treated queens, and occasionally also in male cats.

Fibroadenomatosis is characterized by a rapid proliferation of mammary stroma and duct epithelium of one or more glands and predominantly affects younger female cats. The clinical picture is generally variable and ranges from mild enlargement to extremely pronounced hyperplasia of all of the mammary glands (Feldman and Nelson 2004). The clinical signs usually include skin ulceration, painful mammary glands, lethargy, anorexia and tachycardia (Görlinger et al., 2002).

Since this condition is progesterone-dependent, progestagens should not be administered to queens with a history of mammary gland enlargement or to queens prior to their first oestrus. Queens with a history of mammary gland enlargement should ideally be spayed since endogenous progesterone can also produce this condition.

Treatment

Treatment options include the withdrawal of progestagen treatment, surgical removal of the ovaries (ovariectomy) or the administration of a progesterone receptor blocker or a dopamine agonist (Görlinger et al., 2002).

If the condition is severe, radical surgery or euthanasia may be necessary. For more moderate cases, spaying may be effective, but the condition will usually resolve spontaneously with regression of corpora lutea or withdrawal/elimination of the progestagen.

Subcutaneous administration of the progesterone-receptor blocker aglepristone on one day (20 mg/kg), or two consecutive days (10 mg/kg/day) every week for 1-4 weeks has been reported to be effective (Görlinger et al., 2002). The dopamine agonist bromocriptine (0.25 mg once daily for 5-7 days, orally) has also been reported to be effective, but is associated with marked side-effects (Feldman and Nelson 2004).

8.7.2 Tom cats

8.7.2.1 Spraying (Inappropriate sexual behaviour)

It has been reported that 10% of all cats spray in adulthood (Dehasse 1997). Veterinarians need to distinguish carefully between inappropriate urination and urine spraying. Tom cats spray urine as a chemical means of communication and to mark their territory. This activity, which may be undertaken by both entire and castrated males (and can also be seen in female cats), should be differentiated from normal micturition and abnormal urination associated with feline lower urinary tract disease (FLUTD).

Behavioural training
Once a correct diagnosis has been reached, the key to successful treatment is the introduction of environmental and behavioural changes. Behavioural training aims to reduce stress and decrease territorial behaviour and marking, and foster a positive relationship with the cat.

Additional treatment
Castration of entire males usually causes spraying to diminish or stop, and will, at the same time, make the urine less pungent. However, this is not universally effective: efficacy rates have been reported to be around 78% (Hart and Barrett 1973).
The administration of progestagens is sometimes effective in both entire and neutered cats (Christiansen 1984). Medication can be given continuously or intermittently. The mode of action is thought to be through negative feedback on the hypothalamus and by a calming effect via the cerebral cortex. Progestational compounds are associated with a wide range of side-effects, including mammary hyperplasia and/or neoplasia, diabetes mellitus and others such as depression and increased

appetite, in both male and female, intact and neutered cats. Depression and increased appetite have been reported to occur more commonly following MA treatment (Hart 1980) and this agent should probably be avoided for behavioural indications.

A number of sedative or psychoactive drugs have also been reported to be of help. The benzodiazepine diazepam has been used successfully in the short term but is not effective over the long term, with more than 90% treated cats resuming spraying or marking when treatment was gradually discontinued (Cooper and Hart 1992). The non-benzodiazepine anti-anxiety drug buspirone has been reported to be more effective than diazepam; 50% of cats resumed spraying after treatment ceased at the end of 2 months (Hart et al., 1993). Long term treatment with buspirone has been reported to be safe in cats (Hart et al., 1993). The tricyclic anti-depressant clomipramine (0.25-0.5 mg/kg twice daily) has been reported to be effective in more than 75% of cases (Dehasse 1997).

Pheromone treatment has been reported to be effective in a similar percentage of cases when delivered by spray (Frank et al., 1999) or diffuser (Mills and Mills 2001). The selective serotonin re-uptake inhibitor fluoxetine hydrochloride has also been reported to be an effective treatment but was associated with a reduction in food intake in almost half of the cats treated (Pryor et al., 2001).

8.7.2.2 Cryptorchidism or testicular remnants

In tom cats the testicles have usually descended and are present in the scrotum at birth (Feldman and Nelson 2004, Verstegen 2000) and can be readily palpated at 6-8 weeks of age. Unilateral or bilateral cryptorchidism occurs but it is relatively rare in tom cats. The retained testicle(s) may be situated intra-abdominally or in the inguinal canal. The condition is considered to be hereditary and for that reason, and because there is some risk that retained testicles will become neoplastic, surgical removal is the treatment of choice.

GnRH or hCG stimulation test

A GnRH of hCG stimulation test can be performed to check for functional testicular tissue. A significant positive increase in testosterone 60 minutes after intravenous injection of 0.001-0.002 mg/kg of a GnRH agonist or 50-100 IU hCG per cat is diagnostic for the presence of testicular tissue (Verstegen 2000). The absence of hormone-dependent keratinised spines on the penis, a test which is quick and easy to perform, is also suggestive of prior castration (Verstegen 2000).

8.8 References

Axnér E., Gustavsson T., Ström Holst B. Estradiol measurement after GnRH-stimulation as a method to diagnose the presence of ovaries in the female domestic cat. Theriogenology 2008;70:186-191.

Christiansen IBJ. In Reproduction in the dog and cat. London: Bailliere Tindall 1984

Cline EM., Jennings LL., Sojka NL. Breeding laboratory cats during artificially induced estrus. Lab Anim Sci 1980; 30(6): 1003-1005

Concannon P., Hodgson B., Lein D. Reflex LH release in estrous cats following single and multiple copulations. Biology Repro 1980;23:111-117.

Davidson AP., Feldman EC., Nelson RW. Treatment of pyometra in cats, using prostaglandin $F(_{2\alpha})$: 21 cases (1982-1990). J Am Vet Med Assoc 1992;200:825-828.

Dehasse J. Feline urine spraying. Appl Anim Behav Sci 1997;52:365-371.

Donoghue AM., Johnston LA., Goodrowe KL., O'Brien SJ., Wildt DE. Influence of day of oestrus on egg viability and comparative efficiency of in vitro fertilization in domestic cats in natural or gonadotrophin-induced oestrus. J Reprod Fertil 1993;98:58-90.

Erünal-Maral N., Aslan S., Findik M., Yüksel N., Handler J., Arbeiter K. Induction of abortion in queens by administration of cabergoline (Galastop™) solely or in combination with the $PGF_{2\alpha}$ analogue Alfaprostol (Gabbrostim™). Theriogenology 2004;61:1471-1475.

Feldman EC., Nelson RW. Feline reproduction. In Canine and Feline Endocrinology and Reproduction. Philadelphia: WB Saunders, 2004:3rd edn:pp. 1016-1043.

Fieni F., Martal J., Marnet PG., Siliart B., Guittot F. Clinical, biological and hormonal study of mid-pregnancy termination in cats with aglepristone. Theriogenology 2006;66:1721-1728.

Frank DF., Erb HN., Houpt KA. Urine spraying in cats: Presence of concurrent disease and effects of a pheromone treatment. Appl Anim Behav Sci 1999;61:263-272.

Georgiev P., Wehrend A. Mid-gestation pregnancy termination by the progesterone antagonist aglepristone in queens. Theriogenology 2006;65: 1401-1406.

Goodrowe KL., Howeard JG., Schmidt PM., Wildt DE. Reproductive biology of the domestic cat with special reference to endocrinology, sperm function and in vitro fertilisation. J Reprod Fert Suppl 1989;30:73-90.

Görlinger S., Kooistra HS., Van Den Broek A., Okkens AC. Treatment of fibroadenomatous hyperplasia in cats with aglepristone. J Vet Intern Med 2002;16:710-713.

Gudermuth DF., Newton L., Daels P., Concannon P. Incidence of spontaneous ovulation in young, group-housed cats based on serum and faecal concentrations of progesterone. J Reprod Fertil Suppl 1997;51:177-184.

Hart BL. Objectionable urine spraying and urine marking in cats: Evaluation of progestin treatment in gonadectomized males and females. J Am Vet Med Assoc 1980;177:529-533.

Hart BL., Barrett RE. Effects of castration on fighting, roaming, and urine spraying in adult male cats. J Am Vet Med Assoc 1973:163:290-292.

Hart BL., Eckstein RA., Powell KL., Dodman NH. Effectiveness of buspirone on urine spraying and inappropiate urination in cats. J Am Vet Med Assoc 1993;203:254-258.

Hecker BR., Wehrend A., Bostedt H. Treatment of pyometra in cats with the progesterone-antagonist aglepristone. Kleintierpraxis 2000;45:845-848.

Jöchle W., Jöchle M. Reproduction in a feral cat population and its control with a prolactin inhibitor, cabergoline. J Reprod Fertil Suppl 1993;47:419-424.

Johnson LM., Gay VL. Luteinizing hormone in the cat. II. Mating-induced secretion. Endocrinology 1981;109:247-252.

Johnston SD., Root MV., Olson PNS. Ovarian and testicular function in the domestic cat: clinical management of spontaneous reproductive disease. Anim Reprod Sci 1996;42:261-274.

Kenney KJ., Matthiesen DT., Brown NO., Bradley RL. Pyometra in cats: 183 cases (1979-1984). J Am Vet Med Assoc 1987;191:1130-1132

Kutzler M., Wood A. Non-surgical methods of contraception and sterilization. Theriogenology 2006;66:514-525

Lawler DF., Johnston SD., Hegstad RL., Keltner DG., Owens SF. Ovulation without cervical stimulation in domestic cats. J Reprod Fertil Suppl 1993;47:57-61

Levy JK., Miller LA., Cynda Crawford P., Ritchet JW., Ross MK., Fagerstone KA. GnRH immunocontraception of male cats Theriogenology 2004;62:1116-1130.

Levy JK., Mansour M., Crawford PC., Pohajdak B., Brown RG. Survey of zona pellucida antigens for immunocontraception of cats. Theriogenology 2005;63:1334-1341.

Leyva H., Madley T., Stabenfeldt GH. Effect of light manipulation on ovarian activity and melatonin and prolactin secretion in the domestic cat. J Reprod Fert Suppl 1989a;39:125-a33.

Leyva H., Madley T., Stabenfeldt GH. Effect of melatonin on photoperiod responses, ovarian secretions of oestrogen and coital responses in the domestic cat. J Reprod Fert Suppl 1989b;39:135-142.

Mills DS., Mills CB. Evaluation of a novel method for delivering a synthetic analogue of feline facial pheromone to control urine spraying by cats. Vet Rec 2001;149:197-199.

Onclin K., Verstegen J. Termination of pregnancy in cats using a combination of cabergoline, a new dopamine agonist, and a synthetic PGF2 alpha, cloprostenol. J Reprod Fertil Suppl 1997;51:259-263.

Olson PN., Kustritz MV., Johnston SD. Early-age neutering of dogs and cats in the United States (a review). J Reprod Fertil Suppl 2001;57:223-232.

Pineda MH., Dolley MP. Surgical and chemical vasectomy in the cat. Am J Vet Res 1984;45:291-300.

Potter K., Hancock DH., Gallina AM. Clinical and pathologic features of endometrial hyperplasia, pyometra, and endometritis in cats: 79 cases (1980-1985). J Am Vet Med Assoc 1991;198:1427-1431.

Pryor PA., Hart BL., Cliff KD., Bain MJ. Effects of a selective serotonin reuptake inhibitor on urine spraying behavior in cats. J Am Vet Med Assoc 2001;219;1557-1561

Robbins SC., Jelinski MD., Stotish RL. Assessment of the immunological and biological efficacy of two different doses of a recombinant GnRH vaccine in domestic male and female cats (Felis catus). J Reprod Immunol 2004;64:107-119.

Root Kustritz MV., Olson PN. Early spay and neuter. In SJ Ettinger, EC Feldman Eds Textbook of Veterinary Internal Medicine 5th edn. Saunders 2000; pp. 1539-1541.
Root MV., Johnston SD., Olson PN. Estrous length, pregnancy rate, gestation and parturition lengths, litter size, and juvenile mortality in the domestic cat. J Am Anim Hosp Assoc 1995; 31: 429-433.
Saxena BB., Clavio A., Sigh M., Rathnam P., Bukharovich EY., Reimers Jr TJ., Saxena A., Perkins S. Effect of immunization with bovine luteinizing hormone receptor on ovarian function in cats. Am J Vet Res 2003;64:292-298.
Schmidt PM., Chakrborty PK., Wildt DE. Ovarian activity, circulating hormones and sexual behaviour in the cat. II. Relationship during pregnancy, parturition, lactation and the post-partum oestrus. Biol Reprod 1983;28:657-671.
Swanson WF., Wolfe BA., Brown JL., Martin-Jimenez T., Riviere JE., Roth TL., Wildt DE. Pharmacokinetics and ovarian-stimulatory effects of equine and human chorionic gonadotropins administered singly and in combination in the domestic cat. Biology Reprod 1997;57:295-302.
Van Os JL., van Laar PH., Oldenkamp EP., Verschoor JSC. Oestrus control and the incidence of mammary nodules in bitches, a clinical study with two progestagens. Vet Q 1981;3:46-56.
Verhage HG., Beamer NB., Brenner RM. Plasma levels of oestradiol and progesterone in the cat during poly-oestrus, pregnancy and pseudo-pregnancy. Biol Reprod 1976;14:579-585.
Verstegen J. Feline Reproduction In SJ Ettinger, EC Feldman Eds Textbook of Veterinary Internal Medicine 5th edn. Saunders 2000; pp. 1585-1598.
Verstegen JP., Onclin K., Silva LD., Wouters-Ballman P., Delahaut P., Ectors F. Regulation of progesterone during pregnanct in the cat: studies on the roles of corpora lutea, placenta and prolactin secretion. J Reprod Fertil Suppl 1993;47:165-173.
von Heimendahl A., Cariou M. Normal parturition and management of dystocia in dogs and cats. In Practice 2009;31:254-261.
Wildt DE., Chan SYW., Seager SWK., Chakraborty PK. Ovarian activity, circulating hormones, and sexual behavior in the cat. I. Relationships during the coitus-induced luteal phase and the estrous period without mating. Biology Repro 1981;25:15-28.
Wildt DE., Kinney GM., Seager SWJ. Gonadotrophin-induced reproductive cyclicity in the domestic cat. Lab Anim Sci 1978;28:301-307.
Wildt DE., Seager SWJ. Ovarian response in the estrual cat receiving varying dosages of hCG. Hormone Res 1978;3:144-150.

9 Reproduction in the Buffalo

9.1 Introduction

The domestic buffalo, *Bubalus bubalis*, is a distinct species within the Bovidae family. The buffalo population is increasing all the time. It was estimated at over 160 million in 2002 (FAO, 2003), more than 95% of which is located in Asia where buffaloes play a prominent role in rural livestock production, providing draft animals, and milk and meat. In recent decades, buffalo farming has expanded widely in Mediterranean areas and in Latin America. The swamp buffalo of Southeast Asia (Indonesia, Malaysia, Thailand and Australia) has 48 pairs of chromosomes. It is mainly used for draft work, being only a poor milk producer.
The Murrah and Surti river buffaloes (India, Pakistan) have 50 pairs of chromosomes and a much higher milk yield with a very high fat content (8%). The majority of animals are kept in small village farms under traditional management systems. However, in some countries, such as Italy and Brazil, there are farms engaging in the large-scale production of buffalo milk, and benefiting from the overall control of production and reproduction.

9.2 Physiology

The reproductive organs of buffaloes are smaller, but quite similar to those of cows. The uterine body is much shorter (1-2 cm) than that of the cow (2-4 cm). The cervix of the water buffalo is smaller (length 3-10 cm, diameter 1.5-6.0 cm) and its canal is more tortuous, which probably accounts for the lesser degree of dilation of the external orifice during oestrus. Water buffaloes have three cervical folds on average (Drost 2007).
The smaller buffalo ovary is more elongated than in the cow, and the corpus luteum is not only smaller but also often more deeply embedded in the ovarian stroma.

Puberty in buffalo is later than in cattle, with the age of puberty varying widely, ranging from 16-22 to 36-40 months in different countries. Under field conditions, the first oestrus occurs at

15-18 and 21-24 months in river and swamp buffalo, respectively. In well-fed animals, puberty may be reached before 20 months, and is significantly affected by breed, season, climate, feeding systems and growth rate, with the body weight of the female being the strongest determining factor, as observed in cattle. The average age at first calving is therefore between 3 and 4 years, but many buffalo cows calve much later.

Buffalo may be considered to be seasonally polyoestrous and a short day breeder. In river buffalo, the female is active from July until the end of February. The peak of first matings occurs during autumn and winter (Nasir Hussain Shah et al., 1989). The most likely reasons for this seasonality are the hot and dry conditions during the summer, and nutrition may also play a part. The swamp buffalo cycles continuously throughout the year, but a crop-associated seasonal pattern is observed. In Thailand, breeding is concentrated between December and February - the post-harvest season - when the animals are allowed to graze in the paddy fields.
The average length of the oestrous cycle is 21-22 days; for river buffaloes, and 19-20 days for swamp buffaloes (Singh et al., 2000).

On average, oestrus lasts 12 to 28 hours. Buffalo oestrus behaviour is less intense than that of cows and is consequently much more difficult to detect. Mucosal vaginal discharge, swollen vulva, mounting behaviour (far less frequent than in cattle) and the standing reflex are the main signs of oestrus.

The works of Baruselli et al. (1997), Manik et al., (2002) and Ali et al., (2003) confirmed that, as in cattle, the follicular development during the oestrous cycle also occurs in waves. Two-wave cycles are most common (63.3%) followed by three-wave cycles (33.3%) and those featuring a single wave (3.3%). Buffalo cows tend to have two or three follicular wave cycles, whereas in buffalo heifers there is a prevalence of two-wave cycles. The number of waves influences the length of the luteal phase and the oestrous cycle. Oestrous cycles with two follicular waves are somewhat shorter than three-wave cycles (21 vs. 24 days). Buffaloes that exhibit three waves of follicular

growth show a longer luteal phase (12.6 ±2.9 vs. 10.4 ± 2.1 days), inter-ovulatory interval (24.5±1.8 vs. 22.2±0.8 days) and oestrous cycle (24.0±2.2 vs. 21.8±1.01 days) (Rensis et al., 2007).
The ovulatory follicle reaches a diameter of 10 mm. The diameter of the mature CL ranges from 10 to 15 mm as compared with 12.5 to 25.0 mm in the bovine. Ovulation occurs approximately 10 hours after the end of oestrus.

The patterns of hormone activity of buffaloes and cows appear to be basically identical, but the progesterone concentrations during the cycle and pregnancy are much lower in buffaloes, especially in the swamp type. Circulating concentrations of LH reach a peak at the onset of oestrus, followed by a sharp decrease, and thereafter remain low during the luteal phase. The duration of the LH surge has been estimated to be 7–12 hours.
During the oestrous cycle, progesterone levels are at basal levels immediately after ovulation, increase during the following 4–7 days and reach peak levels at about day 15 after the onset of oestrus.

The gestation period of buffaloes is longer than that of cows, between 310 and 330 days. Murrah tend to have a shorter gestation period (315 days) than swamp buffaloes (330 days). The corpus luteum of pregnancy is invariably located ipsilaterally with the gravid horn.

The calving interval for buffaloes varies between 400 and 600 days, although longer intervals are certainly no exception. Seasonal, nutritional and managerial factors play important roles. The first ovulation in river buffaloes does not usually occur before 55 days post partum, but may be delayed up to day 90 post partum when suckling a calf. The first oestrus is detected after 130 days post partum in suckled cows, but may be delayed much longer depending on nutritional and climate conditions.

9.3 Reproduction management

Reproductive efficiency is the primary factor affecting productivity and is hampered, in the female, by the late attainment of puberty, seasonality of calving, extended post partum anoestrus and the subsequent calving interval. Pregnancy rates following artificial insemination (AI) are similar (>60%) to those obtained in cattle, indicating that the procedures for collection, processing and cryo-preservation of buffalo semen have been well established.

Nonetheless, although of great value for genetic improvement and disease prevention, AI is still not carried out on a large scale in buffalo, because of the weak expression of oestrus and the variability in its length, which make detection very difficult. Moreover, due to the high incidence of silent heat, large numbers of buffaloes are not bred at all, which contributes substantially to the overall figure for 'days open'.

Covert or silent oestrus is the single largest factor responsible for poor reproductive efficiency in buffalo. Additionally, the skills required for effective heat detection are often very limited on many buffalo farms, especially in developing countries. Some of the methods used in cattle can be adopted in buffaloes to enhance oestrus detection. Pedometers have proved to be efficient but the installation of the system itself is often way beyond the financial means of many smaller buffalo farms. On the other hand, the simpler and cheaper methods such as heat-mount detectors are less useful as mounting behaviour in oestrus is rare in buffaloes.

That is the reason for pharmacological oestrus management often being the only realistic possibility for increasing the accuracy of AI timing and improving reproductive performance in buffalo herds.

All of the pharmacological systems for oestrus management currently in use in buffaloes have been adapted, on an empirical basis, from those used in cattle, and are supported by an increasing amount of data reported in the literature. The cattle products are being used in buffaloes, although few of them have the indication for buffalo specifically stated in their user leaflets.

Prostaglandins

As in cattle, the corpus luteum of the buffalo is sensitive to the luteolytic action of exogenous prostaglandins from the 5th day of the oestrous cycle onwards. In cyclic animals, oestrus can be induced with a single injection of $PGF_{2\alpha}$ (e.g. Estrumate®) provided a functional corpus luteum is present (Fig 1).

Figure 1 Treatment schedule for oestrus induction with a single prostaglandin injection

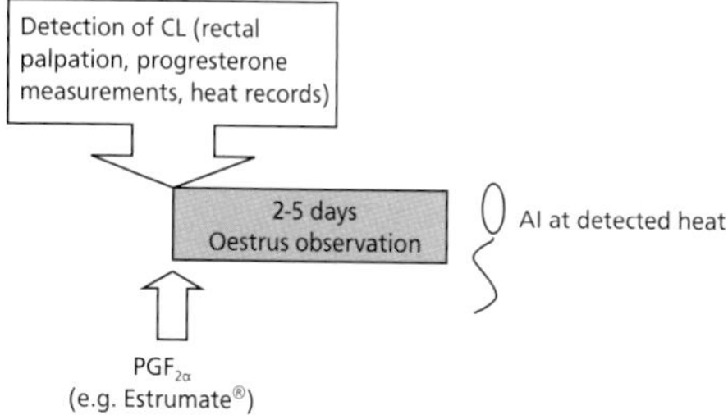

Alternatively, a double injection regime can be adopted with an 11-14 day interval (Fig 2) (Singh et al., 2000; Rensis et al., 2007).

Figure 2 Treatment schedule for oestrus induction with double prostaglandin injection

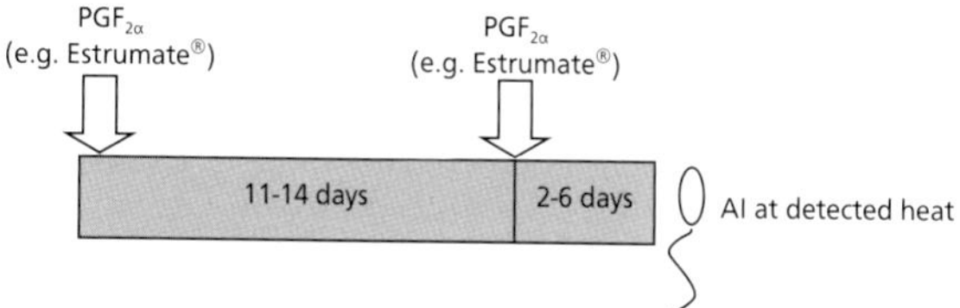

Warriah and Ahmad (2007) evaluated the follicular dynamics in Nili-Ravi buffaloes during spontaneous and $PGF_{2\alpha}$-induced oestrous cycles. Their results indicated that in most buffaloes

treated with $PGF_{2\alpha}$ on day 9, the static phase dominant follicle of the first wave was capable of further growth and ovulation. Moreover, the follicular dynamics during the 3 days before oestrus was similar in buffaloes undergoing spontaneous and $PGF_{2\alpha}$ induced luteolysis.
The interval from $PGF_{2\alpha}$ treatment to oestrus reported by Brito et al. (2002) ranged from 48 to 144 hours, with three quarters of the animals showing heat within 72 to 96 hours post injection. The time from treatment to ovulation ranged in these studies from 60 to 156 hours with over 80% of animals ovulating within 84 to 108 hours post injection. In buffaloes, much as in cows, the onset of oestrus and the timing of ovulation after $PGF_{2\alpha}$ treatment are variable, so insemination at the observed heat is recommended.

It is generally thought that both the oestrus response and fertility rates obtained in buffalo are lower than in cattle after prostaglandin treatment. The most probable reasons for these differences are poor body condition (often encountered post partum in buffalo cows, affecting the follicular growth), and low oestrus detection rates. However during the reproductive season, and with good body condition, single or double $PGF_{2\alpha}$ treatment in buffalo should induce oestrus and ovulation in about 60-80% of animals. In such favourable conditions, pregnancy rates following prostaglandin treatment can reach 45-50% on average and appear to be similar to those obtained after natural oestrus.
El-Belely et al. (1995) observed 77% overall oestrus rate after two $PGF_{2\alpha}$ treatments, but there was only 25% response to the first treatment, and Phadnis et al. (1994) observed a 55.7% oestrus rate after two doses.
It should be borne in mind that season will have a dramatic influence on the results of insemination in prostaglandin-induced oestrus, with conception rates reported to fall below 25% in the non-breeding season, even if the oestrus response to treatment appears fairly good.

In spite of these limitations, oestrus management with prostaglandins should be recognised as the most readily available and valuable tool to facilitate artificial insemination and improve reproductive efficiency in buffalo.

Alternative routes of prostaglandin administration in buffaloes
In the search for possible savings in the management of reproduction in buffaloes, the intra-vulval submucosal injection of prostaglandins has been tested by various researchers and practitioners (Chohan 1998). This route of administration is reported to allow the $PGF_{2\alpha}$ dose to be reduced by 50%. However, care should be taken when using such a reduced dose, because the decline in progesterone concentration and the onset of oestrus were reported to be slower in cows treated with a reduced dose by this route, than in those treated with a standard dose intramuscularly (Chauhan et al., 1986; Canizal et al.,1992).

Ovsynch type of synchronization programmes
In cyclic buffalo cows good results are obtained with the classical Ovsynch protocol (Berber et al., 2002; Baruselli et al., 1999; Neglia et al., 2003; Paul and Prakash 2005). Some authors, however, point out the beneficial effect of two inseminations at 12-18 hours and 24 hours after the second-GnRH treatment (Neglia et al., 2003; Paul and Prakash 2005). De Arujo Berber et al. (2002) reported pregnancy rates of 56.5% under field conditions when the Ovsynch protocol was used in buffalo cows. In the trial reported by Paul and Prakash (2005), the Ovsynch protocol synchronized ovulation effectively in Murrah buffaloes, and resulted in conception rates (to two fixed time inseminations) comparable with those achieved with a single AI after an observed oestrus.

Figure 3 Ovsynch protocol used in buffaloes

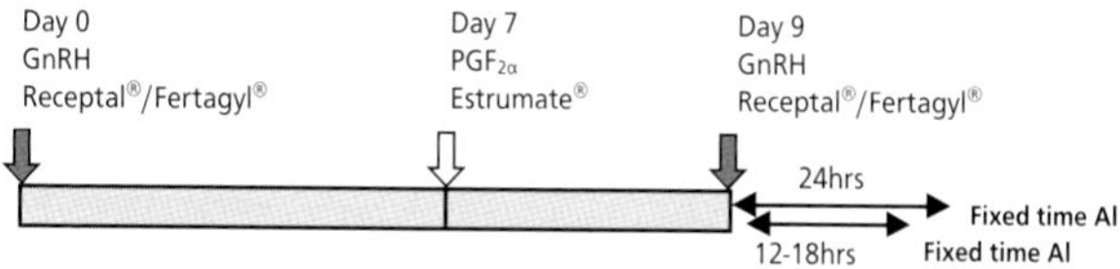

Ali and Fahmy (2007) evaluated the ovarian dynamics and milk progesterone concentrations in cycling and non-cycling buffalo cows during an Ovsynch program (Tab 1).

Table 1 Ovarian response to the Ovsynch protocol in cyclic and non-cyclic buffalo cows (Ali and Fahmy 2007).

Ovarian response	Cyclic cows	Non-cyclic cows
Ovulation to the 1st GnRH	90%	62,5%
Luteolysis after $PGF_{2\alpha}$	80%	87,5%
Ovulation to the 2nd GnRH	80%	100%

Conception rates recorded in this study were 60% for cyclic and 37.5% for non-cyclic cows. It seems that the lower conception rates observed in the latter group could be due to early/asyn chronous ovulation and poor luteal function after induced ovulation.
In a study reported by Warriah et al. (2008), pregnancy rates in buffaloes bred at an observed oestrus (62.5%) or after the Ovsynch protocol (36.3%) during the height of the breeding season did not differ significantly from those of animals inseminated during the low breeding season, (55.5%) and (30.4%), respectively.

The works of Baruselli et al. (1999) suggest that in order to obtain optimum results with the Ovsynch protocol in buffaloes, the animals should be treated during their breeding season and must be in good body condition (>3.5).

Ovsynch is of special interest for reproduction management in buffalo because most of them are located in high temperature zones, where heat stress can affect reproductive performance. As in cattle, treatment with the Ovsynch protocol should bring the benefits of the additional GnRH, and thus LH support for follicular growth and corpus luteum formation.

Progestagens

The high incidence of post partum anoestrus and difficulties with oestrus detection make progestagens a very interesting option for the induction of oestrus and ovulation in buffaloes.

Both progesterone-impregnated intravaginal devices and subcutaneous implants releasing norgestomet (Crestar®) have been used in this species, either alone or combined with the Ovsynch protocol (Singh et al., 1988; Hattab et al., 2000; Bartolomeu et al., 2002; De Rensis et al., 2005; De Rensis 2007). Examples of the treatment protocols are given in Figures 4 and 5.

Figure 4 Oestrus synchronization system with the use of Crestar®

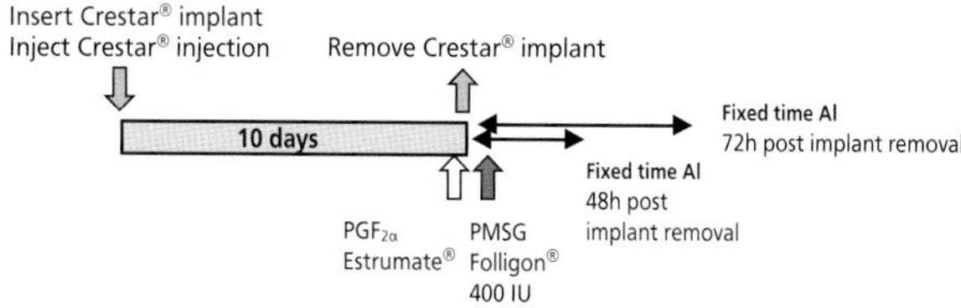

Figure 5 Example of oestrus synchronization protocol combining progesterone releasing intravaginal device and PMSG/eCG

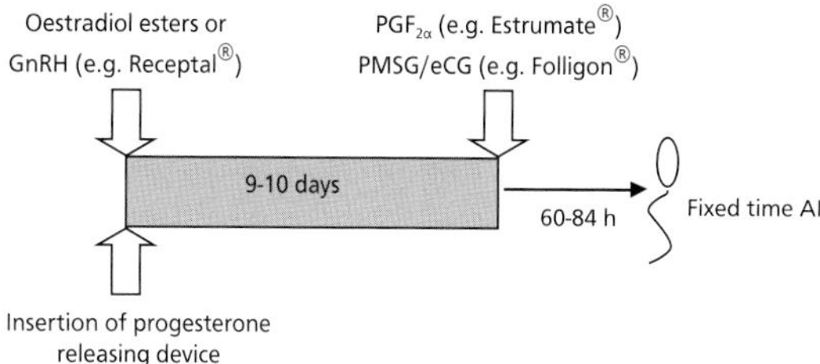

Oestradiol, PMSG/eCG and/or prostaglandin have been used successfully to improve the synchrony of oestrus, as well as conception rates, in progestagen-based protocols. Treatment with oestradiol esters or GnRH at the start of the progesterone/ progestagen therapy ensured adequate follicular turnover and improved conception rates, when used in buffaloes in the transitional period or cycling cows with no CL present at the start of treatment. Additional treatment with PMSG/eCG at the time the progesterone/progestagen source is removed, proved to be especially beneficial in non-cycling buffalo cows and outside the peak of the breeding season. Such a combination can induce the resumption of oestrus in buffalo cows in anoestrus, yielding pregnancy rates close to 30% (Zicarelli 1997; Hattab et al., 2000; Neglia et al., 2003). Barile et al. (2001) used PMSG/eCG at the time the progesterone device was removed followed by two timed artificial inseminations at 72 and 96 h later with a resulting conception rate of 51%.

Although the results of such protocols during the low breeding season are lower than in cyclic buffalo cows, and can be variable, it should be stressed that the use of progesterone-based protocols during the non-breeding season allows for insemination and the establishment of pregnancy in animals that would otherwise be non-productive.

9.4 Reproductive disorders

9.4.1 Uterine disorders

Abattoir surveys suggest that the incidence of endometritis in buffaloes is higher than in cows. The data on the frequency of delayed uterine involution in post calving buffaloes are very variable, but suggest that a considerable percentage of buffalo cows develop uterine infections and endometritis in the post partum period (El-Wishy, 2007a). Buffaloes are highly prone to dystocia, especially uterine torsion, frequently requiring obstetrical intervention which subsequently leads to post partum uterine infection.

Poor hygiene, vaginal stimulation for milk let-down and, possibly, wallowing, may be additional contributory factors.

As in cows with puerperal metritis, *E.coli* seems to be the prevalent pathogen (Jadon et al., 2005; Azawi et al., 2008a,b).

Buffalo cows suffering from endometritis later in the post partum period are mostly infected with *Arcanobacterium pyogenes, Fusobacterium necrophorum, Prevotella melaninogenicus* and other anaerobic bacteria (Jadon et al., 2005; Azawi et al., 2008c).

Diagnosis of uterine infections should be based on clinical examination, preferably including vaginoscopy and/or endometrial cytology, supported by bacterial culture and antibiotic sensitivity tests. However, in the areas where most buffaloes are reared, access to the more sophisticated diagnostic methods may be severely limited, especially by the lack of funds. That is the reason for the use of such simple techniques as exploration of the vagina with a gloved hand, and the use of tools such as Metricheck™ (see Chapter 2; 2.4.3) which can lead to a dramatic increase in the detection rate of uterine infections in buffaloes. Adequate treatment could then be applied in a higher percentage of animals with a reduced incidence of repeat breeding and better reproductive performance.

Recent publications have confirmed the existence of negative effects of uterine infections on the ovarian function of post partum buffalo cows (Hanafi et al., 2008) similar to those found in cattle (Opsomer et al., 2000; Shelton et al., 2002).

Local antibiotic therapy is the treatment of choice. As endometritis is associated with the presence of persistent luteal tissue in a high percentage of buffalo cows, additional treatment with $PGF_{2\alpha}$ is recommended to improve the uterine tone, evacuate the uterine debris and remove the immunosuppressive effect of progesterone.

9.4.2 Ovarian disorders

The most important ovarian problem in the buffalo is true anoestrus, i.e. inactive ovaries. This is observed particularly during the hot summer months.
Other problems are suboestrus/silent oestrus, delayed ovulation and persistence of the corpus luteum.
Compared with dairy cows, the incidence of cystic ovarian disease is low (1.8%).

True anoestrus

Inactive or non-functional ovaries are the most important causes of anoestrus and poor reproductive performance in buffaloes. In a review by El-Wishy (2007b), it was reported that ovarian inactivity is more frequent (30%) in buffaloes on low levels of feeding than in those (3%) on a high plane of nutrition, and also more frequent in summer calvers (41-46%) than in those calving in other seasons (7-33%). In the literature, a wide range of frequency of true anoestrus is reported, from 8% to 80%.

The administration of a GnRH analogue (e.g. Receptal®, 2.5ml) at 14 days post partum supports the early resumption of ovarian activity. Induction of ovarian activity can also be achieved by the application of a Crestar® progestagen implant over 9-10 days in combination with 600-700IU of PMSG/eCG (e.g Folligon®) at implant removal. Fixed time insemination at 48 and 72 hours after implant removal is recommended (Virakul et al., 1988; Nasir Hussain Shah et al., 1990).

Suboestrus, oestrus synchronization and induction

Silent heat is the factor most commonly responsible for poor reproductive efficiency in buffalo. Based on the results of rectal palpation of the ovaries and/or progesterone analysis, a wide variation in the frequency of suboestrus (between 15% and 73%) was reported in anoestrus buffaloes 60-240 days postpartum (summarised in El-Wishy, 2007b).

Suboestrus is more frequent in the early post partum period, during the humid and low breeding seasons and also in undernourished and suckled buffaloes and those calving in the hot season (reviewed in El-Wishy, 2007b).

The artificial control of the oestrous cycle has provided an effective means of increasing the reproductive capacity of this species, eliminating the need for frequent visual inspection for oestrus detection. For a review of available methods see section 9.3.

Delayed ovulation

If delayed ovulation is suspected, ovulation can be induced with the administration of a GnRH analogue (e.g. Receptal®, 2.5ml) or hCG (e.g. Chorulon®, 1.500IU). As in cattle, an injection of GnRH or hCG can be administered at the time of artificial insemination. Alternatively, the complete Ovsynch protocol can be used, with the second GnRH administration inducing ovulation.

Persistent corpus luteum

The results of rectal palpation of the ovaries, twice with a 10 day interval, together with progesterone analysis, revealed prolonged luteal activity in 8% of buffaloes not exhibiting oestrus before 60-90 days post partum (Shah et al., 1990). Endometritis was diagnosed in 45% of these cases.

Regression of the persistent corpus luteum can be achieved with an injection of $PGF_{2\alpha}$ (e.g. Estrumate®). As the condition is often associated with uterine disorders such as endometritis or pyometra, it is recommended that the state of the uterus be assessed and treatment administered as necessary.

9.5 References

Ali A., Abdel-Razek AK., Abdel-Ghaffar S., Glatzel PS. Ovarian follicular dynamics in buffalo cows (Bubalus bubalis). Reprod Domest Anim 2003;38:214-8.

Ali A., Fahmy S. Ovarian dynamics and milk progesterone concentrations in cycling and non-cycling buffalo-cows (Bubalus bubalis) during Ovsynch program. Theriogenology 2007;68:23-28

Azawi OI., Rahawy MA., Hadad JJ. Bacterial Isolates Associated With Dystocia And Retained Placenta In Iraqi Buffaloes. Reprod Dom Anim 2008a;43:286–292

Azawi OI., Omran SN., Hadad JJ. A Study on Postpartum Metritis in Iraqi Buffalo Cows: Bacterial Causes and Treatment. Reprod Dom Anim 2008b;43:556–565

Azawi OI., Omran SN., Hadad JJ. A Study of Endometritis Causing Repeat Breeding of Cycling Iraqi Buffalo Cows. Reprod Dom Anim 2008c;43:735–743

Barile VL., Galasso A., Marchiori E., Pacelli C., Montemurro N., Borghese A. Effect of PRID treatment on conception rate in mediterranean buffalo heifers. Liv Prod Sci 2001;68:283–7.

Bartolomeu CC., Del Rei AJM., Madureira EH., Souza AJ., Silva AO., Baruselli PS. Timed insemination using synchronization of ovulation in buffaloes using CIDR-B, CRESTAR and Ovsynch. Anim Breed Abstr 2002;70:332.

Baruselli PS., Mucciolo RG., Visintini JA., Viana WG., Arruda RP., Madureira EH., Oliveira CA., Molero-Filho JR. Ovarian follicular dynamics during oestrus cycle in buffalo (Bubalus bubalis). Theriogenology 1997;47:1531-1547

Baruselli PS., Madureira EH., Visintin JA., Barnabe VH., Barnabe RC., Amaral R. Timed insemination using synchronization of ovulation in buffalo. Rev Bras Reprod Anim 1999;23:360–2.

Berber RC de A., Madureira EH., Baruselli PS. Comparison of two Ovsynch protocols (GnRH versus LH) for fixed-timed insemination in buffalo (Bubalus bubalis). Theriogenology 2002;57:1421–30.

Brito LFC., Satrapa R., Marson EP., Kastelic JP. Efficacy of $PGF_{2\alpha}$ to synchronize estrus in water buffalo cows (Bubalus bubalis) is dependent upon plasma progesterone concentration, corpus luteum size and ovarian follicular status before treatment. Anim Reprod Sci 2002;73:23–35.

Canizal A., Zarco L., Lima V. Luteolytic failure of areduced dose of prostaglandin $F_{2\alpha}$ injected in the vulvular submucosa of Holstein heifers. Proc of 12th Cong Anim Reprod 1992;4:1109-1111

Chauhan FS., Mgongo FOK., Kessy BM., Gombe S. Effects of intravulvosubmucosal cloprostenol injections on hormonal profiles and fertility in subestrus cattle. Theriogenology1986;26:69-75

Chohan KR. Estrus synchronization with lower dose of $PGF_{2\alpha}$ and subsequent fertility in subestrous buffalo.Theriogenology 1998;50:1101-8
De Rensis F., Lopez-Gatius F. Protocols for synchronizing estrus and ovulation in buffalo (Bubalus bubalis): A review. Theriogenology 2007;67:209-216
Drost M. Bubaline versus bovine reproduction. Theriogenology 2007; 68:447–449
El-Belely MS., Eissa HM., Omaima HE., Ghoneim I.M., Assessment of fertility by monitoring changes in plasma concentrations of progesterone, oestradiol-17β, androgens and oestrone sulphate in suboestrus buffalo cows treated with prostaglandin $F_{2\alpha}$. Anim Reprod Sci 1995;40:7–15.
El-Wishy AB. The post partum buffalo: A review. I. Endocrinological changes and uterine involution. Anim Reprod Sci 2007a;97:201–215
El-Wishy AB. The post partum buffalo. II. Acyclicity and anestrus. Review. Anim Reprod Sci 2007b;97: 216-236
FAO (Food and Agricolture Organization of the United Nations), FAOSTAT Agricolture Data, 2003.http://apps.fao.org/default.htm.
Hanafi EM., Ahmed WM., Abd El Moez SI., El Khadrawy HH., Abd El Hameed AR. Effect of Clinical Endometritis on Ovarian Activity and Oxidative Stress Status in Egyptian Buffalo-Cows. American-Eurasian J Agric Environ Sci 2008;4:530-536
Hattab SA., Kadoom AK., Palme R., Bamberg E. Effect of CRESTAR on estrus synchronization and the relationship between fecal and plasma concentrations of progestagens in buffalo cows. Theriogenology 2000;54:1007–17.
Jadon RS., Dhaliwal GS., Jand SK. Prevalence of aerobic and anaerobic uterine bacteria during peripartum period in normal and dystocia-affected buffaloes. Anim Reprod Sci 2005;88:215–224
Manik RS., Palta P., Singla SK., Sharma V. Folliculogenesis in buffalo (Bubalus bubalis): a review. Reprod Fertil Dev. 2002;14:315-25.
Nasir Hussain Shah S., Wiel DFM van de., Willemse AH., Engel B. Opposite breeding seasons in dairy Zebu cows and dairy River Buffaloes as assessed by First insemination records. Anim Reprod Sci 1989;21:23-35
Nasir Hussain Shah S., Willemse AH., Wiel DFM van de. Reproductive performance of Nili-Ravi buffaloes after single injection of GnRH early post partum. In: Nasir Hussain Shah S. Prolonged calving intervals in the Nili-Ravi buffalo (Thesis). Utrecht 1990
Neglia G., Gasparrini B., Di Palo R., De Rosa C., Zicarelli L., Campanile G. Comparison of pregnancy rates with tow oestrus synchronisation protocols in Italian Mediterranean Buffalo cows. Theriogenology 2003;60:125-133
Opsomer G., Grohn YT., Hertl J., Coryn M., Deluyker H., de Kruif A. Risk factors for post partum ovarian disfunction in high producing dairy cows in Belgium: a field study. Theriogenology 2000;53:841-857
Paul VP and Prakash PS. Efficacy of the Ovsynch protocol for synchronization of ovulation and fixed-time artificial insemination in Murrah buffaloes (Bubalus bubalis). Theriogenology 2005;64:1049–1060
Phadnis YP., Bhosrekar MR., Mangurkar BR. On farm studies on oestrus synchronization in cows and buffaloes. Indian J Anim Sci 1994;64:1151–1154.
Rensis de F., Ronci G., Guarneri P., Nguyen BX., Presicce GA., Huszenicza G., Scaramuzzi RJ. Conception rate after fixed time insemination following ovsynch protocol with and without progesterone supplementation in cyclic and non-cyclic Mediterranean Italian buffaloes (Bubalus bubalis). Theriogenology 2005;63:1824–1831
Shah NH.,Willemse AH., Van de Weil DFM. Descriptive epidemiology and treatment of postpartum anestrus in dairy buffalo under small farm conditions. Theriogenology 1990;33:1333–1345.
Sheldon IM., Noakes DE., Rycroft AN., Pfeiffer DU., Dobson H. Influence of uterine bacterial contamination after parturition on ovarian dominant follicle selection and follicle growth and function in cattle. Reproduction 2002;123:837-845

Singh G., Singh GB., Sharma RD., Nanda AS. Ovarian and uterine response in relation to Norgestomet-PMSG treatment in the true anoestrous buffalo. Anim Reprod Sci 1988;16:71–4.

Singh J., Nanda AS., Adams GP. The reproductive pattern and efficiency of female buffaloes. Anim Reprod Sci 2000;60-61:593-604

Virakul P., Chantaraprateep P., Lohachit C., Prateep P., Demakan T. Synchronisation of oestrus in Swamp buffalo by using norgestomet and norgestomet plus PMSG. Buffalo J 1988;1:95-98

Warriach HM and Ahmad N. Follicular waves during the oestrous cycle in Nili-Ravi buffaloes undergoing spontaneous and $PGF_{2\alpha}$-induced luteolysis. Anim Reprod Sci 2007;101:332–337

Warriach HM., Channa AA., Ahmad N. Effect of oestrus synchronization methods on oestrus behaviour, timing of ovulation and pregnancy rate during the breeding and low breeding seasons in Nili-Ravi buffaloes. Anim Reprod Sci 2008;107:62–67

Zicarelli L. News on buffalo cow reproduction. In: Proceedings of the 5th World Buffalo Congress 1997, vol. 1; p.124–41.

10 Reproduction in Camelidae

There are very few complete accounts of reproduction in the Camelidae. Most of the published articles deal with *Camelus dromedarius* (Arabian camel) but reproduction is comparable across the whole Camelidae family: *Camelus bactrianus* (two-humped camel), *Lama glama* (llama), *Lama pacos* (alpaca), *Lama guanicoa* (guanaco) and *Vicugna vicugna* (vicuna).

10.1 Physiology

Camels

Except for the shape of the ovaries, the genital tract of the female camel is roughly comparable with that of the bovine, with two uterine horns in the abdominal cavity, a short cervix (3.5-5 cm) and a long vagina (30 to 35 cm). The ovaries are relatively small (10 g) and flattened bilaterally, bearing follicles of similar morphology to those of the bovine.

The Arabian camel reaches puberty at the age of 3-4 years, but females are not bred until they are 5-6 years old. Male camels reach puberty at about 3 years, but full reproductive activity is not developed until they are 6-7 years old. The reproductive life of a camel can extend to 20 years.

New world camelids

The majority of reproductive research in South American camelids has been undertaken in the two domesticated species, namely the alpaca (*Lama pacos*) and the llama (*Lama glama*). Far less information is available on the two non-domesticated species, the vicuña (*Vicugna vicugna*) and the guanaco (*Lama guanicoe*).

An excellent review of reproductive physiology in new world camelids was presented by Vaughan et al (2006). New world camelids have a bicornuate uterus with the body approximately 3 cm long and 3 cm in diameter. The left uterine horn is usually larger than the right in pre-pubertal females, and this difference is even more pronounced in multiparous females, because 98% of all pregnancies occur in the left horn. The ovaries of alpaca and llama are round to oval and globular in shape, with an irregular, firm texture and approximately 1.5-2.5 cm×1.2 cm×1.0 cm in size.

Puberty occurs at the age of approximately 6 months, but alpacas and llamas are usually not bred until the age of 12 months. Attainment of puberty is heavily dependent on the body weight of the animal, while conception rate and pregnancy maintenance is affected by the weight of the female at breeding.

10.1.1 Seasonality

The camel is a seasonally polyoestrous animal. The most commonly described season of pronounced sexual activity in the Northern Hemisphere is winter, but it can be altered under zoo conditions. Decreasing day length appears to be the stimulus for the onset of reproductive activity in camels (Musa et al., 1993).

In camels near the equator, factors such as rainfall, nutrition and management may overcome the effects of photoperiod and allow for breeding throughout the year.

Alpacas and llamas are considered non-seasonal breeders. Breeding and parturition are however usually restricted by farmers to the rainy, warmer months of summer in South America (December-April) to ensure the availability of better quality pasture.

Peruvian vicuñas, in their natural habitat, breed in the Southern Hemisphere autumn which is from March to May. In their nonnatural habitat, new world camelids are bred throughout the year (alpacas in Australia and New Zealand), or in seasons determined by climatic or nutritional factors (North America).

10.1.2 The oestrous cycle

Camelids are induced ovulators. Females require coital stimulation and ejaculation to induce ovulation of the dominant follicle, and do not exhibit a luteal phase in the absence of mating.

Camels

Follicular growth takes place in regular waves throughout the breeding season. The oestrous cycle, compared to that of cattle, is incomplete, and consists of proestrus (follicular growth),

oestrus (follicular maturation) and dioestrus (follicular atresia in unmated animals). Heats are observed every 20-25 days.
Oestrus, in which females are agitated and looking for males, lasts about 4-6 days. The external signs of heat are restlessness, bleating, rapid movements of the tail (up and down), mucous vaginal discharge and swelling of the vulva. Luteinizing Hormone (LH) pulses, leading to ovulation, occur approximately 2 hours after mating and end 10 hours later (Driancourt 1991, in: Thibault and Levasseur 1991).
Ovulation in the camel is induced and occurs within 48 hours of mating. Three days after ovulation, serum progesterone rises to 4 ng/ml and remains at that level until day 12 to 14.

New world camelids
Ultrasonographic studies have shown that sexually mature llamas, alpacas, and vicuñas which have not been mated, exhibit a continuous renewal of follicular waves (Vaughan et al., 2006).
Sexual receptivity in South American camelids is associated with a low level of plasma progesterone, females are usually receptive to mating, regardless of the stage of follicular development, and refusal of a male by a female does not necessarily indicate absence of a mature follicle.
The mating behaviour exhibited by a sexually receptive South American camelid female may be divided into courting and copulatory phases. The courting phase occurs when the male actively chases the female. The copulatory phase occurs in sternal recumbency with legs tucked beneath the body. The interval between mating and ovulation is approximately 30 hours (range 24-48 hours) in the alpaca and llama (Tibary and Memon 1999).
Ovulation occurs with equal frequency from the left and right ovary, however most pregnancies are located in the left uterine horn.
Three to 5 days after mating (2-4 days after ovulation) a corpus luteum is formed at the site of ovulation concurrent with rising plasma progesterone levels from 4 to 6 days after mating. The lifespan of the corpus luteum is therefore 8–9 days. Females should be sexually receptive again approximately 12-14 days after mating, if conception does not occur.

10.1.3 Pregnancy and parturition

Camels

The gestation length varies from 355 to 389 days as in most of the Camelidae. The cervical plug has unique properties and seals off the external cervical orifice during pregnancy in the camel (Guyton 1991). The presence of the cervical plug is also an indication of pregnancy in this species.

Parturition occurs either standing or lying down and takes 24 to 40 minutes depending on the size of the foetus. If she had been recumbent, the camel immediately stands up after delivery, and never licks her calf. The placenta is usually expelled at the same time as the calf, though a delay of 15 minutes is considered normal. With good nutrition, heat can occur within a month of parturition, but traditionally it is generally delayed for a year.

New world camelids

The literature reports variable gestation length in South American camelids with strong individual and seasonal variability and longest gestations in spring-mated females (351.0± 4.1), followed by summer (346.7±2.1) autumn (336.9±4.3) and winter-matings (330.6±2.8) (Vaughan 2001). The corpus luteum is the main source of progesterone throughout pregnancy and its presence is necessary to maintain pregnancy.

The interval from parturition to resumption of ovarian follicular activity is about 5-7 days. Mating and ovulation are possible by 10 days post partum. Uterine involution is rapid in camelids and the gross anatomical involution is completed in the majority of the animals by 21 days post partum.

10.2 Management of reproduction

Camels

Reproduction is commonly managed in one of two ways. The traditional one, mainly used in Africa, is based on the pastoral system. It is difficult to compare this with the commercial ranch management found in countries such as Saudi Arabia, Kenya and Israel.

Under commercial conditions (Kenya), most of the births occur in May/June or November/January. Williamson and Payne (in: Mukasa-Mugerwa 1985) noted that the young camel is one of the most fragile of mammals, especially during the first three weeks of life. Under traditional management, the mortality rate during the first year is estimated to be around 50%, of which 26% is in the first 6 weeks (Mukasa-Mugerwa 1985), mainly because the calves are not fed enough colostrum.

New world camelids
There are currently two systems of production for South American camelids around the world. The first is the traditional pastoral system in the dry Andean highlands, where limited financial and labour resources are available, and climatic conditions such as temperature and altitude can be especially challenging.
In the second system, the animals are maintained in a non-native environment (Australia, New Zealand, North America) where these species are bred not only for fibre but also as companion animals. Interest in applying modern reproductive technologies has increased in the last decade because the products from both domestic and wild species have become appreciated internationally, and several programmes to support such sustainable agriculture have been initiated in the Andean region.

10.2.1 Reproductive parameters

In the main, young females are not mated before they are 4 to 6 years old. It can be earlier in domestic vicuñas, but wild vicunas are not fertile before 2 or 3 years of age. Most of the literature records a conception rate of 40 to 50%.
In the majority of females, the interval between successive parturitions is generally around 2 years, but can vary, depending on the management system. Under commercial ranch management, intervals between 14 and 18 months were recorded in some herds by Wilson (1989). In Watson's report (in: Mukasa-Mugerwa 1985), 73% of females were not pregnant for 12 months after calving, and 74% of the calves were not weaned under a year old. See Table 1.

Table 1

Interval between calvings (months)	Number of camels
12	1
14	1
15	1
16	1
24	14
30	1
36	7
Parturition-conception interval (months)	
1-3	1
3	2
6	2
7-11	19
Age at weaning (months)	
3	1
6-11	6
12	17
24	3

from: Mukasa-Mugerwa, 1985

10.2.2 Mating and artificial insemination

Mating

Controlled mating with selected, genetically valuable, males has been practised for a long time in the breeding of both camels and alpacas and llamas. The main drawback of controlled breeding is the fact that males are often selected solely on the basis of their external features or sporting performance (racing camels), while their reproductive ability, especially the quality of their semen, is rarely tested.

Artificial insemination

Much more research is required before the benefits of AI can be fully exploited, including determination of the optimum time for insemination, semen dose and the use of hCG or GnRH to induce ovulation.

Collection of semen from camelids presents many difficulties, due to the nature of their copulatory behaviour and the slow (dribbling) process of ejaculation. The main techniques used are the artificial vagina, electro-ejaculation or post-coital aspiration from a female. Of these, the artificial vagina and electroejaculation are most often used and ensure the higher hygienic standards. Successful collection of semen by artificial vagina has been reported in camels (review: Bravo et al., 2000; Mosaferi et al., 2005), alpacas (Vaughan et al., 2003) and llamas (Lichtenwalner et al.,1996b).

Camel semen has the following characteristics:
volume: 3.5 ml (1-10 ml)
colour: white
appearance: slimy
concentration: 140-760 million/ml
pH: 7.8 (7.2-8.8)
live sperm: 55%
spermatozoa/dose: 400 million

Artificial insemination with fresh semen is a well-established technique in camels, and an increasing number of reports demonstrate good results after insemination with frozen semen (Al Eknah et al., 2000, Aminu et al., 2003).
A major difficulty with artificial insemination in the camel is ensuring that the inseminated females ovulate. Therefore, following AI, ovulation is often induced with either 3000 IU hCG (e.g. Chorulon®) or 20 mcg of buserelin (e.g. Receptal®).
In South American camelids, mostly undiluted or diluted fresh semen is used, with pregnancy rates reaching as high as 68%, while insemination with cooled or frozen semen is still not readily available (Miragaya et al., 2006).

10.2.3 Pregnancy diagnosis

Ultrasound can be used for pregnancy diagnosis (Tinson et al., 1992), but in practice, pregnancy is usually determined by the observation of a dilatation on the camel's right flank (in the sixth month). Some practitioners use rectal palpation (as in the cow) to check for pregnancy and for the presence of a corpus luteum on the ovary. Since the camel is an induced ovulator, a corpus luteum is usually only palpable during pregnancy (Mukasa-Mugerwa 1985).
Bono et al., (1992) proposed a test based on serum levels of oestrone sulphate 15 to 20 days after mating.

Most pregnancies develop in the left uterine horn (Musa and Sineina, 1976 in Mukasa-Mugerwa 1985), early embryo migration being very frequent in the camel (and also observed in the llama; Shalash 1965 in: Novoa 1970). Twin births are reported in only a few studies, recording a twinning rate of only 0.4% (Musa et al., 1976). Multiple ovulations occur relatively frequently, but it appears that either only one ovum is fertilized or further embryos perish very early.

10.3 Control of oestrus

Extensive research and development have been undertaken in oestrus synchronization and controlled breeding in cattle, which is not matched in the Camelidae family.

10.3.1 Induction of oestrus

Both in camels and South American camelids with a functional corpus luteum, oestrus can be induced with an injection of $PGF_{2\alpha}$ analogue.

Various progestagen preparations also have been used in camels and alpacas in order to induce and synchronize oestrus and ovulation. Bono et al. (1992) reported the use of progestagens in combination with eCG/PMSG in the dromedary, as a safe and efficient technique for inducing fertile heats. Bourke et al. (1992) also mentioned the use of implants over a seven-day period in a super-ovulation programme in the llama. eCG/PMSG in doses ranging from 1000 to 8000 IU. has been used to induce oestrus in both the non-breeding and breeding seasons in camel, but the number of pregnancies achieved has been found to be very low (Al Eknah 2000).

10.3.2 Induction of ovulation

Ovulation in the camel has been successfully induced by a single treatment with GnRH or hCG. Skidmore et al (1996) administered 20 mcg of GnRH analogue or 3000 IU hCG when the dominant follicle measured 0.9-1.9 in diameter.

A dose of 8mcg of GnRH (Buserelin, Receptal®) at the time of mating has been tested in llamas with good results (McEvoy et al., 1992). Ovulation occurred 29 hours after injection. Cooper et al. (1992) observed the same effect in the dromedary using a dose of 20 mcg.

A recent study by Skidmore et al. (2009) compared various pharmacological methods of inducing ovulation in dromedary camels. The reported results indicated that two GnRH (20mcg buserelin, Receptal®) injections 14 days apart, or two GnRH injections 14 days apart with an intervening dose of $PGF_{2\alpha}$ (500mcg cloprostenol, Estrumate®) 7 days after the first GnRH, were the most effective methods of synchronizing ovulation. In a study reported in 2008, Nikjou found the double injection of 20mcg GnRH analogue, buserelin (Receptal®) 14 days apart, to be suitable for synchronizing the emergence of a follicle wave in Bactrian camel (Nikjou et al., 2008).

10.3.3 Superovulation

Super-stimulatory treatments consist of the administration of gonadotrophic hormones, eCG/PMSG or porcine follicle stimulating hormone (pFSH) after synchronization of the follicular wave using a natural luteal phase (induction of ovulation) or an artificial luteal phase (with exogenous progesterone).

eCG/PMSG has been tested using doses from 5500 to 8000 IU, 48 to 72 hours before mating. The results showed a 100% calving rate, but the trial only involved 7 animals. In the llama 1000 IU is an appropriate dose for superovulation (Bourke et al., 1992).

Purified ovine FSH has also been tested in the dromedary (Cooper et al., 1992), but with poor results.

10.4 Reproductive disorders

In common with cattle and horses, the camel can suffer from uterine infections in the post partum period, with an incidence varying from 53% to 71% (using the bovine classification). The organisms isolated are the same as in the bovine (Wernery et al., 1992).

Both abortion and stillbirth are known to occur in the camel. The incidence of Brucellosis (*B. melitensis* and *B. abortus*) varies between countries (1-26%). Other important infective causes of abortion are Trypanosomiasis, Pasteurellosis and Salmonellosis. In new world camelids, the most common reasons for presenting infertile females for examination are repeat breeding (75%) pregnancy loss (18%), visible abnormalities of the genitalia (5%) and continuous rejection of the male (2%) (Tibary 2004a,b; Tibary et al., 2001)

Persistent luteal activity

Persistent luteal activity is encountered relatively frequently in practice. Affected females show a high level of serum progesterone, and reject the male. Injection of $PGF_{2\alpha}$ analogues, such as cloprostenol (175mcg i.m. for alpacas, 250 mcg for llamas), are recommended although commercially available products are rarely licensed for use in these species. Dinoprost tromethamine should be used with extreme caution, as signs of toxicity (respiratory distress and death) have been reported in some animals (Fowler 1998).

Ovulation failure

Failure of ovulation occurs commonly both in camels and new world camelids. GnRH analogues (e.g. Buserelin, Receptal®, 4mcg) or hCG (e.g. Chorulon®, 1500 IU) are used in practice, either as a means of prevention, or in order to increase pregnancy rates in alpacas and llamas, while the doses of 20 mcg of buserelin or 3000 IU hCG are used in camels.

Uterine infections

Uterine infection is the most commonly acquired reproductive problem resulting in infertility in camelids. Uterine infection should be suspected in females that have a history of repeat breeding, early embryonic death or dystocia and/or retained foetal membranes during their most recent parturition.

Post partum metritis may be accompanied by systemic signs, while chronic endometritis may go undetected. There are no well-established treatment schedules for uterine infections in camelids, as few antibiotic preparations are licensed in these species.

Prostaglandins and oxytocin are sometimes used, but with variable success.

Embryonic loss

Early embryonic mortality is common in camelids and is estimated to affect 10-15% of all pregnancies in the first 60 days of pregnancy (Vaughan et al., 2006). The incidence of embryonic loss can be much higher in extreme conditions, since nutritional and climatic factors seem to have a profound effect on the maintenance of pregnancy in camelids.

So far, little is known of the efficacy of pharmacological attempts to support luteal function with progesterone, GnRH or hCG in these species.

10.5 References

Al Eknah MM. Reproduction in Old World camels. Animal Reprod Sci 2000;60-61:583-592

Aminu D., Sumant V., Sahani MS. Semen collection, cryopreservation and artificial insemination in the dromedary camel. Animal Reproduction Science 2003;77:223–233

Bono G., Bolelli GF., Moallin Dahir A., Sciajno R., Parini C. The early appearance of oestrone sulphate in peripheral blood of pregnant she-dromedaries. Proceedings of the 12th International Congress on Animal Reproduction; The Hague 1992;4:568.

Bourke DA., Adam CL., Kyle CE., Mc Evoy TG. Superovulation and embryo transfer in the llama. Proceedings of the 1st International Camel Symposium; Dubai 1992:50.

Bravo PW., Skidmore JA., Zhao XX. Reproductive aspects and storage of semen in Camelidae. Anim Reprod Sci 62;2000:173–193

Cooper MJ., Skidmore J., Allen WR., Wensvoort S., Billah T., Chaudhry MA., Billah AM. Attempts to stimulate and synchronize ovulation and superovulation in dromedary camels for embryo transfer. Proceedings of the 1st International Camel Symposium; Dubai 1992:51.

Al Eknah MM. Reproduction in Old World camels. Animal Reproduction Science 2000;60–61:583–592

Fowler ME., Bravo PW. Reproduction. In: Fowler, M.E (Ed.), Medicine and Surgery of South American Camelids, second ed. Iowa State University Press, Ames, USA, 1998:pp. 381–429.

Guyton AC. In: Textbook of Medical Physiology. Saunder. London, UK, 1991, p. 915 **Lichtenwalner AB., Woods GL., Weber JA.** Seminal collection, seminal characteristics and pattern of ejaculation in llamas. Theriogenology 1996;46:293–305.

McEvoy TG., Kyle CE., Young P., Adam CL., Bourke DA. Aspects of artificial breeding and establishment of pregnancy in South American camelids. Proceedings of the 12th International Congress on Animal Reproduction; The Hague 1992;4:573.

Miragaya MH., Chaves MG., Aguero A. Reproductive biotechnology in South American camelids. Small Rum Res 2006;61:299–310

Mosaferi S., Niasari-Naslaji A., Abarghani A., Gharahdaghi AA., Gerami A. Biophysical and biochemical characteristics of bactrian camel semen collected by artificial vagina. Theriogenology 2005;63:92–101

Musa EE., Abusineina ME. Some observations on reproduction in the female camel (Camelus dromedarius). Acta Vet 1976;26:63-69

Musa BE., Siema H., Merkt H., Hago BEO., Willmen T. Artificial insemination of dromedary camel. Proceedings of the 1st International Camel Symposium; Dubai 1992:35.

Musa BE., Siema H., Merkt H., Hago B., Cooper M., Allen WR., Jochle W. Manipulation of reproductive functions in male and female camels. Anim Reprod Sci 1993;33:289-306

Mukasa-Mugerwa E. Le chameau (Camelus dromaderius): Etude bibli ographique. Cipea monographie. Addis-Abeda, Ethiopie 1985.

Nikjou D., Niasari-Naslaji A., Skidmore JA., Mogheiseh A., Razavi K., Gerami A., Ghanbari A. Synchronization of follicular wave emergence prior to superovulation in Bactrian camel (Camelus bactrianus). Theriogenology 2008;69:491–500

Novoa C. Reproduction in Camelidae. Review. J Reprod Fert 1970;22:3-20.

Skidmore JA., Allen WR., Cooper MJ., Wensvoort S., Ali Chaudhry M., Billah T., Billah AM. Attempted recovery and transfer of embryos in dromedary camels: results of preliminary experiments. Proceedings of the 1st International Camel Symposium; Dubai 1992:52.

Skidmore JA., Adams GP., Billah M. Synchronisation of ovarian follicular waves in the dromedary camel (Camelus dromedarius).
Anim Reprod Sci 2009;114:249-255

Tibary A., Memon M.A. Reproductive physiology in the female South American camelidae 1999;6:217–233.

Tibary A., Anouassi A., Memon AM. 2001. Approach to infertility diagnosis in camelids: retrospective study in alpacas, llamas and camels. J Camel Pract
Res 2001;8:167–179.

Tibary A. Infertility in female camelids 2: causes and treatment.In: Proceedings of North AmericanVeterinary Conference, Orlando, Florida,17-21 January 2004, pp. 287–289

Tinson AH., McKinnon. Ultrasonography of the female dromedary camel reproductive tract. Proceedings of the 1st International Camel Symposium; Dubai 1992:36.

Thibault C., Levasseur MC. La reproduction chez les mammiferes et l'homme. INRA ellipses 1991.

Vaughan JL. Control of ovarian follicular growth in the alpaca (*Lama pacos*). Ph.D. Thesis. Central Queensland University, 2001.

Vaughan JL., Galloway D., Hopkins D. The development of artificial insemination technology in alpacas (*Lama pacos*).
A report of the Rural Inducstries Research and Development Corporation,
RIRDC Publication 2003;No. 03/104.

Vaughan JL., Tibary A. Reproduction in female South American camelids: A review and clinical observations. Small Ruminant Research 2006;61:259–281

Wernery U., Wernery R. A review of uterine infections in the dromedary camel. Proceedings of the 1st International Camel Symposium; Dubai 1992:42.

Wilson RT. Performances de reproduction du dromadaire. Base empirique. Revue Elev Med Vet Pays Trop 1989;42(1):117-25.

11 Reproduction in the Rabbit

Artificial insemination (AI) has been used in rabbits since the 1950s (see for example Murphree et al., 1951). This technique has continued to be the focus of much research, in particular with respect to improving semen storage, which has come a long way since it was first used during the 1960s (see for example O'Shea and Wales 1969).

11.1 Physiology

11.1.1 Buck

The buck has oval-shaped testes within the scrotum that remain in communication with the abdominal cavity and can be withdrawn. The short, backward-slanting penis points forward when erect. The testicles descend at about 2 months of age. Sexual maturity, defined as the moment when daily sperm production ceases to increase, is reached at 32 weeks by New Zealand White rabbits in temperate climates. However, a young buck in these same conditions can be used from the age of 20 weeks. The first manifestations of sexual behaviour appear at days 60-70.

The volume of semen ejaculated is about 0.3-0.6 ml, with a concentration of 150-500 million spermatozoa per ml. 'False mounting', 1-2 minutes before copulation, increases the concentration of the ejaculate. Maximum spermatozoa production is obtained by using the buck regularly once a day.

11.1.2 Doe

The doe has small, oval-shaped ovaries and two independent uteri (about 7 cm long) that open separately through two cervical ducts into the vagina.

The first follicles appear on the 13th day after birth and the first antral follicles at about 65-70 days old. Does are able to mate first at 10-12 weeks, but as a rule this will not produce ovulation. The onset of puberty varies greatly with the breed: sexual precocity is more developed in small or medium breeds (4-6 months) than in large breeds (5-8 months). Sexual behaviour (acceptance of mating) appears long before the ability to ovulate and bear a litter.

The female rabbit does not have an oestrous cycle with regular periods of 'heat' during which ovulation will occur spontaneously. Does are considered to be in oestrus more or less permanently. From October to December in the Northern Hemisphere, rabbits may moult and many does do not conceive during moulting.

The rabbit is an induced ovulator, although spontaneous ovulation is also possible (Morrell 1995). Mating induces a neuro-endocrinological reflex which provokes an LH surge leading to ovulation (Bakker and Baum 2000). The luteinizing hormone (LH) pulse rate increases within 10-15 minutes of sexual stimulation, reaching a plateau for at least 1 hour (Jones et al., 1976). Ovulation takes place 10 to 12 hours after the LH peak. Follicle stimulating hormone (FSH) is released in frequent pulses, while LH returns to basal levels 5-6 hours after mating (Dufy-Barbe et al., 1973) (Figure 1). Simultaneously, the hypothalamus secretes oxytocin and the ovaries secrete prostaglandin facilitating ovulation.

Figure 1 Evolution of FSH and LH secretion after mating (Dufy-Barbe et al., 1973).

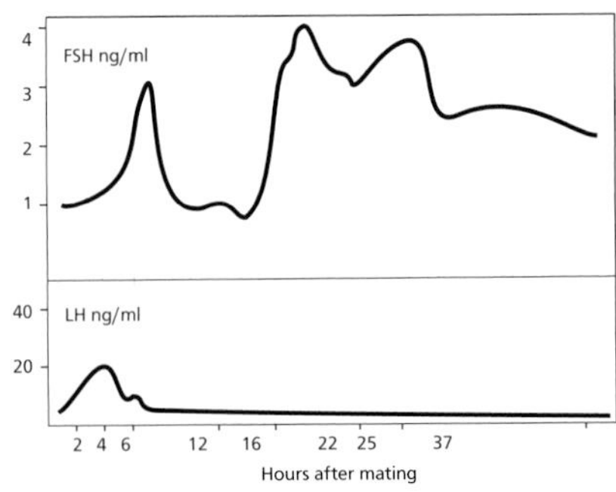

At the same time, the hypothalamus secretes oxytocin and the ovaries prostaglandin, which facilitate ovulation. Muscular activity of the oviductal isthmus (11.7-18.7 contractions/min during oestrus) is increased within 2 hours of ovulation (natural or induced) and this lasts for 2-3 days (Bourdage and Halbert 1980). The periods of elevated and depressed activity correspond closely with the rapid pre-ovulatory transport of sperm (which reach the fertilization area (in the distal ampulla, near the isthmus) 30 minutes after coitus) and slow postovulatory transport of ova through the isthmus (which reaches the uterus 72 hours after ovulation), suggesting the possibility of the regulation of gamete transport by the oviductal musculature (Bourdage and Halbert 1980). Implantation proper takes place 7 days after mating, at the blastocyst stage.
Progesterone concentrations increase from day 3 to 15 post mating and remain elevated until just before parturition.

Fertility is influenced by a large number of factors in the doe: temperature, light and feeding are the three main contributors to the seasonal effect. Increasing daily light exposure may improve litter size in pubertal does (Kamwanja and Hauser 1983). Rabbit does born in summer reach puberty later than those born in other seasons (Kamwanja and Hauser 1983). Does fed *ad libitum* reach puberty 3 weeks earlier than similar does receiving only 75% of the same daily feed (Lebas et al.,1986). In practice, does are usually mated when they reach 80-85% of the mature weight for their breed. Another important factor influencing fertility is the receptivity (the willingness to allow mating) of the doe. This can be measured by the colour of the vulva (an external sign of oestrogen phase) at the time of mating (Caillol et al., 1983). The influence of receptivity on fertility is presented in Table 1.

Table 1 Influence of receptivity (measured by the colour of the vulva) on fertility at AI (Theau-Clement and Roustan 1991)

Colour of the vulva	White	Pink	Red	Dark red
Fertility	35%	55%	75%	40%

Pregnancy in the rabbit lasts 31 days (range of 30-33 days). If gestation is shorter than 29 days, the kits are usually not viable. A minimum of four corpora lutea may be necessary for the successful maintenance of pregnancy in breeds such as the New Zealand White rabbit (Feussner et al., 1992). The minimum number of corpora lutea required may be strain-dependent and may bear a relationship to the normal litter size of the strain (Feussner et al., 1992).

At the end of gestation the doe makes a nest for the litter with her own fur and any other materials available, such as straw and shavings. This behaviour is linked with an increase in the oestrogen/progesterone ratio and with the secretion of prolactin.

Parturition (kindling) lasts for 15-30 minutes, depending on the size of the litter. On average there are 7-9 kits per litter (range 3-12). Weaning of the young usually takes place at 30-42 days of age.

Pseudopregnancy is a normal physiological event that follows an unsuccessful or infertile mating and lasts for 15-19 days before resolving spontaneously. Initially, the corpus luteum and uterus develop as in an ordinary pregnancy, however these changes start to regress at around day 12, due to the action of a luteolytic factor secreted by the uterus. Pseudopregnant does may have mammary gland enlargement and exhibit nesting behaviour. Rabbits for AI should be housed separately for at least 19 days prior to insemination to avoid the possibility of pseudopregnancy.

11.2 Management of reproduction in commercial rabbits

There are three main systems of rabbit reproduction.

- The extensive system, in which does are mated when the young are weaned (5-6 weeks after parturition), common among hobby rabbit-keepers.
- The semi-intensive system, in which the does are mated 10-12 days after parturition, and weaning takes place at 4-5 weeks of age, the most widely used system in commercial rabbit production.
- The intensive system in which the does are mated 2 days after parturition. Weaning takes place at 4 weeks at the latest. In

this system, the interval between litters is around 5 weeks. The conception rate and the litter size are usually somewhat lower than for the semi-intensive system, but the annual number of weaned young can be higher, due to the greater number of litters per doe per year.

Some producers employ a combination of the semi-intensive and intensive systems. Does with small litters (<5) are mated 2 days after parturition, while those with normal litter sizes are mated 10-12 days post partum. Semi-intensive systems appear to be better in terms of doe reproductive performance and litter viability than intensive management systems (Rebollar et al., 2009). In intensive reproduction in European rabbit farms, a single doe can produce 50-60 weaned young annually. At the same technological level, 45-55 rabbits can be produced in a semi-intensive reproduction system. Using the extensive system the best breeders obtain 30-35 weaned young per doe per year. The reproductive life of the doe is generally around one year with an average of six pregnancies (Rosell and de la Fuente 2009) while the male can remain sexually active for 5-6 years in the wild. In selection programs, focusing on the length of the productive life of does and the number of inseminations after the first fertile natural mating or AI, could increase reproductive longevity and decrease the replacement rate (Piles et al., 2006). Under farmed conditions, bucks are usually replaced after one year, mostly due to lack of libido.

11.2.1 Natural mating

Young females are usually mated for the first time at 16-17 weeks of age, but puberty is generally reached earlier (12 weeks) (Rommers et al., 2001). Consequently it is important to take males away from the litter before 10 weeks of age.
Natural mating, based on mating on one or two fixed days every week, is widely used in rabbit farming, generally with high fertility rates. Breeders select the lactating does for mating 10 days after parturition. This is a semi-intensive system with a 42 day cycle (31 days of pregnancy plus 10 days before the next mating). It means that, in favourable conditions, a doe is mated on the same day of the week once every six weeks.

11.2.2 Artificial insemination

Conception rates following AI can be equivalent to, or better than, those achieved by natural mating. Additionally, AI offers the same benefits as in other species: the control of genetic diversity, rapid progress in genetic improvement, establishment of pregnancy in does that refuse to mate and reducing the spread of infectious diseases.
The main limitation to the use of AI in rabbits is the ability to preserve rabbit semen (Roca et al., 2000). Frozen-thawed sperm can be used but careful attention to the cryopreservation technique is required to ensure good conception rates (Morrell 1995).
There is no real effect of season on semen quality (volume, raw motility, individual motility, number of living spermatozoa), although ejaculates collected in March are better than those collected in November (Théau-Clément et al., 1991). There is a significant correlation between kindling rate and the percentage of total motile cells (assessed by computer-assisted sperm analysis), linearity index and the percentage of abnormal sperm in the sample (Lavara et al., 2005).
Reproductive performance is predominantly influenced by the physiological status of the doe (lactation stage and receptivity) at the time of insemination (Brun et al., 2002). Rabbit does mated in July and October have significantly lower fertility (Théau-Clément and Vrillon 1991). Pregnancy rates (74%) and litter sizes at birth (9 kits) are similar whether 16 million or 4 million sperm are used for AI (Viudes de Castro and Vicente, 1997).

Semen is collected for AI with an artificial vagina and has the following characteristics:
- volume 0.5 ml
- concentration 500 million/ml
- pH 6.8 to 7.3

Artificial insemination can be used in the semi-intensive system at 42 days, as in natural mating, but is equally appropriate in the intensive system at 33 days. Between 34 and 40 days, the female is not receptive and cannot be inseminated successfully.

Fresh semen

If fresh semen is to be used, i.e. on the day of collection, semen quality needs to be evaluated. A subjective assessment of the proportion of motile sperm and the motility pattern allows for identification and exclusion of poor quality ejaculates. Fresh semen usually averages 84% live (unstained) spermatozoa, 88% with normal acrosomes (Chen et al., 1989). After quality assessment, the ejaculate is diluted with a suitable semen extender (e.g. Dilap 2000, saline) and can be stored for a few hours at 18°C.

Cooled semen

Semen can be preserved for 24 to 36 hours at 5°C in a special diluent, producing fertility rates of around 64% (Théau-Clément and Roustan 1991). Semen can be preserved effectively for up to 96 hours at 15°C using Tris-buffer extenders (Roca et al., 2000). More recently glucose- and fructose-based extenders containing gelatin (1.4g/100 ml) have been tested in a controlled study after storage of semen at 15°C for up to 5 days (Lopez-Gatius et al., 2005). Kindling rates for does inseminated with gelatin-supplemented semen stored for 48 hours (88%) or 72 hours (83%) were similar to those recorded for controls (81%), whereas rates significantly decreased when the semen was solid and stored for longer (Lopez-Gatius et al., 2005).

Frozen semen

In the past, semen frozen in liquid nitrogen (44% live sperm, 54% normal acrosomes) gave poorer results than fresh semen (Chen et al., 1989). Recently it was reported that fertility rates with frozen semen are similar to those achieved with fresh semen (Si et al., 2006), with fertility and kindling rates of 73.9% and 56.5% for a single freeze-thaw cycle. However, the choice of male (differences in freezing resistance of sperm) may affect the outcome (Moce et al., 2005). Interestingly, the number of spermatozoa inseminated does not appear to affect the reproductive performance (Castellini et al., 2006).

Despite much research, the results obtained after AI of rabbit does with cryopreserved sperm mean that it is not useful in commercial rabbits due to decreased reproductive performance, compared to fresh sperm (Mocé and Vicente 2009). A complex medium containing cryoprotectants is required for the freezing of rabbit semen.

Many protocols and extenders (usually with egg yolk and DMSO or acetamide) have been developed for rabbit sperm cryopreservation (Mocé and Vicente 2009). Most of the protocols include slow cooling and cryopreservation in liquid nitrogen (Mocé and Vicente 2009).

11.2.3 Pregnancy diagnosis

Pregnancy diagnosis is usually performed by abdominal palpation on day 12 to 14 after mating or AI. It has been shown that enzyme-linked immunoassay (ELISA) kits developed for the assay of plasma progesterone in other species can be used with rabbit plasma and serum (Morrell 1990 and 1993). With proper pregnancy diagnosis, pregnant females can be housed and fed appropriately during late pregnancy while non-pregnant females can be removed and put with the next batch to be mated.

11.3 Control of reproduction

Pharmacological methods of controlling receptivity and ovulation have been developed to improve the results of AI in the rabbit.

11.3.1 Induction of receptivity

Receptivity is one of the major problems in the doe. Photoperiod manipulation is used commonly to improve receptivity and synchronise oestrus (Quintela et al., 2001). A photoperiod of 12 hours light/12 hours dark until 6 days before AI produces better sexual receptivity than 8 hours light/16 hours dark (Quintela et al., 2001). Receptivity can also be improved by temporarily separating the doe from her litter (Ubilla et al., 2000), which results in a reduction in prolactin concentrations and an increased response to GnRH administration.

A protocol has been developed using pregnant mare serum gonadotrophin/equine serum gonadotrophin (PMSG/eCG, Folligon®, 40 IU) 48 hours before the expected day of natural mating or AI and a gonadotrophin releasing hormone (GnRH) agonist (Receptal® or Fertagyl®, 0.2-0.35 ml) at the time of AI (Molina et al.,1991, Parez and Chmitelin 1992, Remmen et al.,1979) (Figure 2). The results achieved with this protocol are particularly interesting in females mated for the second time (primiparous) and in lactating does (Parez 1992) as shown in Tables 2 and 3. More recently protocols tend to use lower doses (20 IU) of PMSG/eCG prior to mating (Castellini et al., 2006) PMSG/eCG (20 IU 48 h before AI) has also been used successfully (Remmen et al., 1979), along with photoperiod manipulation, to improve receptivity and synchronize oestrus (Quintela et al., 2001). Oestrus was better synchronized when PMSG/eCG was used with either of the two lighting programs mentioned above. Global productivity (number of weaned rabbits per 100 inseminated does) was better when was used along with either lighting schedule.

Separating does from their litters (for 24 or 48 h) before insemination on day 4 post-partum can be just as effective as PMSG/eCG treatment (25 IU), especially for the first four inseminations (Rebollar et al., 2006). Recently, improved sexual receptivity (76.3%, compared to 58.2% in the control group) and fertility (63.1% compared to 48.4% in the control group) was demonstrated using temporary doe-litter separation (closed nesting box on day 9, and 10 minutes of nursing on days 10 and 11 post partum) before AI, without adverse effects on litter growth (Rebollar et al., 2008). This yielded similar results (77.5% receptivity and 64.1% fertility) to PMSG/eCG (20 IU) administration on day 9 post partum (Rebollar et al., 2008).

Figure 2 Protocol to control receptivity

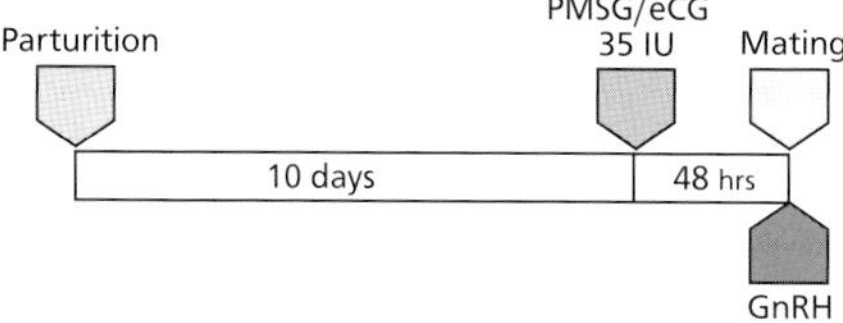

Table 2 Results of the use of the Folligon®/Fertagyl® protocol in primiparous and multiparous does presented for AI (Parez and Chmitelin 1992)

	Primiparous		Multiparous	
	Controls	Treated	Controls	Treated
Number of AI	38	34	166	179
Fertility (%)	29.4*	57.6*	76.6	79.6
Total born/doe	10.56*	13.29*	10.35	11.03
Born live/doe	9.80*	12.59*	9.47	10.19

** significant difference ($p < 0.05$) between controls and treated animals*

Table 3 Results of the use of the Folligon®/Fertagyl® protocol in lactating and non-lactating does presented for AI (Parez and Chmitelin 1992)

	Lactating does		Non lactating	
	Controls	Treated	Controls	Treated
Number of AI	200	212	56	43
Fertility (%)	68.3*	76.5*	85.7	79.1
Total born/doe	10.37*	11.29*	10.36	11.23
Born live/doe	9.49*	10.46*	9.66*	10.54*

** significant difference ($p < 0.05$) between controls and treated animals*

11.3.2 Induction of ovulation

The induction of ovulation is an essential element in artificial insemination in rabbits. Ovulation can be induced reliably by the presence of a vasectomised buck, or the administration of a GnRH agonist (buserelin (e.g. Receptal®), gonadorelin (e.g. Fertagyl®) or human chorionic gonadotrophin (hCG, e.g. Chorulon®).

hCG

Acting directly on the ovaries, hCG (e.g. Chorulon®, 25 IU) is very efficient at inducing ovulation in the doe, but is no longer used because, irrespective of dose, the effectiveness decreases after five injections. In addition, hCG treatment produces a higher percentage of degenerate embryos (Molina et al., 1991).

GnRH agonists
This method is used in the field in both AI and natural mating (to increase the stimulating effect of mating). GnRH acts on the pituitary to induce an immediate release of both LH and FSH. The plasma concentration of LH reaches its maximum 10-30 minutes after the intramuscular injection of a GnRH agonist (e.g. Receptal®, 0.2 ml / 0.0008 mg; Fertagyl®, 0.020 mg). If the preparation is injected subcutaneously at the time of insemination, then ovulation occurs approximately 10-12 hours later.

Improvement of conception rates after natural mating can also be achieved by inducing ovulation with GnRH. Recently, buserelin included in the seminal dose (0.0016 mg per doe intravaginally) was shown to yield similar kindling rates (87.5%) to, but better prolificacy (11.7 kits) than, intramuscular administration (0.0008 mg) (91.7% and 9.4 kits, respectively) (Quintela et al., 2004). More recent work in this area has involved a lower dose (0.0005 mg) administered intravaginally, which also appeared to yield reasonably good results in terms of pregnancy rate, kindling rate and average kits born live (79.5%, 74.8% and 9.5, respectively) compared to the control group (0.001 mg buserelin intramuscularly, 79.5%, 78.6% and 9.4, respectively) (Viudes de Castro et al., 2007).

11.4 Induction of parturition

Oxytocin
Oxytocin concentrations remain low in rabbits throughout gestation and rise only once uterine contractions start during parturition (Fuchs and Darwood 1980; O'Byrne et al., 1986). Injections of synthetic oxytocin (e.g. Intertocine S®, 0.15-0.2 ml) caused a dose-dependent increase in plasma oxytocin and uterine activity (Fuchs and Darwood, 1980). An injection of oxytocin can induce parturition on day 31 (Ubilla and Rodriguez 1990). Some authors report a high incidence of dystocia and a mortality rate of 5.7% in the resultant litters. Nonetheless, this is still used successfully on some rabbit farms.

Prostaglandins
The main use of prostaglandins is to induce luteolysis and to control the timing of parturition. No side-effects have been reported. None of these products are registered for this indication.
The following doses are used in practice:
- Luprostiol 0.5 mg/kg
- Cloprostenol 0.0015 mg/kg (Partridge et al., 1985)
- Etiproston 0.050 mg/doe (Ubilla and Rodriguez 1990)

11.5 Reproduction in pet rabbits

11.5.1 Bucks

Neutering (castration) of bucks is used to prevent aggressive behaviour and urine spraying (territory marking), as well as to avoid pregnancy in does. Bucks are best neutered shortly after they reach sexual maturity (from 4-6 months of age; up to 9 months of age in giant breeds). Neutered bucks should not be put with intact females for at least 3 weeks after neutering, as live sperm may still be present in the vas deferens, and testosterone levels drop slowly.

11.5.2 Female pet rabbits

Ovariohysterectomy
Rabbit does can be spayed (ovariohysterectomy), from about 4 months of age, to prevent unwanted pregnancy, aggressive behaviour and urine spraying (territorial marking behaviour) (Brower 2006).
Ovariohysterectomy is also the treatment of choice for a number of conditions in does (Redrobe 2000) including:
- Endometrial polyps/cystic hyperplasia and uterine neoplasia occur in intact does over 2-3 years of age
- Pyometra and endometritis are common problems in does (including virgin does), with *Pasteurella multocida* and *Staphylococcus aureus* isolated commonly.

Hormonal control of oestrus

There are few reports of the use of progestagens to control oestrus/ovulation in does. One study showed that medroxyprogesterone acetate inhibited mating-induced ovulation for 40-65 days and prevented fertilisation following hCG-induced ovulation from 15 days up to 83 days post-treatment (Chang 1985). Proligestone is used at dose rates around 33 mg/kg in rabbit does. This product is not registered for use in rabbits.

Mismating

The progesterone-receptor antagonist aglepristone has been shown to induce abortion (19-72h post-treatment) in does when administered on days 15 and 16 post mating (Ozalp et al., 2008). Reported side-effects included a short non-receptive period and short period of decreased food consumption (Ozalp et al., 2008).

Dystocia

Dystocia is rare in rabbits (Redrobe 2000). Obesity, nutritional deficiency and foetal deformities, foetal oversize, uterine inertia, narrow pelvic canal (congenital or as a sequel to fractures) may all contribute to dystocia. In cases of non-obstructive dystocia and when uterine inertia is suspected, 5-10 ml of calcium gluconate 10% followed by oxytocin (1-2 units intramuscularly) 30 minutes later, can stimulate uterine contractions. The doe should be placed in a dark, quiet area and left undisturbed for 40-60 minutes. A caesarean section or ovariohysterectomy may be performed if no young are produced, depending upon the viability of the foetuses and state of the uterus.

11.6 References

Bakker J., Baum MJ. Neuroendocrine regulation of GnRH release in induced ovulators. Front Neuroendocrinol 2000;21:220-262.

Bourdage RJ., Halbert SA. In vivo recording of oviductal contractions in rabbits during the periovulatory period. Am J Physiol 1980;239:R332-R336.

Brower M. Practitioner's guide to pocket pet and rabbit theriogenology. Theriogenology 2006;66:618–623

Brun JM., Théau-Clément M., Bolet G. The relationship between rabbit semen characteristics and reproductive performance after artificial insemination. Anim Reprod Sci 2002;70:139-149.

Caillol M., Dauphin-Villemant C., Martinet L. Oestrous behaviour and circulating progesterone and oestrogen levels during pseudopregnancy in the domestic rabbit. J Reprod Fertil 1983;69:179-186.
Castellini C., Pizzi F., Theau-Clément M., Lattaioli P. Effect of different number of frozen spermatozoa inseminated on the reproductive performance of rabbit does.Theriogenology 2006;66:2182-2187.
Chang MC. Inhibition of fertilization in the rabbit long after injection of Depo-Provera. Fertil Steril 1985;43:652-655.
Chen Y., Li J., Simkin ME., Yang X., Foote RH. Fertility of fresh and frozen rabbit semen inseminated at different times is indicative of male differences in capacitation time. Biol Reprod 1989;41:848-853.
Dufy-Barbe L., Franchimont P., Faure JM. Time-courses of LH and FSH release after mating in the female rabbit. Endocrinology 1973;92:1318-1321.
Feussner EL., Lightkep GE., Hennesy RA., Hoberman AM., Christian MS. A decade of rabbit fertility data: study of historical control animals. Teratology 1992;46:349-365.
Fuchs AR., Darwood MY. Oxytocin release and uterine activation during parturition in rabbits. Endcrinology 1980;107:1117-1126.
Jones EE., Bain JB., Odell WD. Postcoital luteinizing hormone release in male and female rabbits as determined by radioimmunoassay. Fertil Steril 1976;27:848-852.
Kamwanja LA., Hauser ER. The influence of photoperiod on the onset of puberty in the female rabbit. J Anim Sci 1983;56:1370-1375.
Lavara R., Moce F., Lavara F., Viudes de Castro MP., Vicente JS. Do parameters of seminal quality correlate with the results of on-farm inseminations in rabbits? Theriogenology 2005;64:1130-1141.
Lebas F., Coudert P., Rouvier R., De Rochambeau H. Reproduction In: The rabbit husbandry, health and production FAO, Rome, 1986;Chapter 3.
Lopez-Gatius F., Sances G., Sancho M., Yaniz J., Santolaria P., Gutierrez R., Nunez M., Nunez J., Soler C. Effect of solid storage at 15 degrees C on the subsequent motility and fertility of rabbit semen. Theriogenology 2005;64:252-260.
Mocé E., Vicente, J. S. Rabbit sperm cryopreservation: A review. Animal Reproduction Science 2009;110:1–24.
Molina I., Pla M., Vicente JS., Martin A., Romeu A. Induction of ovulation in rabbits with pure urinary luteinizing hormone and human chorionic gonadotrophin: comparison of oocyte and embryo quality. Hum Reprod 1991;6:1449-1452.
Morrell JM. Use of an ELISA for plasma progesterone to facilitate rabbit husbandry. Vet Rec 1990;127:521-524.
Morrell JM. Preliminary investigation of an ELISA kit as a qualitative assay for rabbit progesterone. Vet Rec 1993; 132: 434-436.
Morrell JM. Artificial insemination in rabbits. Br Vet J 1995;151:477-487.
Murphree R., Black WG., Otto G., Casida LE. Effect of site of insemination upon the fertility of gonadotrophin-treated rabbits of different reproductive stages. Endocrinology 1951;49:474-480.
O'Byrne KT., Ring JP., Summerlee AJ. Plasma oxytocin and oxytocin neurone activity during delivery in rabbits. J Physiol 1986;370:501-513.
O'Shea T., Wales RG. Further studies of the deep freezing of rabbit spermatozoa in reconstituted skim milk powder. Aust J Biol Sci 1969;22:709-719.
Ozalp GR., Seyrek-Intaş K., Calişkan C., Wehrend A. Mid-gestation pregnancy termination in rabbits by the progesterone antagonist aglepristone. Theriogenology 2008;69(9):1056-1060.
Parez V., Chmitelin F. Effect of a PMSG treatment on reproduction in the rabbit. Proc 12th International Congress Animal Reproduction, The Hague. 1992:1166.
Partridge GG., Lamb IC., Finlay M. The use of a synthetic prostaglandin analogue (cloprostenol) to control parturition in the commercial rabbit. Anim Prod 1985;42:281-286.

Piles M, Garreau H, Rafel O, Larzul C, Ramon J, Ducrocq V. Survival analysis in two lines of rabbits selected for reproductive traits. J Anim Sci 2006;84:1658-1665.
Quintela L., Pena A., Barrio M., Vega MD., Diaz R., Maseda F., Garcia P. Reproductive performance of multiparous rabbit lactating does: effect of lighting programs and PMSG use. Reprod Nutr Dev. 2001;41:247-257.
Quintela LA., Pena AI., Vega MD., Gullon J., Prieto MC., Barrio M., Becerra JJ., Maseda F., Herradon PG. Ovulation induction in rabbit does submitted to artificial insemination by adding buserelin to the seminal dose. Reprod Nutr Dev 2004;44:79-88.
Rebollar PG., Milanés A., Pereda N., Millán P., Cano P., Esquifino AI., Villarroel M., Silván G., Lorenzo PL. Oestrus synchronisation of rabbit does at early post-partum by doe-litter separation or ECG injection: Reproductive parameters and endocrine profiles. Anim Reprod Sci 2006;93:218-230.
Rebollar PG., Bonanno A., Di Grigoli A., Tornambè G., Lorenzo PL. Endocrine and ovarian response after a 2-day controlled suckling and eCG treatment in lactating rabbit does. Anim Reprod Sci 2008;104:316-328.
Rebollar PG., Pérez-Cabal MA., Pereda N., Lorenzo PL., Arias-Álvarez M., García-Rebollar P. Effects of parity order and reproductive management on the efficiency of rabbit productive systems. Livestock Science 2009;121:227–233.
Redrobe S. In: Manual of Rabbit Medicine and Surgery, Ed. PA Flecknell, BSAVA 2000;160 pp.
Remmen JL., van de Steen G., Vente JP. Some results obtained in artificial insemination on a large rabbit farm. Tijdschr Diergeneeskd 1979;104:301-307.
Roca J., Martinez S., Vazquez JM., Lucas X., Parrilla I., Martinez EA. Viability and fertility of rabbit spermatozoa diluted in Tris-buffer extenders and stored at 15 degrees C. Anim Reprod Sci 2000;64(1-2): 103-112.
Rommers JM., Kemp B., Meijerhof R., Noordhuizen JP. The effect of litter size before weaning on subsequent body development, feed intake, and reproductive performance of young rabbit does. J Anim Sci 2001;79:1973-1982.
Rosell JM, de la Fuente LF. Culling and mortality in breeding rabbits. Prev Vet Med. 2009;88(2):120-127.
Théau-Clément M., Vrillon C A. L'insémination artificielle chez la lapine. El et Ins 1991;245:3-12.
Théau-Clément M., Thebault RG., Bolet G., de Rochambeau H. Reproduction of French Angora rabbits: ovulation in the female, semen production in the male. Reprod Nutr Dev 1991;31:667-673.
Théau-Clément M., Roustan A. A study on relationships between receptivility and lactation in the doe, and their influence on reproductive performances. J. Appl. Rabbit Res. 1992;15:412–421.
Ubilla E., Rebollar PG., Pazo D., Esquifino AI., Alvarino JM. Pituitary and ovarian response to transient doe-litter separation in nursing rabbits. J Reprod Fert 2000;118:361-366.
Ubilla E., Rodriguez JM. Induction hormonale de la mise bas et la production de la lapine. Cuniculture 1990;17:171-174.
Viudes de Castro MP., Vicente JS. Effect of sperm count on the fertility and prolificity rates of meat rabbits. Anim Reprod Sci 1997;46:313-319.
Viudes de Castro MP., Lavara R., Marco-Jiménez F., Cortell C., Vicente JS. Ovulation induced by mucosa vaginal absorption of buserelin and triptorelin in rabbit. Theriogenology 2007;68:1031-1036.

12 Fish Reproduction

12.1 Introduction

The propagation of fish has been practised from time immemorial in different parts of the world. Aquaculturists, especially those involved in the rearing and propagation of fish, often have the disadvantage of cultivating species whose seed supply depends largely on capture from the wild.
Techniques for the production of adequate quantities of high quality fish seed from captive broodstock are necessary for the continuation and large-scale expansion of aquaculture. The lack of such techniques has been an important constraint in the controlled and successful culture of several cultivable species. The development of such techniques would provide the opportunity to develop a closed cycle production system which does not need to rely on catching wild broodstock and/or offspring, and would open the door for genetic improvement programmes and better disease control.
Top class fish reproduction management must aim to achieve the physiological potential of each fish species to produce offspring of high quality, quantity and desired gender, including sterile fish.
This review has a dual purpose. Firstly, to discuss briefly the reproductive physiology of fish with the emphasis on cultivated species and, secondly, to indicate areas of reproductive physiology in which artificial intervention is required in order to breed cultivated fish successfully in captivity. This evaluation takes into account the teleost fish as a group, without reference to the large variation in reproduction parameters between species.

12.2 Physiology and conditioning

As in mammalian species, the hormonal pathway of reproduction revolves around the hypothalamic-pituitary-gonadal axis (Figure 1). The hypothalamus is stimulated by environmental and chemical factors such as pheromones.

Following this stimulation, different neuropeptides [gonadotrophin-releasing hormones (GnRH)] are synthesized and released. Different fish species possess different forms of GnRH (Somoza et al., 2002; Sherwood and Wu 2005), ranging between two and three forms per species. Despite the multiplicity of GnRH forms in the fish, only one regulates the production and release of gonadotrophins (GtH) by the pituitary. This species-specific form of GnRH is produced in the brain's pre-optic area, and is the only one which projects directly into the pituitary through neurosecretory fibres. The pituitary gland produces two GtH (GtH-I and GtH-II) that act directly on the gonads (Suzuki et al., 1988a). Because of a significant degree of homology with mammalian luteinizing hormone (LH) and follicle-stimulating hormone (FSH) (Suzuki et al.1988b; Itoh et al., 1990), GtH-I is now clearly identified as fish FSH and GtH-II as fish LH (Yaron et al., 2003).

Figure 1 Hormonal pathway in the hypothalamic-pituitary-gonadal axis and levels of external intervention which can be utilised to induce maturation and ovulation/spermiation in teleost fish.

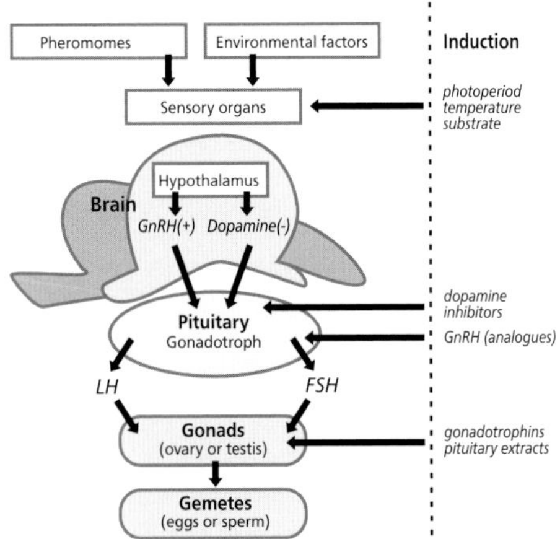

The seasonality of the reproductive cycle is determined by the environmental conditions to which fish are exposed. The environmental cues are transduced into endocrine changes that control gametogenesis.
In poikilothermic species such as fish, there is interaction between water temperature and photoperiod for the control of the reproductive cycle. Depending on the species, one of these factors is the primary transduction mechanism. In cyprinids, temperature plays the major role whereas, in salmonids and other fish families, photoperiod regulates the endocrine activity (Bayarri et al., 2004). It is assumed that photoperiodicity is perceived in fish both through the eyes and the photoreceptors of the pineal gland, the endocrine organ located on top of the brain. The pineal gland synthesizes and secretes the hormone melatonin, which participates in determining the timing of gonadal development (Bromage et al., 1996). However, data on the relationships between gonadotrophin secretion and melatonin in fish are rather scarce. Generally, melatonin stimulates LH secretion but its effect depends on the phase of the day-night cycle (Khan and Thomas 1996).

Figure 2 Reproduction and the environment in fish

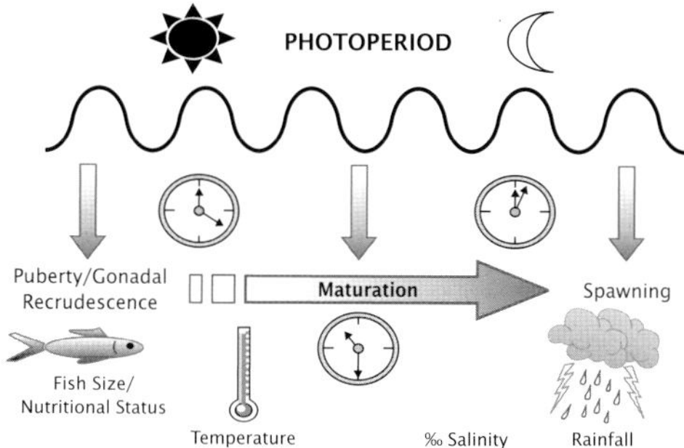

Reproductive cycles

The majority of teleost fish are seasonal breeders, while a few species breed continuously. Among the seasonal breeders, there is wide variation in the time of year when breeding occurs.

Freshwater temperate zone fish spawn in spring and early summer, while others, such as most salmonids, do so in autumn (Billard 1992), the timing of spawning being programmed in order to allow the liberation of offspring into the wild to coincide with optimal food availability.
The seasonality of spawning is a major problem in broodstock management of most fish species. Environmental factors such as photoperiod, temperature, salinity, seasonal rainfall and several features of the stimuli involved in the interaction between males and females, such as tactile, visual, auditory and electrical signals, interfere with the reproductive cycle of teleost fish (Chadhuri 1994; Weerd et al., 1990). In the African catfish, *Clarias gariepinus*, year-round endogenous rhythms of gonadal recrudescence and regression occurring in nature, can be avoided in captivity by raising the broodstock from egg to maturity under a constant high temperature (Richter et al., 1995). In salmonids, the programming of long and short photoperiod sequences in the culture of different strains (spring or autumn spawners) can allow reproduction at any time of the year.

Hypothalamus
As already noted, it is believed that only one form of GnRH regulates the release of GtH. The relevant GnRH induces the release of both FSH and LH (Zohar 1996); however, there are conflicting data showing that GnRH cannot stimulate FSH secretion (Breton et al., 1998a). The neuro-endocrine regulation of LH secretion in teleost fish is mainly under the control of a dual neurohormonal system. LH release is stimulated by GnRH and inhibited by dopamine, which functions as a Gonadotrophin-Release Inhibitory Factor (GRIF).
Dopamine acts directly on the pituitary to modulate the actions of GnRH, as well as the spontaneous release of LH, and also inhibits the release of GnRH (Peter et al., 1993). This tonic inhibition by dopamine on GnRH depends on oestradiol, high levels of which during vitellogenesis (yolk accumulation) prevent LH release. The drop in oestradiol concentration at the end of this process results in the removal of dopamine inhibition (Saligaut et al., 1998).

Pituitary gland (Hypophysis)

One of the main reasons for the lack of ovulation and spawning in a number of cultured fish is the failure of the pituitary to release LH (Lin and Peter 1996). Both FSH and LH induce steroidogenesis in specific gonadal cells. FSH is believed to be mostly involved in regulating earlier stages of gametogenesis, i.e. vitellogenesis in females and spermatogenesis in males. Once these processes end, the levels of FSH in the blood decrease, while LH levels rapidly increase. LH is believed to be mainly involved in regulating final oocyte maturation and ovulation in females and spermatogenesis and spermiation in males (Swanson 1991; Breton et al., 1998a; Chyb et al., 1999).

Ovary, oocyte maturation and ovulation

The ovary in most teleost fishes is a hollow sac-like organ into which extend numerous folds lined with germinal epithelium. The germ cells, the endodermally-derived oogonia, multiply mitotically and are transformed into non-yolky primary oocytes, with meiosis being arrested at the prophase of the first meiotic division until maturation. Primary oocytes undergo vitellogenesis when yolk is deposited in the ooplasm. During maturation, the first polar body is removed and the second meiotic division is arrested at the metaphase. The eggs are spawned at this stage and the second polar body is only released after fertilization. In some fish species, ovulation and spawning occur almost at the same time, whereas in rainbow trout and milkfish, ovulated oocytes are retained in the ovarian cavity and spawning takes place later (few days) (Billard 1992).

Hormonal regulation

As mentioned above, the gonadotrophins act on steroidogenesis in the gonads (Nagahama 1994). In females, the major reproductive steroids are oestrogens (mainly oestradiol-17β), which induce vitellogenin production (yolk) in the liver. Vitellogenin is transported by the blood to the ovaries where it is incorporated into the yolk granules of vitellogenic oocytes.
Progestagens (mainly 17α, 20β dihydroxy-4-pregnen-3-one and 17α, 20β, 21 trihydroxy-4-pregnen-3-one), induce final oocyte maturation. LH is significantly more active than FSH in stimulating ovarian 17α hydroxy, 20β dihydroxy progesterone (Maturation Inducing Steroid; MIS) production for the re-initiation of meiosis at the end of the female sexual cycle.

A surge of LH is necessary for the *in vivo* production of MIS (Suzuki et al., 1988c). MIS stimulates the production of Maturation Promoting Factor (MPF). This non-steroidal factor involves two components: cdc2 kinase and cyclin B (Nagahama et al., 1993). MPF triggers the cellular mechanism of germinal vesicle breakdown (GVBD), the re-initiation of meiosis and the hydration of the oocytes just before ovulation.

Fecundity and egg quality

A major difference between fish and many other domestic animals is their high level of fecundity. There are also significant differences between fish species in this regard. For example, flatfish and other marine fish species produce millions of eggs at a single spawning whilst other species, such as salmonids, produce only thousands (Bromage 1988). These species differences are of profound importance to the planning and management of broodstock facilities, with the less fecund species requiring far more fish, and more facilities, to produce the same number of eggs as the marine species.

A number of biotic and environmental factors have been shown to influence fecundity, as well as egg size and quality. Generally, as the size of the species increases, so do both fecundity and the diameter of the eggs produced. The age of the fish seems to be less important (Bromage 1995). Egg quality is defined as those characteristics of the egg that determine its capacity to survive (Bromage et al., 1992). Many factors have been identified as important in relation to egg quality, e.g. diet (the ration and its formulation), spawning methods, husbandry, manipulations, induced spawning, environment, selection and culture conditions.

Testes, spermatogenesis and spermiation

The testes of teleost fish are in most cases a pair of elongated structures composed of branching seminiferous tubules embedded in the stroma. These thin-walled tubules or lobules contain germ cells, the spermatogonia.

Primary spermatogonia, which are present throughout the year, divide mitotically to give rise to secondary spermatogonia which are transformed into primary spermatocytes. These divide by meiosis giving rise to spermatids from which the spermatozoa are formed. The seminiferous tubules are packed with spermatozoa in the pre-spawning and spawning periods (Winkoop et al., 1995).

Hormonal regulation
Testosterone is the main regulator of spermatogenesis while 11-ketotestosterone and 17α, hydroxy 20β, dihydroxy progesterone are involved in spermiogenesis and spermiation.

12.3 Reproductive management by using hormone preparations

In most cultivated species, gametogenesis generally develops normally in captivity, if fish are kept under the appropriate conditions of temperature and photoperiod, but the final important physiological steps often do not take place spontaneously, leading to poor sperm production in males and the blockade of ovulation in females. This is linked to a lack of environmental stimuli necessary for the release of GnRH and/or a decrease in the inhibitory influence of dopamine to allow for the induction of an ovulatory LH surge.

The most logical point at which to intervene in fish reproduction is at the environmental level, i.e. adjusting the environmental conditions to induce spawning. However, while this approach has been successful in some species, in many others it has failed. In the course of improved broodstock management, there are four areas that can be manipulated to provide the industry with the required quality and quantity of offspring at any given period of the year.

Maturation and ovulation
Induced ovulation involves the induction of final oocyte maturation (germinal vesicle migration and breakdown) in the female. Various hormones and other pharmaceutical compounds are used to induce maturation and ovulation of post-vitellogenic oocytes. These processes can be induced by fish pituitary extract (FPE), human chorionic gonadotrophin (hCG), 17α hydroxy 20β dihydroxy progesterone, GnRH analogues and dopamine antagonists (Chaudhuri 1994; Zohar and Mylonas 2001). Most species require manual stripping (artificial spawning) after induced ovulation.

Spermiation

For most male teleost fish broodstock, spermatogenesis and spermiation are usually adequate and need no hormonal treatment. However, many salmonid hatchery owners encounter the problem of either early or late spermiation in relation to ovulation in the female, leading to a lack of sperm, low availability of milt or poor sperm production, which is generally the case in numerous marine species which require the rearing of large numbers of mature males. Goren et al. (1995) showed that GnRH analogue implants resulted in improved milt volume in Atlantic salmon (70 ml per fish in the treated group compared with 12 ml per fish in the controls).

Synchronization

Synchronization of a population of broodfish reduces the period in which spawning occurs when compared with untreated groups of female broodfish (for review, see Zohar and Mylonas 2001). When salmonids are treated with GnRH several weeks prior to normal spawning, up to 90-100% of them can ovulate within 12-15 days of treatment. In the untreated group, often only about 10% ovulate in the same period, while the remaining controls ovulate in an unsynchronized manner over 30-60 days (Breton et al., 1990; Goren et al., 1995; Haffray et al., 2005).

Figure 3 Synchronization and induction of ovulation in fish

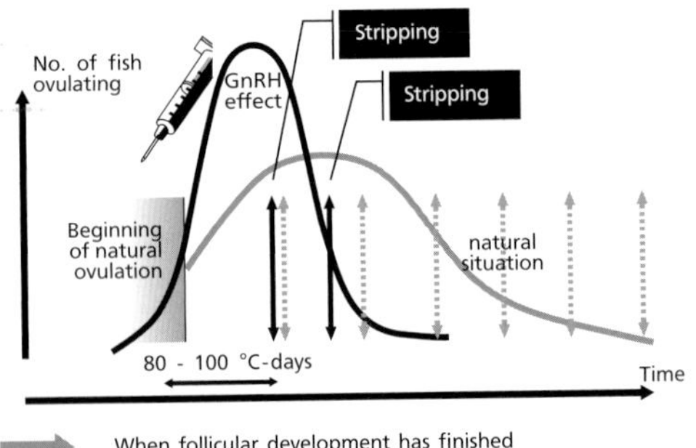

Out of season spawning
Of great practical application for altering the rate of maturation and the time of spawning is the use of modified light or photoperiod regimes, and temperature manipulation. In Atlantic salmon in particular, even a modest 4- to 6-week advancement in spawning constitutes a considerable commercial advantage, because fry are available and can become S1s (1-year smolts that can be released into the sea) (Bromage 1995). In general, while egg quality may suffer slightly, GnRH agonists are effective in inducing and advancing spawning, when administered as early as 6 weeks prior to natural spawning. An acceleration of maturation of up to 4 weeks can be achieved (Goren et al., 1995; Haffray et al., 2005).

Figure 4 Cumulative ovulation in Atlantic salmon after single injection of the spawning aid, Gonazon®. Scotland, injected Dec. 7, brackish water 9°C, 0% natural ovulation at the time of injection,

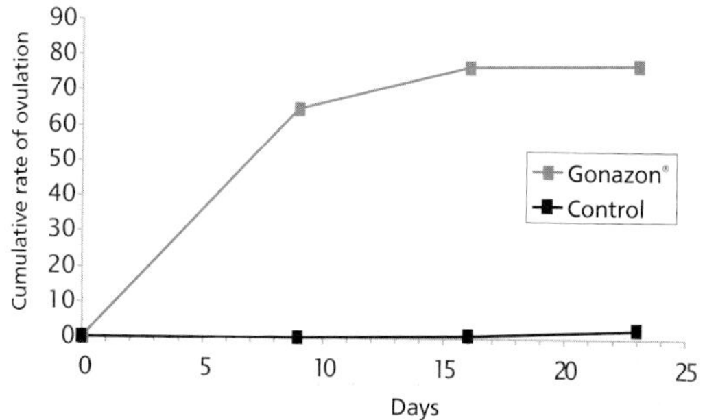

12.4 Induction of spawning

The experimental work on controlled reproduction in fish, for the purpose of seed production in aquaculture practices, can be divided into those studying environmental parameters and those studying the effect of various hormones (of both piscine and mammalian origin).

Environmental manipulation

It is well known that environmental factors influence the reproduction of many animals, including fish. Those factors believed to influence maturation and spawning in fish are temperature, light (photoperiod), salinity, pH, turbidity, and meteorological factors such as rainfall, flood, water current and lunar periodicity (for review, see Bromage et al., 2001; Glasser et al., 2004).

The seasonality of spawning imposes considerable constraints on trout and salmon farming because the consequent restrictions on the supply of eggs and fry make it difficult for rearing farms to maintain a continuity of production of fish of a suitable size for eating, throughout the year (Bromage et al., 1992). Long days early in the reproductive cycle, and short days at any time in the 3-4 months before the summer, advances sexual maturation, whereas short days during the first few months of the cycle, or long days after the summer solstice, delay sexual maturation in rainbow trout (Bromage et al., 1982).

Hormonal treatment

The hormonal induction of spawning is usually carried out in fish that do not normally spawn spontaneously in captivity. For the species which spawn naturally in confinement, hormonal manipulation is undertaken in order to synchronize the spawning of a group of females for the mass production of fry (Ayson 1991; Yaron 1995; Peter and Yu 1997).

Hypophysation

The term 'hypophysation' in this context means the injection of crude fish pituitary extracts (FPE). This method was developed in Argentina many years ago (Houssay 1930). FPE includes gonadotrophic hormones which stimulate the maturation of gonads and reproduction in fish. In many countries, pituitary extracts are used extensively, although periodically there are problems with purity, specificity, continuity of supply, potency and microbiological safety.

Gonadotrophin-releasing hormones (GnRH/LHRH)

GnRH (a linear chain of 10 amino acids) is a potent inducer of GtH release. In practice, synthetic analogues of GnRH are used because they are more potent or because they have a longer-lasting action than the naturally-occurring hormone (i.e. they are better able to withstand enzymatic degradation) (Zohar 1996). In addition to the induction or release of GtH by GnRH, there is evidence that, in teleost fish, LH secretion is under the control of an inhibitory hormone, dopamine (Peter et al., 1988).

Depending on the species, the inhibitory influence of this hormone can block GnRH action, as in most cyprinids and silurids, whereas, in other species, such as in salmonids and most of the marine species, it is not potent enough to block GnRH action.

When necessary, treatment with antagonists of dopamine, such as pimozide or domperidone, together with GnRH, leads to an enhanced release of GtH as compared to the effect of GnRH alone (Sokolowska et al., 1985; Lin et al., 1986; Mikolajczyk et al., 2004).

Human Chorionic Gonadotrophin (hCG)

From the early 1960s, hCG has been largely used for inducing gonadal maturation and spawning in fish. HCG has one big advantage over several of the other hormones and FPE, namely that its potency can be standardised in International Units (IU), so that the results of different investigations can be properly compared.

Chaudhuri (1994) provided quite a long list of positive results obtained by administration of hCG to various fish species.

Sex steroids, pheromones, prostaglandins

It is known that gonadotrophins stimulate the production of sex steroids, which in turn induce maturation and ovulation in fish (Resink et al., 1987; Weerd et al., 1990). Experiments on gonadal steroids have not been very encouraging so far. In addition, progestagens, such as 17α, hydroxy 20β, dihydroxy progesterone, are very expensive.

Pheromones are substances secreted by an individual that may provoke a specific reaction in the opposite sex of the same species. They occur in fish, just as in mammals, and may exert strong influences. For example, Weerd et al. (1990) showed a significant effect of male pheromones on the gonadosomatic index (GSI) of female African catfish.

Prostaglandins have been implicated in the ovulation of oocytes from the follicles in some species (Stacey and Goetz 1982).

12.5 Mode of administration

There are basically two routes by which to administer different endocrine products to teleost fish. The most common technique is injection of the product (typically the active dissolved in a solvent), whereas newer methods, such as the injection of impregnated implants or oral administration, are either not widely used (i.e. not widely registered) or still under evaluation.

Injection

The majority of the fish species treated with hormone preparations are injected with a solution either intramuscularly or intraperitoneally. The latter method, unless performed by an experienced operator, risks damaging or infecting the intestine of the fish. Depending on the species, the rapid clearance of injected GnRH analogue from the circulation may require multiple injections in order to achieve an effective response. Excessive handling of fish receiving multiple injections can lead to stress-related injuries, mortalities and suppression of reproductive processes.

A relatively new method is the implantation of controlled-release delivery systems (Zohar 1996; Zohar and Mylonas 2001). The prolonged diffusion of the implant prevents the problems associated with multiple injections (Goren et al., 1995). However, such implants and indeed many other GnRH or GnRH-dopamine antagonist-containing solutions, may not be approved for commercial use in many countries.

Dietary treatment

Certain fish species are especially susceptible to the stress of handling when they are in a spawning condition. They may fail to ovulate or may even die if they are not anaesthetised prior to netting, handling and injection, particularly if the environmental conditions are sub-optimal (Thomas et al., 1995). Thomas and Boyd (1989) administered 1.0-2.5 mg of a GnRH analogue per kg body weight orally, which resulted in spawning of sea trout after 32-38 hours with high rates of fertilization and hatching. Similar results were obtained in African catfish and common carp (Breton et al., 1998b; Mikolajczyk et al., 2002), Thai carp (Sukumasavin et al., 1992) and sable fish (Solar et al., 1990). This method has some disadvantages as it is usually impossible to achieve the correct dose per individual and some species do not accept feed during the spawning season.

12.6 Propagation

The propagation of fish starts with the collection of eggs and sperm. Generally these gametes are obtained by 'stripping' the ripe spawners or by collecting the fertilised eggs after mating in artificial enclosures (Huisman 1976).

Collection of eggs
To secure the maximum control over the eggs, most species are manually stripped using one of three methods.

a. Eggs are stripped by gently massaging the belly in the direction of the genital pore;
b. The belly is opened surgically and the eggs are removed by hand;
c. A needle is inserted at the posterior end of the belly in order to introduce air to help flush out the eggs from the anterior end.

Collection of sperm
Collection of sperm from male broodstock can be achieved by stripping the male or by removing the ripe testis by surgery. The quality of sperm is highly variable and depends on various external factors such as the feeding regime, the quality of the feed and the rearing temperature of the males. The most commonly used parameters for assessing sperm quality are its motility and survival during storage (Billard et al., 1995).

Fertilization

In general, three different methods of artificial fertilization are in use, all of which involve the manual removal of gametes from the broodfish.

a. Wet method. The gametes are stripped into a pan filled with water;
b. Dry method. Eggs are stripped into a dry pan, dry sperm are mixed with eggs and water is added afterwards.
c. Super-dry. This method is based on (b), but the eggs are stripped onto a sieve to get rid of the ovarian fluid (Huisman 1976). If present, ovarian fluid needs to be removed since it inhibits the movement of sperm. This is very important in the salmonids.

Incubation

After fertilization, eggs can be incubated. Different incubator systems are in use for the various species, depending on the biological requirements of the incubated eggs and local customs. Optimal hatching temperatures vary, e.g. 25-28°C for Chinese carp with hatching after 23-28 hours, but 5°C for halibut eggs, with hatching after 16-19 days (Kjørsvik and Holmefjord 1995). For salmonids, incubation in cold water lasts from about 2 months for rainbow trout and to 6 months for Atlantic salmon or Arctic charr. During incubation, the sensitivity of the eggs varies widely and oxygen supply is of great importance.

Hatching

At the end of egg development the eggs hatch. Hatching can be accelerated by increasing the temperature (Sorensen et al., 1966). However, Lilelund (1967) showed that, for pike, when incubation took place at lower temperatures, birth occurred in a more advanced morphological stage, the larvae being bigger than normal.

12.7 Reproduction-related diseases

Broodstock should be managed to avoid subsequent diseases in progeny resulting in inferior quality offspring.

Vertical transmission
A number of diseases are described that can be transmitted vertically from broodstock to offspring. Bacterial Kidney Disease (BKD) caused by *Renibacterium salmoninarum* is transmitted within the egg. After proper surface disinfection, it was found that 10-20% of the eggs sterile on their surface were still positive for BKD in one study (Evelyn et al., 1984). While the isolation of broodfish may not be critical, the eggs from individual spawners should be quarantined after fertilisation so that the parents can be screened for these pathogens (Pascho et al., 1991).

Contamination
The culture of eggs and larvae of fish in the same environment enhances microbial growth, as a result of the increased volume of available nutrients from the metabolic by-products of the fish, and the increased number of surfaces on which organic debris can be trapped and which micro-organisms can colonise.
Another source of nutrients is the various lipid and protein components of fish eggs that are released at hatching. The most frequently isolated bacteria from the surface of live eggs are members of the genera *Cytophaga, Pseudomonas, Alteromonas, Flavobacterium* and *Aeromonas*. As well as being in the water, these bacteria are often present in the coelomic fluid of the maturing female (Kjørsvik and Holmefjord 1995).

12.8 Gender control

Gender control is of importance for maximising the economic efficacy of production systems (Donaldson 1996). A number of techniques are available, all of them aimed at the development of monosex populations, which have major advantages over mixed populations (such as better growth rate, more homogeneity, lower susceptibility to disease and better meat quality).

Sex reversal

The advantage of 100% monosex cultures also includes reduced gonadal development with no production of offspring during the grow-out phase (Komen et al., 1989). Hand-sorting by gender, hybridisation or hormone treatment are the most common methods of producing monosex stocks in commercial practice (MacIntosh and Little 1995).

For tilapia, hormonal sex reversal by masculinisation of fry with androgens (typically 17-methyl-testosterone) is widely recognised as having significant advantages over both hand-sorting and hybridisation (McAndrew 1993; Lin et al., 1995). However, in some countries (e.g., EU), monosex female populations are produced by indirect feminisation so as to ensure that fish are not exposed directly to steroids.

Gynogenesis

The term gynogenesis implies that the genomic inheritance of the embryo is entirely female. It means that the chromosomes of the fertilising spermatozoon need to be inactivated, without affecting its functional ability to fertilise. Gynogenetic haploid fish do not survive beyond yolk-sac absorption. Diploidy can be restored by interfering with meiosis, by retaining the second polar body with its haploid set of chromosomes, or by interfering with mitosis, by preventing the first cell division (Komen et al., 1988).

Androgenesis

In androgenesis, eggs are irradiated to destroy the female nuclear material. Fertilising these treated eggs using a homozygous sperm donor results in the production of clones (Bongers et al., 1994).

Triploidy

Much of the interest in induced triploidy in fish culture is based on the assumption that triploids would be sterile and may show better growth than diploids at the period of maturation and reproduction of diploids (Purdom 1976; Johnstone et al., 1991). It can also prevent cultured exotic species from forming self-sustaining feral populations. Cold-shocking of eggs is a successful method for inducing triploidy in the African catfish (Richter et al., 1986). Heat shock is applied for inducing of triploidy in salmonid fish (Chevassues et al., 1983; Quillet et al., 1991).

12.9 Transgenesis

Gene transfer has become a very active topic for fish research in recent years (Chen and Powers 1990). The principal approach used to transfer genes into fish eggs is by micro-injection. Cloned DNA sequences are injected into the eggs shortly after fertilization. Transfer of the genes can then be monitored by the presence of the foreign DNA in the progeny or by expression of the foreign genes. The genetic constructs introduced into fish were aimed at antifreeze protein and growth hormones from different sources (Maclean and Penman 1990; Delvin et al., 1995). Public perception and hazards associated with the possible escape of transgenic animals into the wild are the two major elements presently constraining the production and application of transgenic fish in the aquaculture industry (Thorgaard 1995).

12.10 Acknowledgements

The assistance and critical review by Dr. Bernard Breton (formerly of INRA, Rennes, France) and Dr. Tomek Mikolajczyk and Dr. Mirka Sokolowska (University of Agriculture, Krakow, Poland) are very much appreciated.

12.11 References

Ayson FG. Induced spawning of rabbitfish, *Siganus guttatus* (Bloch) using human chorionic gonadotropin (HCG). Aquaculture 1991, 95:133-37.
Bayarri MJ., Rodriguez L., Zanuy S., Madrid JA., Sanchez-Vazquez FJ., Kagawa H., Okuzawa K., Carrillo M. Effect of photoperiod manipulation on the daily rhythms of melatonin and reproductive hormones in caged European sea bass (Dicentrarchus labrax). Gen Comp Endocrinol 2004;136:72-81.
Billard R. Reproduction in rainbow trout: sex differentiation, dynamics of gametogenesis, biology and preservation of gametes. Aquaculture 1992;100:263-98.
Billard R., Cosson J., Crim LW., Suquet M. Sperm physiology and quality. In: Bromage N, Roberts RJ, editors. Broodstock management and egg and larval quality. Blackwell Science, London, UK. 1995, pp. 25-52.

Bongers ABJ., 't Veld EPC., Abo-Hashema K., Bremmer IM., Eding EH., Komen J., Richter CJJ. Androgenesis in common carp (*Cyprinius carpio* L.) using UV-irradiation in a synthetic ovarian fluid and heat shocks. Aquaculture 1994;122:119-32.
Breton B., Weil C., Sambroni E., Zohar Y. Effects of acute versus sustained administration of GnRHa on GtH release and ovulation in the rainbow trout Oncorhynchus mykiss. Aquaculture 1990; 91:373-383.
Breton B., Govoroun M., Mikolajczyk T. GtH I and GtH II secretion profiles during the reproductive cycle in female rainbow trout: relationship with pituitary responsiveness to GnRH-A stimulation. Gen Comp Endocrinol 1998a;111:38-50.
Breton B., Roelants Y., Ollevier F., Epler P., Mikolajczyk T. Improved bioavailability of orally delivered peptides and polypeptides in teleost fish. J Appl Ichthyol 1998b;14:251-257.
Bromage N. Broodstock management and seed quality - general considerations. In: Bromage N, Roberts RJ, editors. Broodstock management and egg and larval quality. Blackwell Science, London, UK. 1995, pp. 1-24.
Bromage N., Whitehead C., Elliot J., Breton B., Matty A. Investigation into the importance of daylength on the photoperiod control of reproduction in the female rainbow trout. In: Richter C, Goos HTh, editors. Reproductive Physiology of Fish. Pudoc, Wageningen. 1982, pp. 233-236.
Bromage N. Propagation and stock improvement. In: Sheppard J, Bromage N, editors. Intensive Fish Farming. Blackwell Science, Oxford, UK. 1988, pp. 103-150.
Bromage N., Porter M., Randall C. The environmental regulation of maturation in farmed finfish with special reference to the role of photoperiod and melatonin. Aquaculture 2001;197:63-98.
Bromage N., Jones J., Randall C., Thrush M., Davies B., Springate J., Duston J., Barker G. Broodstock management, fecundity, egg quality and the timing of egg production in the rainbow trout (*Onchorhynchus mykiss*). Aquaculture 1992;100:141-166.
Bromage NR., Randall CF., Porter MJR., Davies B. How do photoperiod, the pi neal gland, melatonin and circannual rhythms interact to co-ordinate seasonal reproduction in salmonid fish? In: Goetz R, Thomas P, editors. Reproductive Physiology of Fish. The University of Texas, Austin, USA. July 2-8 1995.
Chaudhuri H. History of induced breeding and its applications to aquaculture. Proc Zool Soc, Calcutta. 1994, 47:1-31.
Chen TT., Powers DA. Transgenic fish. Trends in biotechnology 1990;8:209-215.
Chevassues B., Quillet E., Chourrout D. Note technique: obtention d'animaux triploides chez la truite arc-en-ciel. Bull Fr Piscic 1983; 290:161-164.
Chyb J., Mikolajczyk T., Breton B. Post-ovulatory secretion of pituitary gonadotropins GtH I and GtH II in the rainbow trout (Oncorhynchus mykiss): regulation by steroids and possible role of non-steroidal gonadal factors. J Endocrinol1999 ;163: 87-97.
Delvin RH., Yesaki TY., Donaldson EM., Du SJ., Hew CL. Production of germline transgenic Pacific salmonids with dramatically increased growth performance. Can J Fish Aquat Sci 1995;52:1376-1384.
Donaldson EM. Manipulation of reproduction in farmed fish. Anim Reprod Sci 1996;42:381-392.
Evelyn TPT., Ketcheson JE., Prosperiporta L. Further evidence for the presence of *Renibacterium marinum* in salmonid eggs and for the failure of povidone-iodine to reduce the intra ovum infection rate in water-hardened eggs. J Fish Dis 1984;7:173-182.
FAO. Reproductive physiology of teleost fishes. A review of present knowledge and needs for future research. Aquaculture development and coordination programme. Rome. 1981, ADCP/REP/81/16.

Glasser F., Mikolajczyk T., Jalabert B., Baroiller J-F., Breton B. Temperature effects along the reproductive axis during spawning induction of grass carp (Ctenopharyngodon idella). Gen Comp Endocrinol 2004;136:171-179.

Goren A., Gustafson HM., Doering DS. Field trials demonstrate the efficacy and commercial benefit of a GnRHa implant to control ovulation and spermiation in salmonids. In: Goetz R, Thomas P, editors. Reproductive Physiology of Fish. The University of Texas, Austin, USA. July 2-8, 1995, pp. 1-4.

Haffray P., Enright WJ., Driancourt MA., Mikolajczyk T., Rault P., Breton B. Optimization of breeding of Salmonids: Gonazon™, the first officially approved inducer of ovulation in the EU. World Aquaculture, March 2005, pp. 52-56.

Houssay BA. Accion sexual de la hip[ofisis en los peces y reptiles. Rev Soc Arg Bio 1930;106: 686-688.

Huisman EA. Hatchery and nursery operations in fish culture management. In: Huisman EA editor. Aspects of fish culture of fish breeding. Miscellaneous papers, 13. Landbouwhogeschool Wageningen, The Netherlands. 1976, pp 29-47.

Itoh H., Suzuki K., Kawauchi H. The complete amino acid sequences of α. subunits of chum salmon gonadotropins. Gen Comp Endocrinol 1990;78: 56-65.

Johnstone R., MaLay HA.,Walsingham MV. Production and performance of triploid Atlantic salmon in Scotland. Can Tech Rep Fish Aquac Sci 1991;1789:15-36.

Khan I., Thomas P. Melatonin influences gonadotropin II secretion in the Atlantic croaker (*Micropogonias undulatus*). Gen Comp Endocrinol 1996;104:231-242.

Kjørsvik E., Holmefjord I. Atlantic Halibut (*Hippoglossus hippoglossus*) and cod (*Gadus morhua*). In: Bromage NR, Roberts RJ editors. Broodstock management and egg and larval quality, Blackwell science, Oxford, UK. 1995, pp. 169-196.

Komen J., Duynhouwer J., Richter CJJ., Huisman EA. Gynogenesis in common carp (*Cyprinus carpio L.*) I. Effects of genetic manipulation of sexual products and incubation conditions of eggs. Aquaculture 1988;69:227-239.

Komen J., Lodder PAJ., Huskens F., Richter CJJ., Huisman EA. Effects of oral administration of 17a-methyltestosterone and 17b-oestradiol on gonadal development in common carp, *Cyprinus carpio* L. Aquaculture 1989;78:349-363.

Lillelund K. Versuche zur Erbrutung der Eier vom Hecht. *Esox lucius* L. in Abhangigkeit von temperatur und licht. Arch Fish Wiss 1967; 17:95-113.

Lin HR., Peter RE. Hormones and spawning in fish. Asian Fish Sci 1996;9:21-33.

Little DC., Lin CK., Turner WA. Commercial scale tilapia fry production in Thailand. World Aqua Soc 1995;26:21-24.

MacIntosh DJ., Little DC. Nile tilapia (*Oreochromis niloticus*). In: Bromage NR Roberts RJ, editors. Broodstock management and egg and larval quality, Blackwell science, Oxford, UK. 1995, pp. 277-320.

Maclean N., Penman D. The application of gene manipulation to aquaculture. Aquaculture 1990;85:1-20.

McAndrew BJ. Sex control in tilapines. In: Muir JF, Roberts RJ, editors. Recent advances in aquaculture, IV. Blackwell Science, Oxford, UK. 1993, pp. 87-98.

Mikolajczyk T., Roelants I., Epler P., Ollevier F., Chyb J., Breton B. Modified absorption of sGnRH-a following rectal and oral delivery to common carp, *Cyprinus carpio* L. Aquaculture 2002;203:375-388.

Mikolajczyk T., Chyb J., Szczerbik P., Sokolowska-Mikolajczyk M., Epler P., Enright WJ., Filipiak M., Breton B. Evaluation of the potency of azagly-nafarelin (GnRH analogue), administered in combination with different formulations of pimozide, on LH secretion, evulation and egg quality in common carp (*Cyprinus carpio* L) under laboratory, commercial hatchery and natural conditions. Aquaculture 2004;234:447-460.

Nagahama Y. Endocrine regulation of gametogenesis in fish. Int J Dev Biol 1994;38:217-229.

Nagahama Y., Yoshikuni M., Yamashita M., Sakai N., Tanaka M. Molecular endocrinology of oocyte growth and maturation in fish. Fish Physiol Biochem 1993;11:3-14.

Pascho RJ., Elliott DG., Streufert JM. Broodstock segregation of spring chinook salmon *Onchorhynchus tshawytscha* by use of the enzyme-linked immunosorbent assay (ELISA) and the fluorescent antibody technique (FAT) affects the prevalence and levels of *Renibacterium salmoninarum* infection in progeny. Dis Aqua Org 1991;12:25-40.

Peter R., Lin H., Van der Kraak G. Induced ovulation and spawning of cultured freshwater fish in China: Advances in application of GnRH analogues and dopamine antagonists. Aquaculture 1988;74:1-10.

Peter RE., Lin HR., Van der Kraak G., Litte M. Release hormones, dopamine antagonists and induced spawning. In: Muir JF, Roberts RJ, editors. Recent advances in aquaculture IV. Blackwell Scientific Publications, Oxford, UK. 1993, pp. 25-30.

Peter RE., Yu KL. Nueroendocrine regulation of ovulation in fishes: basic and applied aspects. Rev Fish Biol 1997;7:173-197.

Purdom CE. Genetic techniques in flatfish culture. J Fish Res Board Can 1976;33:1088-1093.

Quillet E., Foisil L., Chevassues B., Chourrout D., Liu FG. Production of all-triploid and all-female brown trout for aquaculture. Aquat Living Resour 1991;4: 27-32.

Resink JW., Groenix van Zoelen RFO., Huisman EA., Van den Hurk R. The seminal vesicle as source of sex attracting substances in the African catfish, *Clarias gariepinus*. Aquaculture 1987;63:115-128.

Richter CJJ., Henken AM., Eding EH., Van Doesum JH., De Boer P. Induction of triploidy by cold shocking eggs and performance of triploids in the African catfish, *Clarias gariepinus* (Burchell 1822). Proc. EIFAC/FAO symp. on Selection, Hybridization and Genetic Engeneering in Aquaculture of Fish And Shellfish for consumption and stocking. Bordeaux, France. May 27-30, 1986.

Richter CJJ., Eding EH., Verreth JAJ., Fleuren WLG. African catfish, *Clarias gariepinus*. In: Bromage NR, Roberts RJ, editors. Broodstock management and egg and larval quality. Blackwell Science, Oxford, UK. 1995, pp. 242-276.

Saligaut C., Linard B., Mananos E., Kah O., Breton B., Govoroun M. Release of pituitary gonadotropins GTH I and GTH II in the rainbow trout (*Onchorhynchus mykiss*): modulation by estradiol and catecholamines. Gen Comp Endocrinol 1998;109:302-309.

Sherwood NM., Wu S. Developmental role of GnRH and PACAP in a zebrafish model. Gen Comp Endocrinol 2005;142:74-80.

Sokolowska M., Peter RE., Nahorniak CS. The effects of different doses of pimozide and D-Ala6, Pro9-Nethylamide-LHRH (LHRH-A) on gonadotropin release and ovulation in female glodfish. Can J Zool 1985;63:1252-1256.

Sorensen L., Buss K., Bradfort AD. The artificial propagation of Escoid fishes in Pennsylvania. Prog Fish Cul 1966;28:133-141.

Somoza GM., Miranda LA., Strobl-Mazulla P., Guilgur LG. Gonadotropin-releasing hormone (GnRH): from fish to mammalian brains. Cell Mol Neurobiol 2002;22:589-609.

Solar II., McLean E., Baker JJ., Sherwood NM., Donaldson EM. Induced ovulation in sablefish (*Anopoploma fimbria* Pallas), following oral administration of Des Gly10 (D-Ala6) LHRH ethylamid. Fish Physiol Biochem 1990;8:497-499.

Stacey NE, Goetz FW. Role of prostaglandins in fish reproduction. Can Fish Aquat Sci 1982, 39:92-98.

Sukumasavin N., Leelapatra W., McLean E., Donaldson EM. Orally induced spawning of Thai carp (*Puntius gonionotus* Bleeker) following co-administration of Des Gly10 (D-Arg6) sGnRH ethylamide and domperidone. J Fish Biol 1992;40:477-479.

Suzuki K., Kawauchi H., Nagahama H. Isolation and characterisation of two distinct gonadotropins from chum salmon pituitary glands. Gen Comp Endocrinol 1988a;71:292-301.

Suzuki K., Kawauchi H., Nagahama H. Isolation and characterisation of subunits from two distinct salmon gonadotropins. Gen Comp Endocrinol 1988b;71:302-306.

Suzuki K., Nagahama Y., Kawauchi H. Steroidogenic activity of two distinct salmon gonadotropins. Gen Comp Endocrinol 1988c; 71:452-458.

Swanson P. Salmon gonadotropins: reconciling old and new ideas. In: Scott AP, Sumpter JP, Kime DE, Rolfe MS, editors. Reproductive physiology in fish. University of East Anglia Press, UK. 1991, pp. 2-7.

Thomas P., Boyd, NW. Dietary administration of a LHRH analog induces successful spawning in spotted seatrout (*Cyniscion nebulosus*). Aquaculture 1989;80:363-370.

Thomas P., Arnold CR., Holt GJ. Red drum and other sciaenids. In: Bromage NR, Roberts RJ editors. Broodstock management and egg and larval quality. Blackwell Science, Oxford, UK. 1995, pp. 118-137.

Thorgaard GH. Biotechnological approaches to broodstock management. In: Bromage NR, Roberts JR, editors. Broodstock management and egg and larval quality. Blackwell Science, Oxford, UK. 1995, pp. 76-93.

Weerd JH van., Sukkel M., Richter CJJ. An analysis of sex stimuli enhancing ovarian growth in pubertal African catfish *Clarias gariepinus*. Aquaculture 1990;75:181-191.

Winkoop A van., Timmermans LPM., Goos HJTh. Stimulation of gonadal and germ cell development in larval and juvenile carp (*Cyprinus carpio* L.) by homologous pituitary extract. Fish Physiol Biochem 1995;13:161-171.

Yaron Z. Endocrine control of gametogenesis and spawning induction in the carp. Aquaculture 1995;129:49-73.

Yaron Z., Gur G., Melamed P., Rosenfeld H., Elizur A., Levavi-Sivan B. Regulation of fish gonadotropins. Int Rev Cytol 2003; 225:131-185.

Yoshiura Y., Kobayashi M., Kato Y., Aida K. Molecular cloning of the cDNA encoding two gonadotropin β subunits (GTH-Iβ and IIβ) from the goldfish (*Carassius auratus*). Gen Comp Endocrinol 1997;105:379-389.

Zohar Y. New approaches for the manipulation of ovulation and spawning in farmed fish. Bull Natl Res Inst Aquacul 1996;2:43-48.

Zohar Y., Mylonas CC. Endocrine manipulations of spawning in cultured fish: from hormones to genes. Aquaculture 2001;197:99-136.

13 Product Information

13.1 Introduction

This chapter contains general information on the Intervet/Schering-Plough products used in reproduction throughout the world. For each product the description, mode of action, indications, dosage and administration, contraindications and warnings, withholding period for milk and meat, storage conditions and the available presentations are given.

Regarding the withholding period it is important to remember that only an indication can be given. Due to local differences in registration laws, the withholding period can differ from the ones mentioned. It is important to bear in mind that for certain products licensing conditions such as presentations and indications for use may differ in individual countries. Therefore it is advised to consult the leaflet of the product locally purchased.

13.2 Chorulon®

Description

Chorulon® is presented in vials as a white freeze-dried crystalline plug containing either 500, 1500, 2500, 5000 and 10000 IU hCG (human Chorionic Gonadotrophin) together with a vial containing solvent for reconstitution.

Mode of action

The active compound of Chorulon® is hCG, a complex glycoprotein. hCG is a gonadotrophin with Luteinizing Hormone (LH) activities. In the female, hCG can be used to stimulate the developing follicle towards maturation and to induce ovulation to bring about luteinization of the granulosa cells, to maintain the functional life of the corpus luteum and to increase progesterone secretion from luteinized cells. hCG also augments the action of FSH on ovarian growth.

In the male, hCG stimulates testosterone production and thus influences the development and maintenance of primary and secondary male sex characteristics.

Indications

Chorulon® can be used in the following fertility problems in domestic animals:

- cases of repeated failure of conception in cows and heifers
- induction of ovulation in mares and bitches
- cases of cystic ovaries in cows and heifers
- anoestrus in mares and bitches
- delayed ovulation, prolonged pro-oestrus in bitches
- deficiency in libido in male dogs

Dosage and administration

Reconstitute with the solvent provided, ensuring the freeze-dried plug is fully dissolved. Administer by intramuscular or intravenous injection, observing the usual aseptic precautions.

Species	Indication	Dosage	Administration
Cow, heifer	Improvement of conception rate at AI or mating	1500 IU	i.m. or i.v.
	Cystic ovarian disease (anoestrus, prolonged oestrus, nymphomania)	3000 IU	i.v.
Mare	Anoestrus (follicles ≥ 2 cm diameter)	1500-3000 IU repeat if necessary after 2 days	i.m or i.v.
	Induction of ovulation (follicles ≥ 3.5 cm diameter)	1500-3000 IU 24 hours later AI or mating	i.v.
Bitch	Anoestrus	after pre-treatment with Folligon® (PMSG): 500 IU at first day of oestrus	i.m
	Delayed ovulation Prolonged oestrus	100-800 IU/day repeat treatment until vaginal discharge disappears	i.m
Dog	Deficient libido	100-500 IU 6-12 hours before mating	i.m.

Contraindications, warnings

For animal treatment only. Keep out of the reach and sight of children.

In rare cases, as with all protein preparations, anaphylactoid reactions may occur shortly after injection. Adrenalin injection (1:1000) given intravenously or intramuscularly when symptoms appear is the standard treatment. The administration of corticosteroids may also be indicated.

User warning

Care should be taken to avoid accidental self-injection.

If accidental self-injection occurs, seek medical advice immediately and show the doctor the package leaflet. In such circumstances, prompt medication with adrenaline (1:1000) or glucocorticosteroids may be indicated.

Withdrawal period

Tissues/products	Species	Withdrawal periods*
Edible tissues	Cattle	Nil
Edible tissues	Horses	Nil
Milk	Cattle	Nil

** Local regulations should be observed.*

Pharmaceutical precautions

Before reconstitution: Do not store above 25°C. After reconstitution: Protect from light.

Any product not used immediately after reconstitution should be stored refrigerated between +2°C and +8°C. Reconstituted product remaining 24 hours after preparation should be discarded.

Avoid the introduction of contaminants during use.

Dispose of any unused product and empty containers in accordance with local waste regulation authority.

Presentation

Vials of 500, 1500, 2500, 5000 and 10000 IU hCG, together with solvent for reconstitution.

13.3 Chorulon® in fish breeding

Description

Chorulon® is presented in vials as a white freeze-dried crystalline plug containing either 500, 1500, 5000 IU Human Chorionic Gonadotrophin together with a vial containing solvent for reconstitution.

Mode of action

hCG is a gonadotrophin with Luteinizing Hormone (LH) activities, including maintenance of the functional life of the corpus luteum and stimulating the luteinized cells to increase progesterone secretion.
17α-hydroxy-progesterone and 17α-hydroxy-20β-dihydroprogesterone stimulate the maturation, ovulation and water absorption of the oocytes. The steroids produced by the male Leydig cells in the testis are androgens that stimulate spermatogenesis and water absorption of the testis and seminal vesicles.

Indications

An aid to the improvement of spawning function in female and male brood fish.

Dosage and administration

Reconstitute with the solvent provided, ensuring the freeze-dried plug is fully dissolved. Administer by intramuscular or intraperitoneal injection, observing the usual aseptic precautions.
Anaesthesia of brood fish is often needed to avoid stress and to reduce backflow of fluid after withdrawal of the syringe.
Most fish respond to a single injection of Chorulon®, but some species require two injections with an interval ranging from several hours to three days. In the latter case, the first injection is usually 10% of the total dose administered.
Dosages used for the various fish species typically range from 200 – 4000 IU/kg bodyweight (usually lower for males) but higher doses (up to 60000 IU/kg bodyweight) may be required for some species.

Contraindications, warnings

For animal treatment only. Keep out of the reach and sight of children.

Chorulon® contains a natural glycoprotein, free from toxic properties.

Chorulon® does not induce antibodies in fish. Therefore, fish can be treated repeatedly without any loss of efficacy.

User warning

Care should be taken to avoid accidental self-injection.

If accidental self-injection occurs, seek medical advice immediately and show the doctor the package leaflet. In such circumstances, prompt medication with adrenaline (1:1000) or glucocorticosteroids may be indicated.

Withdrawal period

Nil. Local regulations should be observed.

Pharmaceutical precautions

Before reconstitution: Do not store above 25°C. After reconstitution: Protect from light.

Any product not used immediately after reconstitution should be stored refrigerated between +2°C and +8°C. Reconstituted product remaining 24 hours after preparation should be discarded.

Avoid the introduction of contamination during use.

Dispose of any unused product and empty containers in accordance with local waste regulations.

Presentation

Vials of 500, 1500 or 5000 IU hCG, together with solvent for reconstitution.

13.4 Chronogest CR®

Description
Chronogest CR® is a controlled release intravaginal sponge impregnated with 20mg cronolone for use in sheep and goats.

Mode of action
Whilst in the vagina, the sponge releases cronolone, a progestagen which is absorbed and subjects the animal to a level of progestagen comparable with the luteal phase of the oestrous cycle. This artificially imposed progestational phase is ended by the removal of the sponge.
The injection of Folligon® (Chrono-gest PMSG®) induces the start of the follicular phase, culminating in oestrus and ovulation. Application to a number of females synchronizes the onset of oestrus within the group.

Indications
Synchronization and induction of ovulation in sheep and goats.
Attention: Chronogest CR® is licensed in the EU countries only for use in sheep.

Dosage and administration
The dose is one sponge per animal irrespective of body weight, breed, type and season.
The sponge is inserted intra-vaginally using an applicator.
It should remain in place for 12 to 14 days in sheep and 11 days in goats. At the end of this period, the sponge is gently removed by pulling on its string.
To enhance the occurrence and number of ovulations, an injection of PMSG/eCG is recommended at the time of sponge removal in sheep ($PGF_{2\alpha}$ and PMSG/eCG in goats). The animals display oestrus and ovulate between 36 and 72h after the removal of the sponge.

Contraindications, warnings
Do not use in pregnant females.
Do not use Chronogest CR® in sheep and goats with a vaginal discharge or in animals which have just aborted.

Do not use Chronogest CR® in goats under the age of 1 year.
Do not use Chronogest CR® within 60-75 days of lambing or within 150 days of kidding.
Sponges eaten by animals can cause impaction; they should be disposed of safely after use in accordance with local regulations.

Withdrawal period

Tissues/products	Species	Withdrawal periods*
Meat	Sheep, goats	2 days
Milk	Sheep, goats	Nil

** Local regulations should be observed, Chronogest CR® is licensed in the EU countries only for use in sheep.*

Pharmaceutical precautions

Store in a cool, dry place. Protect from light. Keep out of the reach and sight of children.

Presentation

Bags of 25 sponges.

13.5 Covinan® (Delvosteron®)

Description

Covinan®/Delvosteron® is a sterile aqueous suspension of Proligestone 100 mg/ml.

Mode of action

Covinan®/Delvosteron® exerts a long-acting progestagenic effect in both dogs and cats, with a minimal risk of unwanted effects on the endometrium and ovary. It may be administered in both anoestrus and early proestrus.

Indications

A) Postponement and suppression of oestrus in the dog and cat.
B) Pseudo-pregnancy, abnormal lactation, metrorrhagia and dermatitis of hormonal origin in dogs and cats.

Dosage and administration

Oestrus control

1. *Dosage schedule for animals not previously treated with progestagens:*

- 1st treatment during anoestrus or at first signs of proestrus.
- 2nd treatment 3 months after first injection.
- 3rd treatment 4 months after second injection.
- further treatments at 5-monthly intervals.

2. *Dosage schedule for animals previously treated with progestagens:*

- Two or more earlier treatments: inject Covinan®/Delvosteron® at 5-monthly intervals.
- One earlier treatment: 1st Covinan®/Delvosteron® treatment 3 months after previous treatment, next treatment after a further 4 months and then at 5-monthly intervals.

Note:

If the dosage schedule is interrupted by oestrus or proestrus, schedule 1 should be applied. Signs of proestrus will disappear within a few days of injection, provided that Covinan®/Delvosteron® is given as soon as the signs become apparent.

Bitches will usually return to normal cycling within 9 months of the last treatment.

Dosage for oestrus control

Species	Body weight	Dosage	Administration route
Dog	< 5 kg	1.0 - 1.5 ml	s.c.
	5 - 10 kg.	1.5 - 2.5 ml	s.c.
	10 - 20 kg	2.5 - 3.5 ml	s.c.
	20 - 30 kg	3.5 - 4.5 ml	s.c.
	30 - 45 kg	4.5 - 5.5 ml	s.c.
	45 - 60 kg	5.5 - 6.0 ml	s.c.
	> 60 kg	1 ml/10 kg	s.c.
Cat	< 3 kg	1.0 ml	s.c.
	3 - 5 kg	1.0 - 1.5 ml	s.c.

The subcutaneous injection is best given at a site where the skin in the neck region is loose. Briefly massage the injection site. Show animals are best injected in the groin. Discoloration and loss of hair at the injection site and endometritis have been observed occasionally.

Other Indications

The normal dosage recommended for oestrus control can be used. Subsequent treatments should be based on clinical results.

Contraindications, warnings

Dogs and cats treated during proestrus may remain fertile for as long as one week.
In view of the considerable variation in age at which the first proestrus occurs, it is advisable to postpone treatment until these signs are actually noted. Alternatively treatment can be postponed until the following anoestrus phase.
If treatment is given during early or late pregnancy, parturition may be complicated by insufficient relaxation of the cervix. In a few cases, suppression of oestrus after treatment with Delvosteron®/Covinan® may be permanent.
There is no evidence to suggest that Delvosteron®/Covinan® affects the performance of racing greyhounds.

Pharmaceutical precautions

Store at room temperature (15-25°C). Protect from light. Keep out of the reach and sight of children. Shake well before use. Use a sterile needle and syringe for administration. Avoid the introduction of contaminants during use. If the suspension becomes discoloured or any growth becomes apparent within the vial, the product should be discarded.
Use within 28 days of the withdrawal of the first dose. Dispose of any unused product and empty containers in accordance with local regulations.

Presentation

Vials of 20 ml

13.6 Crestar®

Description

Crestar® forms the major part of a system for the control of oestrus in heifers and cows in a planned insemination program.

Crestar® consists of:

- Crestar® implant: containing 3 mg of the progestagen Norgestomet (17α-acetoxy-11β-methyl-19-norpregna-4-en-2.20-dione) and
- Crestar® injection: 2 ml containing 3 mg Norgestomet and 5 mg Oestradiol valerate.

Mode of action

Crestar® injection:

The oestrogen plus the Norgestomet compound shortens the luteal phase of the oestrous cycle if given at an early stage of the cycle, and induces the so-called follicular turnover (ovulation or luteinization of any LH-sensitive follicle present at the time of injection), thus preventing the formation of persistent dominant follicles.

At the same time Norgestomet suppresses oestrus and ovulation by pituitary inhibition.

Crestar® implant:

The continuous release of Norgestomet maintains the suppression of oestrus and ovulation. Removal of the implant, removes the inhibition of the pituitary and a new follicular phase begins.

In non-cycling animals, the priming effect of Norgestomet is enhanced by an intramuscular PMSG/eCG injection when the implant is removed, stimulating synchronized follicular development.

Indications

Oestrus control in both cycling and non-cycling cattle (heifers and cows).

Dosage and administration schedules

Type of animal	Day 0	48h before implant removal	Day 9-10	Artificial Insemination
Beef heifers	Crestar® implant and injection	x	Implant removal Injection of 400-600IU PMSG/eCG (Folligon®)	48h after implant removal
Dairy heifers	Crestar® implant and injection	x	Implant removal	48h after implant removal
Beef cows	Crestar® implant and injection	x	Implant removal Injection of 500-700IU PMSG/eCG (Folligon®)	56h after implant removal
Dairy cows	Crestar® implant and injection	Prostaglandin injection (Estrumate®)	Implant removal Injection of 300-400IU PMSG/eCG (Folligon®)	56h after implant removal

Note

Cows and heifers can be inseminated without oestrus detection. If two inseminations are performed, they should be at 48 and 72 hours after implant removal.
The dose of Folligon® (PMSG/eCG) depends on age, breed, season, post-partum interval, management, etc.

Contraindications, warnings

- Crestar is to be used only in healthy animals.
- Heifers to be treated should have reached at least 65-70% of their adult weight and an age of 15-20 months, depending on breed.
- Cows should not be treated within 45 days of the last calving.

Withdrawal period

Tissues/product	Species	Withdrawal periods*
Edible tissues	Cattle	2 days after removal of implant
Milk	Cattle	Nil

** Local regulations should be observed.*

Pharmaceutical precautions

Store in a dry place at room temperature (15-25° C). Protect from light. Keep out of the reach and sight of children.

Presentation

Box of 5x5 Crestar implants and 5x5 vials of 2 ml Crestar® injection.

13.7 Dexadreson®

Description

Dexadreson® is a clear aqueous solution for injection. Each ml contains 2.63 mg dexamethasone sodium phosphate (equivalent to 2.0 mg dexamethasone). Benzylalcohol 1% v/v is included as a preservative.

Mode of action

The product is a short-acting, highly potent, synthetic glucocorticosteroid with a rapid onset of activity, with minimal mineralocorticosteroid activity. Dexamethasone has ten to twenty times the anti-inflammatory activity of prednisolone. Corticosteroids suppress the immunological response by inhibiting the dilatation of capillaries, the migration and function of leucocytes and phagocytosis. Glucocorticoids affect metabolism by increasing gluconeogenesis. Administration of glucocorticoids mimics the effect of cortisol and therefore provides a signal which initiates the parturition process in ruminants (if the foetus is alive). Glucocorticoids have anti-shock activity.

Indications

Dexadreson® can be used therapeutically for its anti-inflammatory, anti-allergic, anti-shock and gluconeogenic actions, and for the induction of parturition in ruminants.

- Bovine, porcine, equine, caprine, canine and feline: treatment of inflammatory or allergic conditions, and treatment of shock.
- Bovine and caprine: treatment of primary ketosis (acetonemia and pregnancy toxaemia) and induction of parturition.
- Equine: treatment of inflammatory articular syndromes.

Dosage and administration

For intravenous, intramuscular, subcutaneous or intra-articular administration.

Species	Route of administration	Dosage (mg dexamethasone/kg)*
Equine, bovine, caprine and porcine	i.m.	0.06 mg/kg (3 ml/100 kg)
	i.v. (in case of shock)	0.6 mg/kg (30 ml/100 kg)
Canine and feline	i.m., s.c.	0.10 mg/kg (0.5 ml/10 kg)
	i.v. (in case of shock)	1.0 mg/kg (5 ml/100kg)

** Treatment may be repeated once after a 24 to 48-hour interval.*

In equines, the product can also be administered locally by intra-articular injection. The recommended dose is 0.125 to 5 ml per joint, depending on the size of the animal.

Induction of parturition

Bovine: 20 mg (10 ml)
Caprine: 12 to 16 mg (6 to 8 ml)

Contraindications, warnings

Do not use in animals suffering from diabetes mellitus, hyperadrenocorticism, renal insufficiency, cardiac insufficiency, or gastrointestinal ulcer.
Do not use in animals with infectious diseases unless suitable anti-infective therapy is given at the same time.
Because corticosteroids can reduce the immune response, the product should not be used in combination with vaccine administration.

Concurrent use with non-steroidal anti-inflammatory drugs may exacerbate gastrointestinal tract ulceration.
When used for the induction of parturition in ruminants, there is an increased likelihood of retained placenta.
In cases of laminitis in equines, the product should only be used very early in the disease process.
Except in cases of acetonemia and the induction of parturition, corticosteroid administration produces an improvement in clinical signs rather than a cure. Therefore, identification and treatment of the underlying disease is recommended.
When used for the treatment of shock, intravenous fluids should be given to maintain circulating volume and the acid-base balance should be monitored and controlled.

Pregnancy
Laboratory studies in rodents during early pregnancy have shown evidence of foetotoxic effects. During the first two thirds of pregnancy, use only in accordance with a risk/benefit assessment undertaken by the responsible veterinarian.
Administration in late pregnancy may cause early parturition or abortion. Do not use during the last third of pregnancy, except in ruminants to induce parturition.

Lactation:
Administration in lactating ruminants may cause a temporary reduction in milk yield.

Withdrawal period

Tissues	Species	Withdrawal periods*
Edible tissues	Bovine, equine, caprine	7 days
Edible tissues	Porcine	1 day
Milk	Bovine, caprine	4 milkings

** Local regulations should be observed.*

Pharmaceutical precautions
Store at room temperature. Keep out of the reach and sight of children.

Presentation
Vials of 20 ml, 50 ml and 100 ml, in a carton.

13.8 Dexafort®

Description

Dexafort® is an aqueous suspension containing per ml:

- 2.67 mg dexamethasone phenylpropionate (equivalent to 2 mg dexamethasone)
- 1.32 mg dexamethasone disodium phosphate (equivalent to 1 mg dexamethasone)

Mode of action

Dexamethasone is a highly potent glucocorticosteroid with minimal mineralocorticoid activity. It has gluconeogenic, anti-inflammatory and anti-allergenic activity and can induce parturition. Dexafort® has a rapid onset and relatively long duration of activity.

Indications

- Treatment of inflammatory and allergic conditions in horses, cattle, dogs and cats.
- Treatment of ketosis in cattle.
- Induction of parturition in cattle.

Dosage and administration

Horse, cattle:	0.02 ml/kg (0.06 mg/kg) by the intramuscular route.
Dog, Cat:	0.05 ml/kg (0.15 mg/kg) by the intramuscular or subcutaneous routes.

Treatment may be repeated after 7 days.

Contraindications, warnings

Do not use in animals suffering from diabetes mellitus, osteoporosis, hyperadrenocorticism, renal diseases and cardiac insufficiency.
Do not use to treat infectious diseases unless suitable anti infective therapy is given at the same time.
Do not use in animals suffering from gastrointestinal or corneal ulcers, or demodecosis.
In cases of laminitis in equines, the product should only be used very early in the disease process.
Because corticosteroids can reduce the immune response, the product should not be used in combination with vaccine administration.

The induction of parturition using corticosteroids in cattle may be associated with reduced viability of the offspring and an increased incidence of retained placenta.
Corticosteroids such as dexamethasone are known to exert a wide range of side-effects. They may cause Cushingoid symptoms involving significant alteration of fat, carbohydrate, protein and mineral metabolism, e.g. redistribution of body fat, muscle weakness and wastage and osteoporosis may result. Polyuria, polydipsia and polyphagia may occur.
During therapy, effective doses may suppress the hypothalamo-pituitary-adrenal axis.
Use of corticosteroids in lactating cattle may cause a temporary reduction in milk yield.
Administration of dexamethasone may induce hypokalaemia and hence increase the risk of toxicity from cardiac glycosides. The risk of hypokalaemia may be increased if dexamethasone is administered together with potassium-depleting diuretics.
Glucocorticoids antagonise the effects of insulin.
Concurrent use with phenobarbital, phenytoin and rifampicin can reduce the effects of dexamethasone.
High doses of corticosteroids may cause drowsiness and lethargy in horses.

Use during pregnancy and lactation
Foetal abnormalities have been observed after the administration of corticosteroids during early pregnancy in laboratory animals. During the first two thirds of pregnancy, use only in accordance with a risk/benefit assessment undertaken by the responsible veterinarian, except when the intention is to induce parturition. Administration in late pregnancy may cause early parturition or abortion.

Withdrawal period*

Tissues/product	**Species**	**Withdrawal times****
Edible tissues	Cattle	53 days
Edible tissues	Horse	47 days
Milk	Cattle	11 milkings

** These withdrawal periods apply following intramuscular injection.*
*** National regulations should be observed.*

Pharmaceutical precautions
Shake well before use.
Store at room temperature. Keep out of the reach and sight of children.

Presentations
Vials of 50 ml in a carton.

13.9 Estrumate®

Description
Estrumate® is a clear, colourless aqueous solution for injection, containing Cloprostenol Sodium, equivalent to 250 mcg/ml cloprostenol. Also contains 0.1% Chlorocresol as a bactericide.

Indications
Cloprostenol is a synthetic prostaglandin analogue structurally related to Prostaglandin $F_{2\alpha}$ ($PGF_{2\alpha}$), for use in cattle and horses. As a potent luteolytic agent it causes functional and morphological regression of the corpus luteum (luteolysis) in cattle and horses followed by return to oestrus and normal ovulation.

Note:
There is a refractory period of four to five days after ovulation when cattle and horses are insensitive to the luteolytic effect of prostaglandins. Estrumate® has a good safety margin and does not impair fertility. No deleterious effects have been reported on the progeny conceived at the oestrus following treatment.

CATTLE
Therapeutic:
Suboestrus (or non-detected oestrus - NDO):
This condition occurs in high yielding cows, usually at peak lactation, which have normal ovarian cyclicity but in which the behavioural manifestation of oestrus is either very poor or absent. Such animals can be treated following the diagnosis of a corpus luteum and then closely observed for oestrus. Those showing heat should be inseminated. Animals not seen in heat

should be re-examined 11 days later and may receive a further single injection and be bred at oestrus or at fixed times (see Controlled breeding cattle)).
When re-examination is carried out 14 days later to fit in with routine fertility visits, animals should be bred on detection of oestrus rather than at fixed times.

Induction of parturition:
Estrumate® induces parturition in the period around term. Induction should be attempted as close to the predicted calving date as possible and not more than 10 days before. Induction should not be attempted before 270 days after the day of conception except in pathological conditions (see below).
All treated animals must receive adequate supervision.
In common with other methods of shortening the gestation period, a higher than usual incidence of retention of the foetal membranes is to be expected.

Termination of normal pregnancy:
Normal pregnancy can be terminated in cattle from one week after conception until the 150th day of gestation. Before 100 days of gestation, abortion can be induced rapidly and efficiently but between 100 and 150 days of gestation results are less reliable, probably because a proportion of cattle become progressively less dependent upon the corpus luteum for the maintenance of pregnancy. Abortion should not be attempted after day 150 of gestation. Treated animals should be kept under observation and examined in order to ensure that expulsion of the foetus and the placental membranes is complete. Termination of more advanced pregnancy requires more complex treatment regimes and greater post-treatment care.

Termination of abnormal pregnancy
Mummified foetus
Death of the conceptus may be followed by its dehydration and degeneration. Induction of luteolysis at any stage of pregnancy will result in the expulsion of the mummified foetus from the uterus into the vagina, from which manual removal may be necessary. Normal cyclical activity should then follow.

Hydrops of the foetal membrane
Pathological accumulation of placental fluids - hydramnion or hydrallantois - can cause severe physiological complications and death. Surgical drainage is not usually successful in alleviating the condition.
A single dose may be used to induce parturition in such cases; success has been achieved as early as the sixth month of pregnancy.

Chronic endometritis (Pyometra):
This condition may be successfully treated with a single dose. In longstanding cases treatment may be repeated after 10 - 14 days.

Ovarian luteal cysts:
When cystic ovaries are diagnosed associated with persistent luteal tissue and absence of oestrus, Estrumate® has proved effective in correcting the condition and bringing about a return to cyclicity.

Controlled breeding in cattle:
The luteolytic activity of Estrumate® can be harnessed to control the breeding pattern of cattle.
A variety of treatment regimes exist from which to choose the most appropriate for the characteristics and objectives of each particular herd. Individuals or groups of animals can be controlled, as required. Estrumate® can be used to complement the herdsman's oestrus detection, or animals may be bred 'on schedule' during critical times of the breeding season, without reference to oestrus detection, as preferred.

Controlled breeding programs in cattle
Examples of programs which have been used are:

1. A single treatment of cattle with palpable evidence of a corpus luteum, followed by breeding on detection of the subsequent oestrus.
2. Observation for signs of oestrus for 6 days, breeding those animals seen in heat; a single treatment is given to all non-served animals on the 6th day, and these cattle are bred at the subsequent oestrus.
3. Two injections 11 days apart, breeding at oestrus or at fixed times (see below).
4. As 3, above, but breeding any animals showing oestrus before the second injection. Thus the second dose of Estrumate® is given only to those cattle not seen in oestrus during that time and is followed by breeding either on signs of oestrus or at fixed times (see below).

Cattle which respond to a single prostaglandin injection will normally do so within 6 days of treatment. The response time after two injections is more rapid. Animals may be inseminated on detection of oestrus in any of the Estrumate® programs. However, fixed time insemination should only be used following the second of a two injection program (i.e. examples 3 and 4). In the latter case, insemination should be performed either once at 72-84 hours or twice at 72 and 96 hours after the second injection, as preferred.
Double 'fixed-time' insemination may give superior results to a single insemination. However, economic factors in the particular herd may outweigh such a benefit.
For successful treatment, animals should be cycling normally. Rectal examination before treatment should avoid the disappointment of treating non-cycling (anoestrous) or pregnant animals.
Attention should be directed to the diet and condition of the treated animals. Sudden changes in feeding levels, in feed constituents and in housing, etc. should be avoided around the time of the breeding program, as should any other management changes, such as regrouping, which could reasonably be expected to lead to stress.
If artificial insemination is to be used, the quality of semen and insemination technique should be assured beforehand.

Control of the oestrous cycle is of value in the:

Dairy herd

1. To control oestrus in the individual animal giving better control of the individual calving index and reducing the number of cows culled as barren.
2. To control oestrus in groups of cows: to promote management of the herd in groups of suitable size and facilitate the maintenance of a seasonal calving pattern.
3. To permit the use of AI in dairy heifers: allowing the speeding up of the breeding program.

Beef herd

1. To facilitate the use of AI.
2. To enable the most efficient use of available bulls: where natural service is preferred.
3. To permit better herd management at conception and calving: The shape of the calving pattern is improved, resulting in greater average age and weight of calves at weaning. Feeding and other programs can be scheduled more easily.

HORSES

The property of shortening the life-span of the corpus luteum enables Estrumate® to be highly effective in certain conditions in the horse.

Induction of luteolysis following early foetal death and resorption

About 8 to 10 per cent of all mares which conceive lose the conceptus during the first 100 days of pregnancy. Persistence of luteal function in the ovary may preclude an early return to oestrus.

Termination of persistent dioestrus

Non-pregnant mares frequently and spontaneously go into and out of periods of prolonged dioestrus. A very high proportion of mares in this category, i.e. not cycling, are in prolonged dioestrus rather than anoestrus, particularly in the latter part of the breeding season.

Termination of pseudopregnancy
Some mares which are covered at normal oestrus and subsequently found to be empty (but not having lost or resorbed a conceptus) display clinical signs of pregnancy. These animals are said to be 'pseudopregnant'.

Treatment of lactational anoestrus
Failure of lactating mares to cycle again for several months after exhibiting an early 'foal heat' can be avoided.

Establishing oestrous cycles in barren/maiden mares
Some of these animals will be found, on examination, to have a functional corpus luteum and are suffering from abnormal persistence of luteal function or are simply failing to exhibit normal oestrus behaviour ('silent heat') while ovarian cyclicity continues.

As an aid to stud management
Mares may be brought into oestrus on a planned timing schedule (singly or in groups), to facilitate more efficient use and management of stallions during the breeding season.

Dosage and administration

Species	Administration route	Dose
Cattle	i.m.	2.0 ml
Ponies and donkeys	i.m.	0.5-1.0 ml
Thoroughbreds, hunters and heavy horses	i.m.	1.0-2.0 ml

Administer by intramuscular injection. Due to the possibility of post-injection bacterial infections observe normal aseptic precautions. Care should be taken to avoid injection through wet or dirty areas of skin.
Following withdrawal of the first dose, use the product within 56 days. Discard unused material.

Contraindications, warnings

On rare occasions severe life-threatening local bacterial infections may occur associated with clostridial proliferation. It is important to keep treated animals under observation and, if local infection occurs, aggressive antibiotic therapy is a matter of urgency.

Overdose in cattle: At x5 to x10 overdose the most frequent side-effect is increased rectal temperature. This is usually transient, however, and not detrimental to the animal. Limited hypersalivation may also be observed in some animals.
Overdose in horses: The most frequently observed side-effects are sweating and decreased rectal temperatures. These are usually transient, however, and not detrimental to the animal. Other possible reactions are increased heart rate, increased respiratory rate, abdominal discomfort, locomotor incoordination and lying down. If these occur, they are likely to be seen within 15 minutes of injection and disappear within 1 hour. Mares usually continue to eat throughout.
Do not use in horses intended for human consumption.

Operator Warnings

Prostaglandins of the $F_{2\alpha}$ type can be absorbed through the skin and may cause bronchospasm or miscarriage. Care should be taken when handling the product to AVOID SELF-INJECTION OR SKIN CONTACT
Women of child-bearing age, asthmatics and persons with bronchial or other respiratory problems should avoid contact with the product, and/ or wear disposable plastic gloves when administering it.
The incidence of bronchospasm induced by Estrumate® is unknown. Should shortness of breath result from accidental inhalation or injection, seek urgent medical advice and show the doctor this warning.
Accidental spillage on the skin should be washed off immediately with soap and water.

Withdrawal period

Tissues/product	Species	Withdrawal periods*
Edible tissues	Cattle	24 hours
Milk	Cattle	Nil
Meat	Horse	Do not treat horses intended for human consumption

** Local regulations should be observed.*

Pharmaceutical precautions

Store at room temperature, protected from light. Keep out of the reach and sight of children.

Presentation

Multidose vials of 10ml, 20ml and 50ml. Single-dose vials of 2ml.

Attention: In many countries Estrumate® is also licensed for use in pigs. For details please consult your Intervet/Schering-Plough representative and the product data leaflet.

13.10 Fertagyl®*

Description

Fertagyl® is a clear solution of gonadorelin (100 mcg/ml) for injection.

Mode of action

The active compound of Fertagyl® is gonadorelin, a decapeptide identical to the naturally occurring Gonadotrophin Releasing Hormone (GnRH).
Fertagyl® therefore has exactly the same action as endogenous GnRH: it controls the production and secretion of Luteinizing Hormone (LH) and Follicle Stimulating Hormone (FSH) by the pituitary gland.
Injection of Fertagyl® causes the simultaneous release of LH and FSH shortly after administration. Both LH and FSH have a direct effect on the ovary. FSH stimulates follicle development and LH induces ovulation and luteinization.

Indications

CATTLE

Fertagyl® can be used for:

1. *Induction of ovulation during oestrus*
   Delayed ovulation is a common condition especially in high yielding dairy cows. Fertagyl® can be administered at the same time as natural service or alternatively 6 hours before AI. Ovulation occurs in the majority of animals within 24h of treatment.
2. *Therapy of cystic ovarian disease*
   Both follicular and luteal cysts will respond to treatment with Fertagyl®. In 18-23 days post treatment most animals return to oestrus and can be inseminated. The conception rate at this first insemination is normal.
3. *Improvement of fertility*
   Even though clinically normal, a number of animals require 3 or more inseminations for conception. This problem is called 'repeat breeding'. To improve the conception rate Fertagyl® can be administered at the time of insemination or mid-cycle (11-12 days post-oestrus).
4. *Improvement of fertility post-partum.*
   Fertagyl® administered in the early post-partum period (15-40 days post-partum) stimulates the resumption of physiological oestrous cycles, reduces the incidence of cystic ovarian disease and shortens the interval of calving to first oestrus.

RABBIT

In the rabbit Fertagyl® can be used for the induction of ovulation at AI.

Dosage and administration

Species	Indication	Dosage	Administration
Cattle	Ovulation induction at AI	2.5 ml	i.m.
	Cystic ovarian disease	5 ml	i.m.
	Improvement of conception rate (10-12d post AI)	2.5-5 ml	i.m.
	Improvement of fertility post partum (< day 40)	1-2.5 ml	i.m.
Rabbit	Induction of ovulation	0.2 ml	i.m.

Contraindications, warnings
None.

Withdrawal period

Tissues/product	Species	Withdrawal periods*
Edible tissues	Cattle	Nil
Edible tissues	Rabbit	Nil
Milk	Cattle	Nil

** Local regulations should be observed.*

Pharmaceutical precautions
Store at room temperature (15-25°C). Protect from light.
Keep out of the reach and sight of children.

Presentation
Vials of 2.5ml, 5 ml or 50ml containing 100 mcg of gonadorelin per ml.

** Fertagyl® in European Union countries is marketed by Janssen Animal Health B.V.B.A.*

13.11 Folligon® (Chrono-gest® PMSG, Folligonan®)

Description
Folligon® contains the hormone Pregnant Mare Serum Gonadotrophin (PMSG)/Equine Chorionic Gonadotrophin (eCG) as a white freeze-dried crystalline powder together with solvent for reconstitution.

Mode of action
The active constituent of Folligon® is PMSG/eCG, a complex glycoprotein. PMSG/eCG is a gonadotrophin with Follicle Stimulating Hormone (FSH) and Luteinizing Hormone (LH) activities. In females, PMSG/eCG stimulates the growth and maturation of the follicles. In the male, PMSG/eCG stimulates development of the interstitial tissue of the testis and spermatogenesis.

Indications

Folligon® can be used for the management of reproduction and treatment of reproductive disorders in domestic animals:

- Anoestrus (oestrus induction and increase of ovarian activity leading to increased fertility) in the cow, the rabbit, the bitch and mink.
- Induction of multiple ovulation (Superovulation) in embryo/oocyte donors in the cow, the rabbit and deer.
- Increase of fertility rate after progestagen treatment (oestrus induction and synchronisation, increase of ovarian activity) in the cow, the ewe, the goat and deer.

Contraindications, warnings

In rare cases, as with all protein-containing preparations, anaphylactoid reactions may occur shortly after administration. In such circumstances, prompt medication with adrenaline (1:1000) or glucocorticosteroids may be indicated.

Withdrawal period

Tissues/product	Species	Withdrawal periods*
Edible tissues	Cattle, goat, sheep, rabbit, deer	Nil
Milk	Cattle, Goat, Sheep	Nil

* *Local regulations should be observed.*

Pharmaceutical precautions

Store at 8-15°C. Protect from light. Keep out of the reach and sight of children.

Reconstituted product should be used within 12 hours.

Dosage and administration

Female animals	Indication	Dosage and administration
Cow	Anoestrus/oestrus induction*	500-1000 IU, i.m.
	Induction of superovulation	1500-3000 IU, i.m., between day 8-13 of the cycle, followed by PGF_{2a} after 48 hours
	Increase of fertility rate after progestagen treatment	300-750 IU, i.m., at the end of progestagen treatment
Bitch	Anoestrus/oestrus induction	500 IU/animal or 20 IU/kg bodyweight per day for 10 days, i.m. At day 10 injection of 500 IU hCG
Goat	Increase of fertility rate after progestagen treatment (during and out of the breeding season)	400-750 IU, i.m., at the end of progestagen treatment
Sheep	Increase of fertility rate after progestagen treatment (during and out of the breeding season)	400-750 IU, i.m., at the end of progestagen treatment
Rabbit	Anoestrus/oestrus induction	40 IU, i.m. or s.c.
	Induction of superovulation	40 IU, i.m. or s.c.
Mink	Anoestrus/oestrus induction	100 IU, i.m., twice with an interval of 2 days
Deer	Increase of fertility rate after progestagen treatment	200 IU, i.m., at the end of a progestagen treatment
	Induction of superovulation	200 IU, i.m., in combination with 0.5 IU FSH

** Anoestrus is often caused by inadequate feeding and housing. Therefore improvements in nutrition and management are prerequisites for successful treatment.*

Presentation

Folligon®: vials of 1000 and 5000 IU together with solvent for reconstitution.
Chrono-gest® PMSG: vials of 500, 600, 5000 and 6000 IU together with solvent for reconstitution.

13.12 FolliPlan®

Description
FolliPlan® is an oral progestagen for the management of breeding in pigs.

Composition
Pressurised can containing 360 ml of an oily solution of 0.4% Altrenogest.

Indications
Programming and synchronization of heat in cycling gilts.
Synchronization of oestrus and improvement of litter size in primiparous sows.

Dosage and Administration
When pressed and released the valve delivers a single metered 5 ml dose (= 20 mg Altrenogest).

Gilts: One dose of 5 ml per gilt per day for 18 consecutive days given orally with feed for immediate consumption.

Sows: One dose of 5 ml per sow per day for 3 consecutive days given orally with feed for immediate consumption.

Treatment should begin on the day of weaning.

Contraindications
Not to be administered to male animals. Not to be administered to pregnant sows or to those suffering from uterine infection.
Part-consumed feed must be safely destroyed and not given to any other animal.

Withdrawal period
Local regulations should be observed.

Pharmaceutical precautions
Store at room temperature. Keep out of the reach of children.

Presentation
360 ml pressurized container with integral metering valve.

13.13 Incurin®

Description
Each tablet of Incurin® contains 1mg of oestriol.

Properties
Oestriol is a short-acting natural oestrogen. A steady state is reached after the second day of oral treatment. There is no cumulative effect after multiple dosing. Because it is short-acting, oestriol does not induce bone marrow suppression in the dog.

Indications
Incurin® is indicated for the treatment of hormone-dependent urinary incontinence due to sphincter mechanism incompetence in bitches.

Dosage and administration
Incurin® is intended for once daily oral administration.
There is no relationship between the effective dose and body weight. The dose must be adjusted for each dog on an individual basis.

The following schedule is recommended: begin treatment with 1 tablet every day. If this is successful reduce the dose to half a tablet per day. If treatment is unsuccessful increase the dose to 2 tablets per day.
Some dogs do not need daily treatment; once the effective daily dose has been established, treatment every other day may be successful.

Contraindications, warnings
The use of Incurin® is contraindicated during pregnancy and in animals under 1 year old.

Undesirable side-effects
Mild, oestrogenic effects such as swollen vulva, swollen teats and/or attractiveness for males have been observed at dose rates of 2 mg per day. These effects are reversible after reducing the dose. Vomiting has been observed in some dogs.

Pharmaceutical precautions

Store at room temperature (15-25°C). Keep out of the reach and sight of children.

Presentation

Push-through strips of hard PVC film backed by aluminium foil with a heat-seal coating on the side in contact with the tablets. One strip contains 30 tablets. Each strip is packed in a carton.

13.14 Intertocine®-S (Oxytocin-S)

Description

Intertocine®-S is a synthetic oxytocin at a concentration of 10 IU per ml.
The product contains no vasopressor or anti-diuretic impurities.

Mode of action

Intertocine®-S causes contractions of the smooth muscle of the oestrogen-sensitized uterus and mammary gland. It also stimulates uterine involution.

Indications

- Stimulation of uterine contractions, to facilitate parturition.
- To promote the involution of the post-parturient uterus and thus aid the passage of retained placenta and removal of detritus.
- To help control post-partum haemorrhage.
- To promote milk let-down in cases of agalactia.

Dosage and administration

Species	Dosage	Administration
Mare	0.5 - 5 ml (5-50 IU)	s.c. or i.m.
Cow	1.0 - 5 ml (10-50 IU)	s.c. or i.m.
Sheep, Goat, Sow	0.5 - 3 ml (5-30 IU)	s.c. or i.m.
Bitch	0.2 - 1 ml (2-10 IU)	s.c. or i.m.
Queen	0.1 - 0.5 ml (1-5 IU)	s.c. or i.m.

The product is administered by intramuscular or subcutaneous injection: it may be repeated, if necessary, after 40 minutes.
For a very rapid effect, Intertocine®-S may be given by slow intravenous injection at a quarter of the above dose rate, diluted 1 in 10 with water for injection.

Especially during parturition, by any route, a low initial dose is recommended, because repeat administration is permissible. In post-parturient animals larger doses may be employed.

Contraindications, warnings
The use of Intertocine®-S is contraindicated in any form of obstructive dystocia.
Intertocine®-S must only used as an aid to parturition after cervical dilatation has been confirmed.

Excessive doses of Intertocine®-S may delay parturition by producing incoordinated uterine contractions which interfere with the progress of the foetus, especially in multiple pregnancies.

Adrenaline reduces the effect of oxytocin on the uterus or mammary gland. For this reason the animal should not be stressed unnecessarily if the full effect of oxytocin is required.

Withdrawal period

Tissues/product	Species	Withdrawal periods*
Edible tissues	Cattle. Horse, sheep, goats, pig	Nil
Milk	Cattle, sheep, goats	Nil

** Local regulations should be observed*

Pharmaceutical precautions
Store at 2-8°C. Protect from light. Keep out of the reach and sight of children.

Presentation
Vials of 10, 25 and 50 ml, containing 10 IU Oxytocin/ml.

13.15 Metricure®

Description

Each syringe of Metricure intra-uterine suspension contains 500 mg of cephapirin (as benzathine).

Mode of action

Cephapirin - a first generation cephalosporin - is a broad spectrum antibiotic with bactericidal action against Gram-positive and Gram-negative bacteria. Cephapirin is resistant to the action of penicillinase produced by staphylococci, and is active in the anaerobic environment of the uterus.
After a single treatment with Metricure, concentrations of cephapirin in the endometrium tissue above the MIC of sensitive bacteria are maintained for at least 24 hours. The suspension is well tolerated, enables good diffusion of cephapirin into the endometrium and can be infused easily.

Indications

Subacute and chronic endometritis in cattle (> 14 days after parturition).
Treatment of repeat breeder cows at the day after AI.

Dosage and administration

The contents of the Metricure syringe are introduced into the lumen of the uterus using the disposable catheter provided with each syringe.

1. Fix the syringe to the catheter.
2. Take the cervix of the uterus into one gloved hand introduced into the rectum.
3. Introduce the catheter through the cervix into the lumen of the uterus by gentle oscillating movements of the cervix.
4. Inject the contents of the syringe into the lumen of the uterus.

One treatment with Metricure is generally sufficient for complete cure. If necessary, treatment can be repeated after 14 days.
In animals that are inseminated, Metricure can be used at one day after insemination.

In cases of pyometra it is advised to start treatment with an injection of prostaglandin in order to induce regression of the corpus luteum and to remove the debris from the uterine cavity before treatment with Metricure.

Contraindications, warnings
Animals with known allergy to cephalosporins.

Withholding period
Meat: 48 hours
Milk: nil.

Storage conditions
Store at room temperature (15-25° C).

Presentation
Box with 10 syringes plus 10 catheters and 10 gloves.

13.16 PG 600® (Suigonan®)

Description
PG 600® contains 400 IU serum gonadotrophin (PMSG/eCG) and 200 IU chorionic gonadotrophin (hCG) per dose as a white freeze-dried crystalline powder together with solvent for reconstitution.

Mode of action
PG 600® combines the two most important hormones with a role in the development of follicles and their ovulation. The serum gonadotrophin stimulates the development of follicles, the chorionic gonadotrophin promotes ovulation and the formation of corpora lutea. The combination of hormones promotes the development of a fertile oestrous cycle in the pig.

Indications

	Indication	Time of treatment
Sows	Induction of oestrus after weaning	0-2 days post-weaning
	Increasing litter size/ subfertility	0-2 days post-weaning
	Anoestrus/seasonal infertility	8-10 days post-weaning
	Pregnancy diagnosis	Within 80 days post-service or AI
Gilts	Treatment of delayed puberty	At the age of 8-10 months
	Oestrus induction in prepuberal gilts	At the age of 5.5-6.5 months and/ or a body weight of 85-100 kg

The use of PG 600® for all indications mentioned induces oestrus 3-6 days post treatment.

Dosage and administration

Reconstitute the freeze-dried powder and inject the contents of a single dose vial (5 ml) or one dose (5 ml) of the 5-dose vial subcutaneously or intra-muscularly behind the ear.

Contraindications, warnings

As with all protein-containing preparations, in rare cases anaphylactoid reactions may occur shortly after administration. In such circumstances, prompt medication with 2-3 ml adrenaline (1:1000) or glucocorticosteroids may be indicated.

Withdrawal period

Tissues/product	Species	Withdrawal periods*
Edible tissues	Pigs	Nil

** Local regulations should be observed.*

Pharmaceutical precautions

Store at 8-15° C. Protect from light. Reconstituted product should be used within 12 hours.
Keep out of the reach and sight of children.

Presentation

Single dose presentation:	5 vials + solvent 5 x 5 ml
	25 vials + solvent 25 x 5 ml
5 doses presentation:	1 vial + solvent 1 x 25 ml

13.17 Planate®

Description

Planate® is a colourless injectable solution. Each 2 ml contains 184 micrograms of Cloprostenol Sodium, a synthetic analogue of $PGF_{2\alpha}$, equivalent to 175 micrograms of cloprostenol. Chlorocresol 0.1% w/v is added as a preservative.

Indications

Planate® is indicated for use in pigs as a luteolytic agent to induce farrowing in sows and gilts, thus providing an opportunity for more efficient and convenient management under a variety of systems.

- Allows batch management of sows and gilts to be achieved effectively.
- Minimises the number farrowings at weekends, public holidays and during the night.
- Facilitates the supervision of farrowing and fostering between sows and litters.
- Enables farrowing and labour schedules to be planned for convenience.
- Prevents the pregnancy of sows and gilts going over term.
- Allows the optimal use of farrowing quarters, equipment etc.

Planate® should only be used where accurate service records are kept. If used too early in pregnancy induction of farrowing may lead to non-viable piglets being born. It is therefore essential that the average gestation length is calculated on each farm from past records (using the first day of service as Day 0), so that sows can be induced at the required time. In most situations, gestation length varies between 111 and 119 days (average around 115 days).

Dosage and administration

A single 2 ml dose by deep intramuscular injection. The use of a 1½ inch needle is recommended.
Having calculated the average gestation length for each farm, sows and gilts may be injected two days before the calculated date or on any date thereafter to suit the requirements of the particular management system. Trials have shown that 95% of animals will usually commence farrowing within 36 hours of treatment. The majority of animals can be expected to respond within 24 ± 5 hours following injection, except in those cases when farrowing is already imminent.

Contraindications, warnings

An increase in the number of non-viable piglets may result if Planate® is used more than two days prior to the average gestation length calculated from farm records.

Operator Warnings

Prostaglandins of the $F_{2\alpha}$ type can be absorbed through the skin and may cause bronchospasm or miscarriage. Care should be taken when handling the product to AVOID SELF-INJECTION OR SKIN CONTACT.
Women of child-bearing age, asthmatics and persons with bronchial or other respiratory problems should avoid contact with the product, and/ or wear disposable plastic gloves when administering it.
Should shortness of breath result from accidental inhalation or injection, seek urgent medical advice and show the doctor this warning.
Accidental spillage on the skin should be washed off immediately with soap and water.

Withdrawal period

Animals must not be slaughtered for human consumption during treatment. Pigs may be slaughtered for human consumption only after 2 days from the last treatment.

Pharmaceutical precautions

Store at room temperature, protected from light. Keep out of the reach and sight of children.

Presentation

Multidose vial containing 10 doses (20 ml).

13.18 Receptal®

Description

Gonadotrophin-Releasing Hormone Analogue.

Composition

Solution for injection: 1 ml contains 0.0042 mg buserelin acetate equivalent to 0.004 mg buserelin.

Indications

Reduced fertility caused by ovarian dysfunction, induction of ovulation and improvement of conception rate.

Cows:

Cystic ovaries with and without symptoms of nymphomania.
Anoestrus.
Delayed ovulation.
Anovulation.
Improvement of conception rate after artificial insemination and oestrus synchronization.
Prophylaxis of fertility disorders by the early induction of post-partum cycling.

Mares:

Anoestrus.
Induction of ovulation.
Fixed time ovulation and service.
Improvement of conception rate.
Prolonged or continuous oestrus.

Rabbits:

Induction of ovulation at post-partum insemination.
Improvement of conception rate.

Dosage and Administration

Species	Indication	Dose
Cattle (cows and heifers)	Cystic ovaries with and without symptoms of nymphomania	5.0 ml
	Anoestrus	5.0 ml
	Delayed ovulation	2.5 ml
	Improvement of conception rate after artificial insemination	2.5 ml
	Prophylaxis of fertility disorders by the early induction of post-partum cycling	5.0 ml
Mares	Anoestrus	2 doses of 5.0 ml, with 24 h interval
	Induction of ovulation (when a follicle ≥3.5cm is present)	10 ml
	Fixed time of ovulation and service (when a follicle ≥3.5cm is present)	10 ml
	Improvement of conception rate	10 ml
	Prolonged or continuous oestrus	10 ml
Rabbit does	Induction of ovulation at post-partum insemination	0.2 ml
	Improvement of conception rate	0.2 ml

The preferred route of administration for Receptal® is intramuscular injection, but it may also be injected intravenously or subcutaneously.

Withdrawal period

Tissues/product	Species	Withdrawal periods*
Edible tissues	Cattle, horse, rabbit	Nil
Milk	Cattle	Nil

** Local regulations should be observed.*

Pharmaceutical precautions

Store at room temperature. Keep out of the reach and sight of children.

Contraindications
None.

Presentation
Vials of 2.5ml, 10ml and 50ml.

13.19 Regumate Equine®

Description
Regumate Equine® contains altrenogest, a synthetic progestagen.

Composition
Vegetable oil solution, containing 2.2 mg altrenogest per ml.

Target species
Horses.

Indications
In mares with significant follicular activity during the transitional period between seasonal anoestrus and during the breeding season (follicles of at least 20-25 mm present at the beginning of treatment):

- Suppression/prevention of oestrus (usually after 1 to 3 days of treatment) during the prolonged oestrus periods occurring during this period.
- Control of the time of initiation of oestrus (approximately 90% of mares show signs of oestrus within 5 days following the end of treatment) and synchronization of ovulation (60% of mares ovulate between days 11 and 14 following the end of treatment).

Dosage and administration
The recommended dose of Regumate Equine® is 1 ml per 50 kg bodyweight by the oral route, which corresponds to 0.044 mg altrenogest/kg bodyweight.

Duration of treatment depends on the indication:
Induction of ovulatory oestrus 10 consecutive days.
Suppression of prolonged oestrus 10 consecutive days.
Suppression of oestrus in normally cycling mares 15 consecutive days.
Control of the cycle in breeding mares 15 consecutive days.

Method of administration
The product should be added to the mare's feed, at one feed per day, or directly administered into the mouth using a syringe. Medicated feed should be offered to mares being treated as soon as the product has been added, and should not be stored.

To withdraw the volume of product corresponding to the mare's bodyweight:
150, 300 and 1000ml bottles
Wearing gloves, remove the original cap and screw on the luer lock cap in its place. Keeping the bottle upright, screw the syringe onto the luer lock cap, turn the bottle upside down, and carefully withdraw the appropriate volume of solution using the syringe. Turn the bottle the right way up before detaching the syringe. Replace the small cap on the luer lock cap securely.

250ml bottles
Wearing gloves, remove the white cap and the aluminium foil seal from the neck of the measuring compartment. Keeping the bottle upright, squeeze the body of the bottle until the required volume of product has been forced into the measuring compartment. Carefully pour the contents of the measuring compartment onto the mare's feed.

Contraindications, warnings
Do not use in mares with endometritis.
Do not use in males.
Adverse reactions, such as uterine infection, are extremely rare.

Operator warnings
Women who are pregnant, or suspected of being pregnant, should not use this product. Women of childbearing age should

handle this product with extreme care. The product should not be handled by persons with known or suspected progesterone-dependent tumours or thrombo-embolic disorders.
Direct contact with the skin should be avoided. Personal protective clothing (gloves and overalls) must be worn when handling the product. Porous gloves may allow the product to reach the operator's skin, and transcutaneous absorption may even be enhanced when the skin is covered by an occlusive material, such as latex or rubber gloves. Accidental spillage on the skin should be washed off immediately with soap and water. Wash hands after treatment and before meals.
In case of accidental contact with the eye, rinse with copious volumes of water. Seek immediate medical attention.

Effects of operator exposure:
Repeated exposure could lead to disruption of the menstrual cycle, uterine or abdominal cramping, increased or decreased uterine bleeding, prolongation of pregnancy and headache.

Withdrawal period
Edible tissues: 21 days.
Not permitted for use in lactating animals producing milk for human consumption.

Pharmaceutical precautions
Store in the dark at room temperature. Keep out of the reach and sight of children.

Presentation
Bottles containing 150, 250, 300 or 1000ml.

13.20 Regumate Porcine®*

Description
Oral progestagen for the management of breeding in pigs.

Composition
Pressurised can containing 360 ml of an oily solution of 0.4% Altrenogest.

Indications

Programming and synchronization of heat in cycling gilts. Synchronization of oestrus and improvement of litter size in primiparous sows.

Dosage and Administration

When pressed and released the valve delivers a single metered 5 ml dose (= 20 mg Altrenogest).

Gilts: One dose of 5 ml per gilt per day for 18 consecutive days given orally with feed for immediate consumption.

Sows: One dose of 5 ml per sow per day for 3 consecutive days given orally with feed for immediate consumption.

Treatment should begin on the day of weaning.

Contraindications

Not to be administered to male animals. Not to be administered to pregnant sows or to those suffering from uterine infection. Part-consumed feed must be safely destroyed and not given to any other animal.

Withdrawal period

Local regulations should be observed.

Pharmaceutical precautions

Store at room temperature. Keep out of the reach of children.

Presentation

360 ml pressurized container with integral metering valve.

** Regumate Porcine in European Union countries is marketed by Janssen Animal Health B.V.B.A.*

Note

Note

Note